THE INFORMED CONSUMER'S PHARMACY

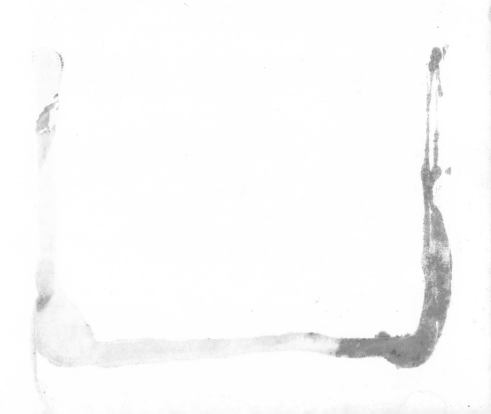

THE INFORMED CONSUMER'S PHARMACY

The Essential Guide to Prescription and Over-the-Counter Drugs

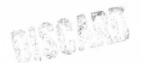
Ellen Hodgson Brown and
Lynne Paige Walker

Carroll & Graf Publishers, Inc.
New York

Copyright © 1990 by Ellen Hodgson Brown and Lynne Paige
Walker

First Carroll & Graf edition 1990

Carroll & Graf Publishers, Inc.
260 Fifth Avenue
New York, NY 10001

Library of Congress Cataloging-in-Publication Data

Brown, Ellen Hodgson.
    The informed consumer's pharmacy : the essential guide to
prescription and over-the-counter drugs / Ellen Hodgson
Brown, Lynne Paige Walker. —1st Carroll & Graf ed.
        p.   cm.
    ISBN 0-88184-586-8 : $12.95
    1. Vegetarianism—Handbooks, manuals, etc.   2. Drugs—
Handbooks, manuals, etc.   3. Self-care, Health—Handbooks,
manuals, etc.
I. Walker, Lynne Paige.   II. Title.
RM236.B688   1990
613.2'62—dc20   90-1701
                                                              CIP

Manufactured in the United States of America

Notice to the Reader

This book is not intended to replace good medical diagnosis and treatment. Its purpose is to help you work with your doctor in making informed treatment decisions.

Contents

Tables

Preface

THE INFORMED CONSUMER

The desire to take medicine is perhaps the greatest fea-
ture which distinguishes man from animals.
—Sir William Osler (1849–1919)

Stories are increasingly featured in the news of drugs and supplements thought to be safe that caused unsuspected reactions in people using them. Sometimes the danger is inherent in the products. Sometimes the products are improperly used—by the wrong people, in the wrong combinations, in the wrong doses. These tragedies can be avoided only by being fully informed of the possible consequences. Being armed with up-to-date information is particularly important today, when drug use is escalating and well-paid advertisers are becoming ever more adept at seducing the unwary. Providing that information is the task of this book.

The well-stocked medicine cabinet that graces nearly every home is a tribute to Madison Avenue advertisers who have convinced us that everything that ails us can be cured by something in a bottle. What these advertisers haven't stressed are the adverse reactions and side effects of their products, the contraindications for use in particular combinations and by particular people, and how the drugs can interfere with natural bodily processes.

The drug business is so enormously lucrative that it has exploded from a short list of basic drugs to some 25,000 brand-name varieties. Not that science has discovered 25,000 new drugs, but industry-supported researchers have succeeded in developing a myriad of variations on old themes. These near-clones may be only slightly

different, and no better, than the originals. They don't necessarily
serve the interests of the patient. They may simply serve the drug
industry interest of circumventing the patent laws.

Drug knock-offs and combination products can actually be more
dangerous and less effective than the originals. But undaunted manufacturers make up for whatever their products lack in safety and
efficacy with massive advertising campaigns, on which they're pre-
pared to spend about three times as much as the average U.S. manufacturer. It is on this marketing, carried out by drug company
detail men and in medical journals, that the busy doctor often must
depend for his knowledge of the mushrooming market. This means
even your doctor may have become the unwitting pawn of
voracious drug company interests.

Yet drug companies aren't necessarily at fault. They just do what
they must to survive in a highly competitive business: engage in
aggressive sales tactics. *Ultimate responsibility for making reasoned
choices rests with you, the informed consumer.* What can you do to
avoid unnecessary or inappropriate drugs? First, you can be well
informed. Before you reach for the pill bottle, find out how the pills
work and what they can do to you.

This book is designed to help you wend your way through the
maze of drugs and their side effects. One of the authors, in over
twelve years of hospital pharmacy work, has seen hundreds of patients with serious conditions caused by drugs improperly prescribed, prescriptions improperly administered, and products
thought to be harmless that caused unanticipated reactions. The
other author, in eleven years of practice as an attorney, has followed
cases of this type when they wound up in court. This book is intended to help you avoid the ill effects of risky drug use.

Here are some typical cases that illustrate the issues addressed in
the following chapters.

A man in his sixties sought treatment for impotence. The impotence was traced to his blood pressure medication, which
had been prescribed because he had had a stroke. The stroke
was traced to a daily aspirin habit, which had been recommended as a preventative for heart disease.

Issues: Is the popular aspirin-a-day fad for the prevention of heart attacks something to be recommended? What conditions can be caused by drugs, and how should they be treated?

A man with a cold treated himself with his wife's leftover antibiotics. The condition at first seemed to get better. But because the full drug course wasn't taken, the surviving bacteria succeeded in developing an overgrowth of organisms causing symptoms much worse than the original infection. Ironically, the man who developed this "superinfection" was self-treating a simple respiratory ailment that would have gone away by itself if left alone.

Issues: When are antibiotics appropriate? What illnesses can you safely leave untreated? What drugs can you safely take without seeing a doctor first? How long should you wait before seeking drug treatment?

A woman working on a hot day remarked that she felt faint. A second woman, who had a heart condition, offered the first woman her nitroglycerin tablets. The second woman stated the pills worked well when *she* felt faint. The drug dilates the arteries so more blood can flow through. In normal people, this dilation results in a rush of blood to the heart and head. When the woman whose arterial blood was not restricted took the drug, she indeed fainted. Paramedics had to be called. She awoke with a severe headache caused by the undue rush of blood to her head, precipitated by the inappropriate drug.

Issues: How do drugs function? How can they malfunction when improperly used?

A 35-year-old Huntington Beach woman had a bad case of acne. Normally, the condition would have been treated as an infection, with tetracycline or other antibiotics. But the woman's astute dermatologist traced the reaction to the fluoride in her city's water, her toothpaste, and her mouthwash. The woman switched to bottled water and tooth products made without fluoride, purchased at her local health food store. Her skin cleared up dramatically.

Issues: What conditions commonly diagnosed as something else may in fact be due to hidden sensitivities to household products and drugs? What alternatives are there to drug treatment?

To answer these and other questions related to everyday drug use, the authors draw on the latest research in medical journals and texts, then convert this technical information into an easy, comprehensive, and practical guide for the layperson. The text takes a risk/benefit approach. Risks and side effects are weighed against the likelihood that a drug will prolong life and improve its quality.

Special attention is devoted to groups of people who may be particularly vulnerable to adverse drug reactions, including the elderly, diabetics, pregnant women, and people with heart conditions or allergies. If you're in any of these groups, you need to know how to adapt your drug intake to your limitations.

What's the safest course for you as a patient/consumer? How can you minimize adverse drug reactions? What substances are you better off avoiding? What are the alternatives? These questions are answered in the following chapters.

1

YOUR MEDICINE CABINET: FRIEND OR FOE?

> *I firmly believe that if the whole* materia medica *as now used could be sunk to the bottom of the sea, it would be all the better for mankind—and all the worse for the fishes.*
>
> —Oliver Wendell Holmes

Overdosing on drugs is the most popular form of suicide; but drugs in lesser amounts can kill as surely. Like time bombs, they just act more slowly. More Americans are killed each year by drugs than by auto accidents. The American Medical Association estimates as much as one-third of all illness may be "iatrogenic"— caused by drugs and other medical therapies aimed at cure.[1]

It has also been estimated that 70–80 percent of the people who visit doctors have nothing wrong with them that wouldn't be cleared up by a vacation, a raise, or relief from the stresses of their lives. Another 10 percent have diseases for which there is no cure. Only 10 percent would benefit from drugs or surgery. Yet 75 percent or more come away with prescriptions.[2]

Up to one-third of prescription drugs, and a much higher percentage of nonprescription drugs, are thought to act primarily as "placebos." They work because the patient expects them to. Pain is relieved by stimulating the release of endorphins, the body's own pain relievers. The problem with triggering this trick-of-the-mind with chemical agents is the risk of side effects. Doctors now write prescriptions for 1.6 billion drugs a year, and all of them pose the risk of serious side effects. If they didn't, you could get them without a prescription.[3]

Before you put potentially lethal chemicals into your body, it's prudent to be well informed. You should find out what the drugs can do to you and what can go wrong. According to the National Council on Patient Information, inappropriate drug use causes 125,000 deaths a year. Four out of five adverse drug reactions are predictable and preventable.

Various studies have found medication error rates in hospitals ranging from 5.3 percent to 20.6 percent, with an average of 11.6 percent. Since each hospitalized patient receives about ten doses of medication a day, that means a mistake is made on his medication an average of once a day.[4]

Many of the errors are without consequence, except to shake the patient's confidence in the quality of his health care. There was, for example, the case of a hospital attendant who ran out of injectable vitamin B_{12} and attempted to substitute two doses of vitamin B_6.

Other errors, however, are deadly; and they can involve simple mistakes like merely misreading a decimal on a label. Here are some examples that ended tragically:

A patient suffering an acute attack of gout received ten times the intended dose of the antigout drug colchicine, because the nurse failed to see the decimal point in the doctor's prescription for "1.0 mg." The overdose killed him.[5]

A Michigan patient who had undergone minor surgery was given morphine, one of the most commonly used narcotic painkillers. Allergic reactions resulted in his death. Hospital records indicated he was allergic to the drug, but no one in charge had read them.[6]

A woman in protracted labor was given oxytocin (Pitocin), a drug commonly used to stimulate uterine contractions. Administration of the drug was not carefully monitored, and the result was a ruptured uterus.[7]

An 18-year-old boy with a history of asthma suffered a heart attack and died after he was given an anesthetic containing a narcotic analgesic for minor surgery.[8]

An 8-year-old child suffered a heart attack after receiving Demerol, a narcotic painkiller, following administration of a general anesthetic. The child survived but was permanently disabled.[9]

What can go wrong is also illustrated in this case reported by British authors Arabella Melville and Colin Johnson:

Mary was a healthy woman in her late twenties who was under a lot of stress. She started suffering heart palpitations, for which her doctor prescribed a beta-blocking drug called practolol.

The heart palpitations stopped, but Mary's periods became very heavy, and she was often dizzy. Once, she went completely blind for several hours. Her doctor prescribed tinted glasses.

Gradually, it got so Mary ached all over and was in constant pain. Her doctor prescribed painkillers.

She got a severe pain in her neck that kept her in bed for three days. Her doctor prescribed a surgical collar and more painkillers.

Yet Mary's eyes continued to hurt. Her ears ached and rang. Her skin itched and she developed a rash. She cried frequently. She couldn't sleep, although her doctor prescribed a battery of sleeping pills. Her stomach became upset and her nose and throat were sore and dry. When her stomach pains became severe, her doctor finally took her off practolol.

The rash cleared up, but her other troubles persisted. Her stomach grew huge. She had a hysterectomy, and a grapefruit-sized mass of fibrous tissue was removed.

She tried to hold down a job but could not, because she kept falling. She was given medicines for vertigo, along with sleeping pills, painkillers, and tranquilizers.

Mary had to undergo another operation, after which she was kept in the hospital for six weeks of extensive testing. Her doctors diagnosed multiple sclerosis.

Mary knew she didn't have multiple sclerosis, and this suspicion was subsequently confirmed. Her condition has now been diagnosed as systemic lupus erythematosus (or "lupus"), a complicated syndrome resulting from her treatment with the drug practolol. Practolol led her body to reject its own tissues as foreign.[10]

Lupus is a connective tissue disease whose specific cause is unknown. However, an estimated 10 percent of the 500,000 American cases are drug-related. The most common cause of the condition is the drug procainamide, an antiarrhythmic used to regulate erratic heart beats. A definite association has also been shown with the antiarrhythmic quinidine, the blood-pressure-lowering drugs hydralazine and methyldopa, the tuberculosis drug isoniazid, and the tranquilizer chlorpromazine. A probable association has been shown with the antipsychotic lithium, many anticonvulsant agents, antithyroid drugs, penicillamine (used to treat rheumatoid arthritis), sulfasalazine (used to treat ulcerative colitis), and the beta-blockers (used to lower blood pressure). A possible association has been shown with estrogens, the antibiotics penicillin and tetracycline, para-aminosalicylic acid (used to treat tuberculosis), gold salts (used for arthritis), griseofulvin (used for fungal infections), and reserpine (used to lower blood pressure).[11] We'll look at these drugs more closely later.

As for practolol, it's no longer a threat. It was never introduced in the United States; and in Britain, where it was introduced, it's been taken off the market. However, it illustrates what can go wrong. Practolol's dangers weren't detected until its cumulative use totaled one million patient/years, and its victims totaled seven thousand. Mary couldn't walk without support, and had to wear a surgical collar, years after she'd quit taking the drug.[12]

What could she have done to avoid this result? If she'd known how the drug was going to affect her, she would obviously have resisted taking it. But what if she'd merely been given a technical description of its potential side effects? They don't sound so bad when couched in vague, general terms and labeled "remote"—skin rash, joint and neck problems, eye and ear problems, tinnitus.

For most patients, whether they'd choose to take their prescriptions if they knew everything that could go wrong is a moot question, since even general warnings are omitted from the bottles. Unlike over-the-counter drugs, which are boxed with circulars detailing side effects, prescription drugs are removed from their boxes by the druggist. He places them in unmarked bottles and labels them only with the names of the patient, the drug, the doctor's name, and directions for use.

In part, this lack of warnings is merely expedient. The druggist gets his wares in economy-sized containers that include only one warning circular, and he doesn't have enough to go around.

In part, however, the omission is intentional. Doctors know that if their patients were aware of all the known risks of the drugs they prescribe, their patients would never take them. Doctors quite reasonably feel they are more capable than their patients of weighing the risks, and of determining whether the risks are justified in individual cases.

Courts haven't always agreed, and physicians have been held liable for failing to warn their patients of potential side effects. But physicians have no duty to warn of "remote" effects, since these warnings might unnecessarily frighten the patient into refusing to take a useful drug. And what may be an acceptably remote risk to the doctor may not be to the patient—particularly in hindsight, when the patient turns out to be the remote person for whom the risk materializes.

Mary is one example. Another is the man in his sixties described in the preface who sought treatment for impotence. His immediate problem was caused by his blood pressure medication, which he was taking because he'd had a stroke. The stroke was traced to a daily aspirin habit, which had been recommended as a preventative for heart disease.

This man can't sue for either stroke or impotence. Both are risks that are legally considered "remote." What could he have done to avoid this situation? Not much, other than to *take a more active role with his doctor in making the treatment decision.*

The National Council on Patient Information and Education in Washington, D.C., suggests you ask your doctor these questions about any drug he prescribes: What is the name of the drug, and what does it do? How and when do I take it, and for how long? What foods, drinks, other medicines, or activities should I avoid while taking the drug? Are there any side effects, and what should I do if they occur? Is there any written information on the drug?

You can also do some independent research. Your local library is one source of information. Check the *Physicians' Desk Reference.* It contains information supplied by drug manufacturers, at the behest of the FDA, on the side effects of their products. If you're really motivated, you can try your local medical school library. Some now provide computers that will give you printouts including abstracts of the latest research on your subject.

Your pharmacist is another potential source of information. As already noted, your prescription won't come with warning labels. This doesn't make much sense, since prescription drugs can do far more harm than the over-the-counter drugs that are elaborately labeled. Your doctor is supposed to give you the necessary warnings, but you can't count on this. An FDA survey conducted in 1983 found that 70 percent of patients were not told about drug side effects by their doctors. Your pharmacist is required to furnish the warning insert on request. Ask him to see it.

All drugs can have side effects. No drug is entirely specific for the condition for which it's prescribed. Every drug acts by interfering in some manner with natural bodily functions. This means there can always be effects other than those you wanted. To determine whether you should take a drug, you first need to know about these unwanted side effects—both the obvious, short-term ones and the long-term ones that are more insidious and difficult to document. Then you need to weigh the gravity of these unwanted effects against the probability that the drug will also achieve the effect you want.

Most conditions for which people seek medical treatment are self-limiting: they will get better on their own if left alone. You don't want to fool around with side effects in situations that aren't inherently unbearable, or in which your body's own curative powers will work better unaided. Ideally, you should take drugs only in situations that:

(a) threaten to shorten your life or do irreversible bodily harm, where studies have clearly established that your chances of preserving life and limb are substantially improved by taking the drug; or

(b) are so painful or socially embarrassing that you don't mind risking long-term havoc in exchange for short-term relief.

To determine whether your condition fits one of these categories, you need to know the statistics and the risks. As for the statistics, it's not enough to know simply that the drug reverses the *symptoms* of your condition. If the drug doesn't reach its actual cause, your chances of survival may be unaffected or even made worse. A recent example involves certain drugs proven effective in suppressing the symptom of cardiac arrhythmia (irregular heartbeat). The drugs had been approved by the FDA and were already in widespread use, when a long-term study showed they actually *doubled* the risk they were intended to prevent—that of a fatal heart attack.[13]

There's no point in taking a drug and suffering its side effects if it's not going to improve your chances of long-term survival or short-term well-being, even if it does reduce symptoms that are theoretical risk factors. The symptoms themselves may not be what's increasing your risk. The symptoms may merely reflect an underlying unhealthy condition, which a symptom-oriented drug can't correct, and may make worse.

Symptoms can also reflect the side effects of other drugs. Drugs can cause depression, constipation, diarrhea, nervousness, upset stomach, dizziness, weakness, blurred vision, and impotence. If you have any of these symptoms, before you seek treatment with drugs, consider whether they might not be caused by one you're already taking. Then ask your doctor whether you can get by without that drug.

Your depression may not be the result of your personal problems. It may be a side effect of the barbiturates, tranquilizers, heart drugs, beta-blockers, ulcer medications, or antibiotics you're already taking.

Your need for tranquilizers or sleeping pills may be due to other drugs that contain stimulants—including analgesics like Anacin and Excedrin, which contain caffeine; over-the-counter diet aids, nasal decongestants, and asthma products; prescription asthma, cough and cold remedies; amphetamines; thyroid preparations; and even "natural" herb remedies, like ginseng and ma huang (herba ephedra).

The yeast infection for which you had to see your doctor may have been the result of a course of antibiotics prescribed by him earlier. Antibiotics wipe out not only unfriendly but friendly intestinal bacteria, leaving the field wide open for invasion by antibiotic-resistant organisms like the popular yeast *Candida albicans.*

The pivotal question is: Did you need the antibiotic? In 1983, more than three million people visited their doctors for treatment of the common cold. More than half were prescribed antibiotics that couldn't possibly help their condition—since antibiotics kill only bacteria, and *colds are caused by viruses.* [14] Antibiotics not only don't do any good, but can do harm. If you have a bacterial infection and don't take the entire prescription, the drugs can lead to superinfections. The partially used antibiotic wipes out the friendly bacteria and allows the remaining unfriendly organisms to take over.

Antibiotics are wonder drugs, but only in life-threatening situations. And they'll no longer work in those situations if they continue to be used for everyday complaints. Bacteria are notoriously adaptable organisms. They easily become resistant to drugs after repeated exposure. Estimates are that at present rates of adaptation, the antibiotic era will be over in about ten years. [15] To ensure that there will be a drug around that works when you're the victim of a really serious infection, it's best to let your body tackle milder ones without chemical help.

We'll look at when you can do this safely in later chapters. In general, your best bet is to take a conservative approach. Most common complaints will go away by themselves. The body can heal itself. Most drugs actually work to suppress the body's efforts in this direction. Drugs target the coughing, sneezing, fever, and diarrhea we think of as the problem. In fact, these symptoms may be the body's attempt to get rid of the problem—the foreign toxins, microbes, or chemicals that have built up in the tissues. When these reactions are deadened with drugs, the toxins are left to accumulate in the body.

The insidious result is suggested by a recent study of people who never caught colds. Professor Kurt S. Zanker of the University in Witten/Herdecke, West Germany, found that people who suffered less than one cold a year were *six times* more likely than other people to develop cancerous tumors. The cancer patients he studied suffered very few common colds and fevers, not only after developing tumors, but for ten years beforehand. The proposed explanation: colds stimulate the immune system, which sends out killer cells that attack and destroy not only viruses, but cancer cells.[16]

The body is an amazingly complicated system of electrochemical potentials, which work in delicate harmony with each other. All drugs can throw off this careful balance and interfere with the natural flow of energies through the body. That's why their sought-after effects can always be accompanied by unwanted side effects. It is also why you're generally better off living with your symptoms if you can, rather than suppressing them with drugs. Even if you have a symptom that's considered life-threatening, before you take drugs aimed at suppressing it, you need to determine whether the treatment will actually prolong life. Drugs that lower blood pressure and serum cholesterol, for example, don't necessarily increase your chances of survival, as we'll see in part II.

2

THE GENERICS SCANDAL AND THE DRUG APPROVAL PROCESS

The generic drug approval process depends in large measure on the "honor system." Inspections to date have demonstrated that this can no longer be relied upon.

—Inspector General Richard Kusserow,
United States Department of Health
and Human Services[1]

The U.S. prescription drug market is valued at $30 billion annually. Not long ago, it was almost exclusively the territory of brand-name manufacturers, but the generic drug market has mushroomed in recent years. Generic drugs now account for about one-third of all prescriptions, and some analysts predict generics will carry two-thirds of the market by 1995.[2]

One reason for the generics boom is legal. Federal legislation passed in 1984 made the generic drug approval process much easier. It codified requirements for approval by the Food and Drug Administration (FDA) based on premarket testing demonstrating "therapeutic equivalence" to branded counterparts. A further boost to sales is expected from a new law that gives pharmacists an economic incentive to dispense generic drugs to Medicare patients. At the same time, patents for many of the most frequently prescribed drugs have expired, allowing generic competition.

Another reason for the generics boom is economic. Prices of many brand-name drugs have shot out of reach. The cost of prescription drugs rose about 80 percent from January 1980 through 1986, 2½ times faster than consumer goods in general. The elderly are hardest hit, since they use three times as many prescription drugs as the rest of the population. For three out of four elderly people, prescription drugs are their largest out-of-pocket health care expense. According to the FDA, generic drugs generally cost 30–40 percent less, and often as much as 80 percent less, than their brand-name equivalents. A recent comparison of six best-selling drugs found that the brand-name drugs were two to three times as expensive as their generic counterparts.[3] Generic savings for some popular drugs are listed in table 1.

Table 1.   *Generic Savings for Selected Products*[4]

Generic	Brand	Generic savings
allopurinol	Zyloprim	55%
amitriptyline HCL	Elavil	70%
chlorpropamide	Diabinese	75%
clonidine HCL	Catapres	60%
doxycycline hyclate	Vibramycin	80%
imipramine HCL	Tofranil	74%
indomethacin	Indocin	63%
hydroxyzine HCL	Atarax	64%
methyldopa	Aldomet	49%
propranolol HCL	Inderal	55%

A third factor in the generics boom is the test of time. Although 8,000 generic drugs have been approved since 1970, and their use has involved billions of patient exposures, remarkably few cases of product failures have been reported. ("Product failures" are different from "therapeutic failures," which are common to most drug treatment. No drug, generic or brand-name, always works.) The Generic Pharmaceutical Industry Association contends that not a single scientifically documented case of unexpected side effects from generic substitution has ever been reported.[5]

The generics boom, however, recently suffered a major setback from charges of cheating and bribery in the drug approval process. At first, the scandal was limited to a few unscrupulous new firms.

But in September of 1989, it hit the major players. That was whe..
the FDA announced it intended to withdraw its approval of the
only remaining generic version of the antihypertensive Dyazide, the
most widely prescribed drug in the country. The withdrawn generic
was marketed by Bolar Pharmaceutical of Copiague, New York, an
industry leader.[6]

The federal investigations began when Vitarine Pharmaceutical,
Inc., and Par Pharmaceuticals were caught cheating in the drug
approval process. These were only two out of 200 generics manufacturers. But in August of 1989, the FDA began an extensive sam-
pling and analysis of the thirty most-prescribed generic drugs—
representing about 75 percent of all new generic prescriptions—as
well as their brand-name counterparts. The FDA seized more than
two thousand samples of products to test for safety and quality.

Bolar was among the first thirteen companies investigated. The
FDA found that its version of Dyazide was not "of proven therapeutic equivalence to the brand name drug Dyazide," manufactured
by SmithKline. There is evidence that Bolar, which won approval of
its product in an "unusually fast six months," passed off Dyazide as
its own generic drug to pass bioequivalency tests, which determine
whether the bioavailability of a generic drug is the same as that of
the brand-name product being copied. Bolar also allegedly tried to
cheat on tests for its version of thioridazine, a widely prescribed
antipsychotic drug.[7]

This makes generics look bad. The scandals, however, aren't limited to generics firms. They have touched brand-name manufacturers and the approval process in general. In July of 1989, three FDA
employees pleaded guilty to accepting bribes from companies whose
new-drug applications they were reviewing. And in September
1989, FDA investigators reported that Eli Lilly & Co., one of the
biggest makers of brand–name drugs, submitted false or incomplete
data to the FDA on some of the drugs made at its Indianapolis
plant. The investigators said there was no evidence of fraud at Lilly,
but that "a number of objectionable practices" had been found, and
that "callous and cavalier business practices were commonplace" at
the plant. The agents' ninety-page report, which culminated four

months of investigations, detailed problems "in nearly every area inspected."[8]

These scandals have shaken public faith in the drug approval process. They show you can't necessarily rely on it to guarantee safety and efficacy, whether the drug is a generic or a brand-name product. The trouble is that the FDA itself doesn't test drugs. It relies on data submitted by drug companies; and it's difficult to assure that that data is accurate. Even the drug companies may not know for sure. Most retain private laboratories to do their drug testing, and private labs have been caught in corrupt and slipshod practices.[9]

On the plus side, the FDA has responded to the scandals by overhauling its generic drug operations, intensifying its watch of firms and their drug applications, reorganizing the generic drug approval process, broadening current investigations, and seeking greater power to act quickly against improper activities. The FDA, generic drug manufacturers, and Eli Lilly are all quick to point out that there is no evidence that the safety and effectiveness of the drugs investigated has been compromised.

That a few generic firms have cheated in gaining approval of their products doesn't mean therapeutic equivalence tests aren't valid when properly done. Equivalence tests are based on the premise that drugs delivering comparable blood levels of the same active ingredients will produce comparable therapeutic effects, an apparently valid premise. (Generic drugs may, on the other hand, contain different fillers and binders, which can account for differences in perceived effects.) Of the nearly two thousand samples of generic drugs tested by the FDA, only 1.6 percent were found to be deficient in potency or dissolution (the rate at which the drug dissolves in the stomach). This failure rate is considered normal for the industry.[10]

But while generic drug companies must prove that their drugs are absorbed into the blood and maintained at certain levels at comparable rates to brand-name drugs, the FDA allows a variability in this potency of up to 20 percent. For some drugs, for some patients, a variation this wide could be dangerous. However, generic drug industry officials say the average variability is only 3.5 percent, comparable to that between batches of the same brand-name drug.[11]

Should you switch from a brand-name to a generic product? That depends. Doing it on your own can be hazardous, especially with drugs for which the effective dose is very close to the toxic dose. If you want to switch, ask your doctor if there is a generic equivalent available; or tell your pharmacist you want the generic version, and ask him to call your doctor for approval.

Some generics shouldn't be substituted, even though they contain identical active ingredients to the brand-name products. Generic substitution is inappropriate for drugs for which blood levels are critical, like Digoxin (digitalis), Dilantin (phenytoin) and Coumadin (warfarin).

Another drug for which substitution is risky is slow-release theophylline, used for the control of chronic asthma. At least thirty different generic brands are available, but their bioequivalency and interchangeability can't be assumed. Only one generic theophylline product (that made by Theocron, Inwood Laboratories) has been approved by the FDA as bioequivalent to the market leader, Theo-Dur. For the rest, differences in rate and extent of absorption can result in too-low serum concentrations, increasing asthmatic symptoms; or in too-high serum concentrations, producing nausea, vomiting, headache, nervousness, and insomnia. At very high concentrations, life-threatening cardiac arrhythmias, seizures, permanent brain damage, and death can occur.[12] On the other hand, Theo-Dur is much more expensive than its generic counterparts, making substitution attractive. If you want to use a generic version, what's particularly important is to begin with one manufacturer and stay with it. Don't change from one to another.

Other generics may not be equivalent to the "brands." Examples are the topical corticosteroids whose brand-name counterparts are Kenalog, Aristocort, and Valisone. Potencies among these products have been shown to vary.[13] Here, too, however, depending on what the drugs will be used for, the savings may justify generic substitution.

Some drugs generally aren't substituted in practice although generic versions are available, because users can tell the difference.

Estrogen is one example. Slight variations in estrogen products can make a big difference in emotional states and other side effects; so women are usually willing to pay more for the brand-name product.

A list of generic drugs evaluated by the FDA as therapeutically equivalent to their brand-name counterparts is presented in the appendix. It doesn't, however, reflect the FDA's recent investigations, the results of which haven't yet been published.

For most drugs, if you must have them and cost is an object, you might as well go for the cheaper generic version. However, you may not need the drug. In the following chapters, we'll look at the long-term track records for safety and efficacy of the most popular medications. We'll also look at nondrug therapeutic alternatives. While the FDA is revamping its drug approval process and peering more closely at the drugs it has approved, it is prudent to be wary of all medications, and to cut their use to a minimum.

I

Drugs for Infectious Diseases
and Allergies

3

ANTIBIOTICS: THE EXPLOITATION
OF A WONDER DRUG

*Some experts believe that the antibiotic era will end by
the year 2000, when all important bacteria may be resistant to all antibiotics.*
 —K. Butler, L. Rayner, M.D.[1]

Penicillin, the first official antibiotic, wasn't discovered until 1928
or used clinically until 1941. But the treatment of infections with
antibiotics dates back thousands of years. The ancient Chinese
treated boils and other skin infections with moldy soybean preparations. The antibiotic that killed the bacteria was in the mold.

The boils treated by the Chinese, however, can no longer be cured
by antibiotics. In the mere four decades that these drugs have been
aggressively pursued by modern medicine, more than half the
staphylococcal bacteria have become resistant to them, including
those responsible for boils.[2] The problem is that bacteria are notoriously adaptable organisms. After their initial retreat in the face of a
new drug, they can mutate resistant strains. They do this by synthe-
sizing enzymes that render the drug ineffective.

Antibiotics and vaccines are credited with eradicating the major
infectious diseases of the nineteenth century although there is some
dispute about this, since most of these diseases were on their way
out before the drugs came on the scene. In any case, infectious
disease remains number four among the major killers, and antibiotic
overuse threatens to eliminate this once-powerful weapon against
it.[3]

Antibiotics have been heralded as "wonder drugs," and in life-threatening situations they clearly are. The problem is that they've been overused and abused, often rendering them ineffective for the very conditions needing them most.

The treatment of gonorrhea is a case in point. It used to be that if a soldier got the "clap," a quick round of antibiotics would clear it right up. The first antibiotics used against this disease were the sulfonamides (sulfa drugs), which were introduced in the 1930s. But in less than a decade, the wily bacteria outwitted the chemists, and the drugs increasingly failed against the disease.

The chemists responded with penicillin therapy, which was begun in 1943. These drugs worked for thirty years, though it took increasingly higher doses. Eventually, however, the bacteria succeeded in producing a strain that was resistant to even very high doses of penicillin. This strain soon accounted for up to 50 percent of all cases of gonorrhea in the Far East.

In its continuing battle against the disease, the U.S. military added spectinomycin to its arsenal in 1981. Spectinomycin is an antibiotic approved solely for the treatment of gonorrhea. But again the bacteria succeeded in cracking the code, and this time it took a mere three years.[4]

In the past few years, antibiotic-resistant gonorrhea has been accelerating at an alarming rate. The worst areas are those with high background rates of antibiotic abuse. In 1985, 2,455 cases of antibiotic-resistant gonorrhea were reported in a single county in Florida. Unlike former epidemics, this one wasn't linked to prostitution or illicit narcotics; but it was linked to illicit drug use. The illicit drugs were antibiotics, which can easily be purchased without a prescription in Miami. In many cases, men with antibiotic-resistant gonorrhea had previously medicated themselves with these drugs.[5]

In some areas, an antibiotic called ceftriaxone (Rocephin) is reserved for the treatment of gonorrhea. To prevent the development of resistance to the drug, it isn't allowed in the community for general use. The reason is that it's the *only* drug effective in those areas for treating the prevalent variety of gonorrhea bacteria. If resistance develops, sufferers will be out of luck. Treatment with either spectinomycin or ceftriaxone is five to eight times as expensive as treatment with more common antibiotics.

Penicillin-resistant pneumonia is also on the increase, and most cases have occurred in people who have had recent antibiotic therapy. In 1981, deaths from pneumonia outnumbered those from auto accidents for the first time since autos joined the major killers. Most of the antibiotic-resistant strains of pneumonia are impervious not only to penicillin but to other antibiotics. Multiply-resistant strains may well emerge worldwide in the near future.[6]

Food poisoning due to salmonella bacteria is on the increase, along with antibiotic-resistant strains of the disease. This resistance is attributed to antibiotic overuse not only in humans but in animals. A nearly five-fold increase in the disease due to the bacteria known as *Salmonella newport* was reported in California in 1985. Two cases ended in death. The bacterial strains responsible for 87 percent of these cases were resistant to the antibiotic chloramphenicol. This clue allowed researchers to trace the epidemic to cows from dairy farms using chloramphenicol in their animals for growth promotion. Most of the victims had also used penicillin or tetracycline during the previous month, and had eaten ground beef during the previous week.[7]

The livestock industry is a major source of the antibiotic overuse that has led to bacterial resistance. It purchases fully one-half of all antibiotics sold. The drugs are incorporated into feed to kill bacteria that stunt the growth of the animals. But this means resistant bacteria can develop and multiply. When you eat these animals, you can become infected with the resistant strains. Cooking the meat will kill the bacteria, but the antibiotic remains in the flesh and is absorbed into your bloodstream when the meat is eaten. While the doses absorbed are low, they're sufficient to allow the bacteria to develop a resistance to the drug. Your risk is increased if you've taken antibiotics recently yourself, since the normal bacterial population in your intestines will have been reduced, allowing the invading strains to take over more easily. The antibiotic-resistant bacterial infections that result aren't easily treated. This is particularly true if the bacteria have developed a resistance to the "broad spectrum" antibiotics, leaving your doctor with the tricky task of determining which infectious agent he's dealing with.

Other sources of antibiotic overuse are certain common prescribing practices by doctors. Some doctors prescribe antibiotics when no infection is present, just to keep one from occurring. The trouble with this approach is that exposure allows bacteria to develop a resistance to the drug. If an infection does develop, the drug then has no effect on the offending bacteria. Moreover, the normal flora —the "good" bacteria that hold down the fort against invaders— are wiped out at the same time.

Antibiotics may be prescribed just to please the patient or to conform to prevailing practice, in situations where the body can heal itself if left alone. As a Swedish research team observed:

> [A]ntibiotics are increasingly prescribed without reasonable indications—sometimes even at the request over the telephone of unexamined patients. Some colleagues claim to fear that a restrictive attitude in prescribing antibiotics might be regarded as a disclosure of their medical knowledge not being up to date. Others claim that otherwise the patient will go "to another doctor." Several colleagues openly disclose their fear of indictments and law suits and of not being backed up by the medical board in such events, even when no therapeutic effect whatsoever could be expected from treatment with antibiotics.[8]

Acquiring an antibiotic-resistant illness is only one risk of antibiotic overuse. Your odds of an allergic reaction to antibiotics also increase with use, and these reactions can be severe.

Another risk is that of superinfection by resistant bacteria. Antibiotics are nonspecific. Their shotgun attack wipes out friendly intestinal bacteria along with unfriendly ones. Without the friendly bacteria, the intestinal field is left wide open for invasion by antibiotic-resistant organisms. Particularly likely are infections by the ubiquitous yeast *Candida albicans.* Particularly dangerous are superinfections by bacteria that have adapted to the drug.

Friendly intestinal bacteria also help in the synthesis, digestion, and absorption of protein, and in the synthesis of vitamins. Vitamin K, which helps blood coagulate, is one of the vitamins synthesized by bacteria. Marked decreases in these bacteria after antibiotic use can result in a decrease in the vitamin, producing a tendency to excessive bleeding.[9]

Thus while antibiotics are wonder drugs, they are also dangerous drugs, particularly when inappropriately used. Before you start on them, make sure they're necessary and effective for your particular condition. And once you start on them, finish the entire course. Otherwise, you risk killing off your friendly microflora while allowing enough invading survivors to take over. In fact, this can happen even if you do take the entire course. Though the drug gets all the germs it was targeting, removal of the normal residents allows invasion of your intestinal field by any antibiotic-resistant organisms that are left.

4

ANTIBIOTIC AND ANTIMICROBIAL OPTIONS

Medical men all over the world having merely entered into a tacit agreement to call all sorts of maladies people are liable to, in cold weather, by one name; so that one sort of treatment may serve for all, and their practice be thereby greatly simplified.
—Jane Welsh Carlyle (1837)

This nineteenth century comment on the medical treatment of infection is no longer apt. Chemists have now come up with some three thousand different antibiotics and some thirty thousand derivatives. Only about forty, however, are in current general use. The top 25 generic drugs of 1988 included ten antibiotics and other anti-infectives: amoxicillin, penicillin VK, ampicillin, tetracycline, doxycycline, erythromycin (stearate and base), cephalexin, trimethoprim-sulfamethoxazole, and nystatin.[1] These drugs and some other popular anti-infectives are discussed in this chapter.

Penicillins

The penicillins were the first antibiotics to be discovered by modern medicine, and they are still the most popular. The top three generic prescription drugs are all penicillins, and so is the number one brand-name prescription drug, Amoxil.

The penicillins fall into three categories: standard, broad spectrum, and penicillinase-resistant.

Standard penicillins were the original product line, but their effectiveness has been diminished by the development of widespread resistance. Newer, costlier penicillins have been necessitated as infections have become more complicated and difficult to treat.

Broad spectrum penicillins reach bacteria against which the standard penicillins are ineffective.

Penicillinase-resistant penicillins are used against penicillinase, an enzyme developed by clever bacteria to destroy penicillin. Penicillinase-resistant drugs were developed by clever chemists to foil the enzyme.

Penicillins are used to treat pneumonia and meningitis, sexually transmitted infections, and infections of the ears, pharynx, sinuses, urinary tract, stomach and abdomen, skin and soft tissues, and bones and joints. They work by interfering with the synthesis of bacterial cell walls.

Penicillins are relatively safe, except in those unusual cases where serious reactions occur. Then the result can be anaphylactic shock (a severe allergic reaction in which the patient has trouble breathing), coma, and death. Side effects that are less serious but more common include skin reactions, eosinophilia (the formation of an unusually large number of a certain type of white blood cells), drug fever, nausea, vomiting, and diarrhea. Diarrhea is particularly common in children taking ampicillin.[2]

Sulfonamides

Sulfa drugs are synthetic by-products of the dye industry. They were the first effective antibiotics used in humans, but again, familiarity has bred contempt and widespread resistance among bacteria. While sulfonamides were once effective against gonorrhea, pneumonia, and certain ear infections, their use is now limited mainly to urinary tract infections. They are also very popular for treating AIDS-related pneumonia.

Side effects of sulfa drugs can include headache, intestinal complaints, dizziness, and ringing in the ears, as well as more serious blood disorders from bone marrow depression. In susceptible people, the drugs can also produce serious allergic reactions. Hypersensitivity reactions include a condition called "Stevens-Johnson syndrome," characterized by bright red swelling all over the body, sloughing of skin, and a drying of the eyes that can permanently impair vision.

Cephalosporins

Cephalosporins came from humble roots. The first of these popular drugs was produced by a fungus dredged up from sewage off the coast of Sardinia in 1945. The most popular generic version today is cephalexin, while the most popular brand-name versions are Duricef (cefadroxil) and Ceclor (cefaclor).

Cephalosporins work like the penicillins, by preventing bacteria from forming their cell walls. Cephalosporins are also effective against most of the same bacteria as the penicillins, and often work where penicillins fail. They're effective against most streptococci and staphylococci bacteria, making them first-choice drugs for most skin and soft tissue infections.

Cephalosporins are usually good for people who are allergic to the penicillins or who have infections that are resistant to them, but about 5–10 percent of patients who are allergic to penicillin are also allergic to the cephalosporins. Like penicillin, cephalosporins can produce serious allergic reactions. Skin rash is the most common. These drugs can also produce blood disorders, and their long-term use can result in superinfections by invading organisms. Other side effects include nausea, vomiting, and cramps.

Cephalosporins are "beta-lactam" antibiotics, consisting of a four-membered beta-lactam ring bound to another six-membered ring. Modifications of the side chains of this structure have produced a bewildering variety of cephalosporins in recent years. Research has aimed at developing new derivatives with broader effectiveness, increased stability, and slower elimination that allows less frequent dosage. As molecular structures have become more complex, however, novel side effects have also emerged. The objective of once- or twice-daily dosing was achieved, but the price was a marked increase in the risk of diarrhea and, more serious, colitis.

Diarrhea is a risk of all cephalosporins, but it occurs more commonly with the newer ones—especially ceftriaxone and cefoperaxone—which severely suppress the normal intestinal bacteria.[3] The ability of the newer-model cephalosporins to drastically decrease intestinal bacteria can also result in a marked deficiency of vitamin K, producing a tendency to excessive bleeding.[4]

Tetracyclines

Tetracyclines are derived from bacteria that prevent the bacterial synthesis of protein. They are useful against a broad spectrum of microbes. While other agents are available for most routine infections, the tetracyclines remain the antibiotics of choice for infections caused by the bacteria with the Latin names *Chlamydiae, Rickettsiea, Brucella,* and *Borrelia.* The drugs are commonly prescribed for certain pneumonias, urinary tract infections, pelvic inflammatory disease, and inflammations of the urethra and prostate.

As with the cephalosporins, long-term tetracycline use can result in superinfections by resistant organisms. Yeast infections of the mouth and vagina are common. Tetracyclines aren't recommended for children under eight years of age, since in 80 percent of them the drugs produce a permanent yellowing of the teeth. The drugs aren't recommended for pregnant women for the same reason—they can cause discoloring of the teeth and other deformities in their babies.

Other side effects of tetracyclines include allergic reactions, blood disorders, dizziness, and stomach, intestinal, and kidney problems. Kidney problems are especially likely in people with preexisting disease, or when outdated medications are taken. All drugs should be thrown away when their expiration dates have passed, but this is particularly important for tetracyclines. Their degradation products can cause kidney damage; so stick strictly to the dating information on the label. Photosensitivity, or extreme sensitivity to the sun, is another problem with tetracycline use. If you're using these drugs, you shouldn't sunbathe or use tanning booths.

Tetracyclines are very irritating to the gastrointestinal tract, making nausea and vomiting another common side effect. Food diminishes these symptoms, but it also binds the drug and inhibits its absorption. Absorption is decreased particularly by dairy products, antacids, and other products containing calcium. The drugs should be taken at least an hour before, or two hours after, these foods or products.

Gastrointestinal problems from the tetracyclines were thought to have been overcome to some extent when doxycycline, a structural isomer of tetracycline, was introduced to human medicine in 1966. But a 1987 postmarketing follow-up study comparing doxycycline with penicillin VK, ampicillin, and tetracycline found that doxycycline actually produced *three times as much* nausea and vomiting as the other antibiotics. Complaints of skin rash were also four times as frequent. In staff-initiated reports, nausea and vomiting occurred in as many as 31 percent of patients on doxycycline, compared to only 10 percent on other antibiotics.[5]

Despite these side effects, doxycycline remains number seven on the most-prescribed-drug list, and tetracycline remains number five.

Erythromycin and related drugs

Like the tetracyclines, erythromycin and its relatives are derived from bacteria that prevent bacterial protein synthesis. These drugs are among the most frequently prescribed antibiotics for patients who aren't bedridden, ranking number nine and number eleven among most-prescribed generic drugs.

Allergic reactions are less common with erythromycin than with other antibiotics, but nausea, vomiting, diarrhea, and upset stomach are more common and unpleasant. At modest doses, these side effects occur in 7–40 percent of patients, and at high doses they occur in 50–70 percent. Surprisingly, the "enteric-coated" pills, which are covered with a hard candy-like shell for the purpose of easing stomach irritation, seem to be the worst. The side effects can prompt patients to abandon treatment before completing the course.

The drugs are relatively safe, but their range of effectiveness is narrower than the cephalosporins'. They work particularly well against diphtheria, whooping cough, Legionnaire's disease, certain pneumonias, and *Chlamydia* infections.

Erythromycin's relatives, lincomycin and clindamycin, may be used when other drugs don't work, but they're usually reserved for intractable cases, since they can produce severe inflammation of the colon. Colitis is three to four times more frequent with oral administration of these drugs.[6]

Chloramphenicol

Chloramphenicol was once widely used to treat minor infections. In 1960, enough chloramphenicol was sold to give 3.73 million Americans a ten-gram course. That was before the discovery of its most serious side effect—potentially lethal blood disorders, including aplastic anemia and bone-marrow inhibition.

A case involving a healthy 7-year-old boy ended in death. He was given chloramphenicol to treat an infected wound on his knee. He developed severe bone marrow depression, leaving insufficient white blood cells to fight off infection. He first suffered an ear infection that could not be controlled with antibiotics. Then he contracted acute peritonitis and meningitis, which also could not be controlled, and from which he died.[7]

Chloramphenicol can also be responsible for the "grey baby syndrome," which develops in infants three or four days into therapy and results in death in 40 percent of them two or three days later.

These drawbacks aside, chloramphenicol is effective against a wide spectrum of microbes, and the development of resistance to the other options has prompted a resurgence in its use. Serious blood disorders have been documented only for the oral, not the injected, form of the drug. The injected form is a currently popular therapy for meningitis caused by the bacteria *Haemophilus influenzae*. Disturbingly, in some countries oral chloramphenicol is still sold without a prescription, due to its inexpensive production. In this country, the drug is generally limited to use in patients allergic to other agents, or against organisms resistant to them.[8]

Combination antibiotics

Antibiotics are sometimes combined to broaden the usefulness of two otherwise-limited agents. Two new combination antibiotics are Augmentin, composed of amoxycillin and clavic acid, and Unasyn, composed of ampicillin and sulbactam sodium. They're effective against bacteria that have developed resistance to their constituent penicillins used alone.

Another popular combination product is cotrimoxazole (Bactrim or Septra), which combines the sulfa drugs sulfamethoxazole and trimethoprim. Its most universal application is in the treatment of urinary tract infections. It is also used for the type of pneumonia associated with AIDS. However, because the immune systems of AIDS patients are weak, its use for this purpose is linked to a high incidence of side effects, particularly rash, fever, and leukemia (a reduction in white blood cells).

In normal people, adverse effects from cotrimoxazole are uncommon. Yet the German Committee for Medicinal Drugs recorded more than a thousand of them over a 25-year period. Like the sulfa drugs it combines, cotrimoxazole can cause severe allergic reactions, including Stevens-Johnson syndrome. It isn't recommended for pregnant or nursing women, or for infants under two months of age. A rare complication that can be fatal is liver damage.

One case (which wasn't fatal) involved a German farmer who had mixed sulfa drugs daily into the food he fed his hogs. When he was treated with the sulfa drug cotrimoxazole himself, he developed drug-induced liver disease. The reaction was attributed to an acquired hypersensitivity to the drug.[9]

Although using multiple antibiotics in combination is a very common practice, some combination products may do more harm than good. Their combination significantly increases the risk of side effects and the cost of treatment. In some cases, the drugs actually interfere with each other's effectiveness. Penicillin and erythromycin, for example, work in opposite ways and can counter each other's effects. They should never be given together.

Like broad spectrum antibiotics, combination antibiotics are effective in wiping out a wide variety of bacteria. However, frequent use of either combination or broad spectrum antibiotics can lead to increased numbers of organisms that are resistant to multiple antibiotics. Again, the friendly intestinal population dies along with the unfriendly invaders, increasing the risk of superinfection by resistant organisms. The result can be epidemics of nosocomial, or "hospital-acquired," infection. These infections can be much harder to treat than the original versions. For this reason, the safest and most effective antibiotic therapy aims at as narrow a spectrum of bacteria as possible.[10]

Aminoglycosides

Aminoglycosides include gentamicin, tobramycin, neomycin, streptomycin and amikacin. They're generally given only in the hospital by intravenous or intramuscular injection. Even here, however, they are often overused. They may be given prophylactically when no infection is present, or when the type of infection isn't yet known, merely to "cover all bases." The aminoglycosides are powerful antibiotics with powerful side effects, including acute kidney failure and hearing loss.

In two cases that wound up in court, a 36-year-old woman who was given excessive doses of neomycin sulfate lost her hearing; and a man given the aminoglycoside kanamycin sulfate ("Kantrex") along with other drugs suffered a similar fate.[11]

Neomycin is an aminoglycoside contained in the popular topical antibiotics Neosporin and Cortisporin. These drugs can also have unanticipated side effects. In one case, a boy developed glaucoma after fifteen months of treatment with topical Cortisporin that had been prescribed by his ophthalmologist for a rash around his eyes. The child became blind in one eye and partially blind in the other.[12]

The aminoglycoside streptomycin was the first drug used in the treatment of tuberculosis. Its usefulness was limited, however, by its serious side effects and its nonavailability in oral form. It has now been replaced for the most part by newer oral agents, including isoniazid, rifampin, pyrazinamide, and ethambutol. These drugs, too, can have serious side effects, including liver and nervous system toxicity; but they're considered safer than streptomycin.[13]

Quinolones

Quinolones are new broad spectrum antibiotics that are projected to replace the aminoglycosides in many cases. The quinolones currently on the market—ciprofloxacin (Cipro) and norfloxacin (Noroxin)—are expensive, running up to seven dollars a pill. But they have the advantage over the aminoglycosides that they needn't be taken by injection. You can take them at home, thus avoiding the much higher costs of a hospital stay.

Antimicrobial agents to treat infections from viruses, fungi, and other parasites

Few drugs are effective against viruses, and the only one that is widely used is acyclovir. It is not approved for use against oral herpes and works only fairly well in the treatment of genital herpes. Its other drawbacks are its excessive cost and its tendency to produce resistant strains of herpes viruses. These resistant strains can be deadly.[14]

For combatting vaginal infections caused either by bacteria or by the parasite known as *Trichomonas vaginalis,* metronidazole (Flagyl) is the most popular option. It is also effective against infections by amoebic and anaerobic (non-air-breathing) microbes, including the intractable parasite *Giardia lamblia.* Side effects of metronidazole are uncommon, but they can include nausea and nerve damage in the extremities. The drug has also been shown to cause cancer in rats, and it may cause birth defects.[15]

Oral metronidazole is effective for the type of chronic inflammatory facial eruption known as "rosacea," but long-term use can result in toxic side effects. Topical metronidazole has now been approved by the FDA for application directly to the skin. It appears to be effective with fewer side effects than the ingested form of the drug.[16]

The most common parasites are fungi, particularly the wily yeast *Candida albicans*. These yeasts are natural residents of the body, but they're normally found in harmless proportions. The body's natural defense against fungus infection is its resident population of normal flora, which prevents invasion by foreigners. When the friendly bacteria are leveled, the yeasts move in. The yeasts get the edge in an antibiotic attack because the drugs leave them unscathed.

To treat the resulting fungus invasion, you may need another drug. For strictly local infections, nystatin (Mycostatin) is used topically or as a "swish" in the mouth. It is generally safe and nontoxic, although it can produce nausea, vomiting, and diarrhea.

For vaginal yeast infections and topical use on diaper rash, clotrimazole (Lotrimin) is currently the most popular option.

These drugs don't work on more serious systemic (whole-body) fungal infections. Fortunately, systemic infections are uncommon except in people with serious immune deficiencies, caused by AIDS, cancer, or immune-suppressive therapy. For their treatment, the likely drug candidate used to be amphotericin B. It was, however, very toxic and could seriously damage the kidneys. Now there is another option, called Diflucan. It has fewer short-term side effects; and it can be taken orally, where amphotericin B had to be injected. The long-term side effects of Diflucan remain to be determined.

For mild systemic and local infections, a popular option is ketoconazole. It, too, is less toxic than amphotericin B, but it can still cause nausea, liver damage, sexual dysfunction, impotence, and enlarged breasts in men.

Griseofulvin is an antifungal used for infections of the hair and nails. Its potential side effects include headaches, upset stomach, tiredness, insomnia, allergic reactions, blood disorders, and fungal superinfections.

For a natural remedy for yeast infections, try garlic. In laboratory experiments, its antifungal activity has proved to be greater than that of either nystatin or amphotericin B.[17] Health food stores now sell deodorized garlic tablets that make this age-old remedy both easy to take and socially acceptable.

Another remedy that seems to work well for vaginal yeast infections is a homeopathic suppository called Yeast Guard (or in California, "Femicine").

Table 2. *Antibiotics and Antimicrobials Among the Top 500
Bestselling Drugs*[18]

Class	Generic name	Brand name
cephalosporins	cefaclor	Ceclor
	cefadroxil	Duricef
	cephalexin	Keflex
	cephradine	Velosef
erythromycins	erythromycin	E-Mycin, ERYC, PCE
	erythromycin estolate	Ilosone
	erythromycin ethylsuccinate	E.E.S., Pediamycin
	erythromycin stearate	Erythrocin
penicillins	amoxicillin	Amoxil, Larotid, Polymox, Trimox, Wymox
	ampicillin	Omnipen, Principen, Totacillin
	bacampicillin	Spectrobid
	carbenicillin	Geocillin
	cloxacillin sodium	Tegopen
	cyclacillin	Cyclapen-W
	dicloxacillin	
	penicillin G potassium	Pentids
	penicillin V	Ledercillin VK, Pen-VeeK, Robicillin VK, V-Cillin K, Veetids
	penicillin VK-potassium	Beepen VK, Betapen–VK
tetracyclines	doxycycline	Vibramycin, Vibratabs
	minocycline	Minocin
	tetracycline	Achromycin V, Panmycin, Robitet, Symycin
sulfonamides (systemic)	sulfamethoxazole	Gantanol
	sulfasalazine	Azulfidine
	sulfisoxazole	Gantrisin

Class	Generic name	Brand name
sulfonamides (topical, for eyes and vagina)	sodium sulfacetamide — sulfanilamide sulfisoxazole (as diolamine)	Bleph-10 Liquifilm Sulamyd-Ophthalmic AVC Vaginal Cream Gantrisin-Ophthalmic
other topical anti-infectives for the eyes	gentamicin tobramycin	Garamycin-Ophthalmic Garamycin-Dermatologic Tobrex Ophthalmic
combination anti-infectives	amoxicillin + clavulanate potassium	Augmentin
	erythromycin ethylsuccinate + sulfisoxazole	Pediazole
	nystatin + neomycin + gramicidin + triamcinolone (steroid)	Mycolog
	polymyxin B + neomycin + gramacidin	Neosporin Ophthalmic
	sulfamethoxazole + phenazopyridine	Azo Gantrisin, Azo Gantanol
	sulfamethoxazole + trimethoprim	Bactrim, Bactrim DS, Septra, Septra DS
	sulfathiozole + sulfacetamide + sulfabenzamide	Sultrin Vaginal Cream
other antimicrobials	clotrimazole (topical antifungal)	Gyne-Lotrimin, Lotrimin
	miconazole (vaginal antifungal)	Monistat 3, Monistat 7
	lindane (antiparasitic, e.g. for lice)	Kwell
	metronidazole (antiprotozoa, antibacterial)	Flagyl
	nitrofurantoin macrocrystals (urinary tract anti-infective)	Macrodantin
	norfloxacin (urinary tract antibacterial)	Noroxin
	nystatin (antifungal, antibiotic)	Mycostatin (Oral or Topical)

5

ANTIBIOTICS FOR COMMON AILMENTS: EAR INFECTIONS AND STREP

[A]s to how pediatricians selected which antibiotic to give to a particular child . . . the other members of the panel . . . mostly stated that either the drug was picked at random or was selected by the doctor's preference for one drug or another chosen on the basis of available samples or side effects. . . . One physician said that frequently, if the child wasn't better by the end of a period of time, then all drugs were stopped and subsequently the child sometimes did recover. The leader then suggested that possibly the drugs were contributing to the child's illness.
—Frank Disney, M.D.,
Past-president,
American Board of Pediatrics[1]

"Otitis media," or middle ear infection, is the bread and butter of the pediatrician. Its medical and surgical treatment in this country grosses at least $1 billion annually. Despite aggressive treatment, ear problems in American children have reached epidemic proportions.[2]

Chronic middle ear effusion (fluid in the ears) underlies the most frequently performed operations of childhood—myringotomy (surgical incision of the eardrum, with or without the insertion of tubes), tonsillectomy, and adenoidectomy. Yet the condition is generally without pain, redness, or bulging, and eventually clears by itself, presumably because the skull and Eustachian tubes have grown.[3] So why operate? Some parents elect these procedures because they're afraid that reduced hearing in the meantime will impair learning. But recent studies show that the effectiveness of these operations is very limited, and they should be reserved only for children who are severely affected. Operations can mean further trauma to the eardrum, prolonging the time required for the ear to heal; and they don't shorten the duration of pain.[4]

Treatment with antibiotics is equally problematic. Although chronic otitis media is blamed on acute infection by bacteria, the condition often fails to respond even to repeated courses of antibiotics.[5] The widespread use of antibiotics for treating ear infections is based on only a handful of studies, and their results have been questioned.[6]

One question is whether the treatment is necessary. In studies of preschool children in Pittsburgh and 7-year-olds in Denmark, all having otitis media with fluid in the ears, about 65 percent of the cases resolved without treatment by the following month.[7]

Another question is whether the benefits of treatment are worth its costs. The drugs may not work, and they may subject the child to unnecessary side effects and repeated bouts of the disease.

The children of one of the authors were cases in point. They had recurring ear infections when they were small, and they saw a lot of the pediatrician. The children invariably got antibiotics. Sometimes they got the drugs when they just went in for checkups, with no visible symptoms. The doctor would peek in their ears, spy the telltale signs, and whip out his prescription pad. One child developed a second ear infection while she was taking a six-week course of antibiotics for a prior infection. The drugs didn't seem to be doing much good. The problem resolved itself spontaneously when the children quit seeing the pediatrician.

A landmark Swedish study reported in 1974 showed that antibiotics not only aren't necessary for the majority of ear infections, but can actually contribute to their recurrence. The study sample covered 2,975 ears attached to 2,145 patients.[8] The hospital records showed that ear infections went away no faster in those patients treated with antibiotics than in those not treated. More important, patients treated with antibiotics were *30 percent more likely to have a recurrence of the infection.* For children treated with antibiotics from the first day of the disease, recurrences were *40 percent* more likely. The chance of a repeat infection within a month of the previous one was more than twice as great in children treated with antibiotics as in those not treated. And in those children treated with antibiotics from the first day of the disease, the chance of recurrence was nearly three times as great.[9]

The researchers noted that ear infection recurrences are on the increase and concluded that routine early administration of antibiotics may be responsible. Antibiotics apparently depress the immunological response to bacteria. This means they prevent the development of natural antibodies and interfere with the development of natural immunity. Thus, the earlier they're given, the more frequent are relapses of the disease.[10] Other researchers suggest the problem is related to infections by the yeast *Candida.* Antibiotics permit overgrowths by these resistant microbes, which then produce toxins that can weaken the immune system and reduce the child's resistance.[11]

The ineffectiveness of antibiotics was confirmed in a study reported in the *New England Journal of Medicine* in February of 1987. Five hundred and eighteen children aged seven months to twelve years with middle ear infection were divided into three groups. One group received an antibiotic alone (the popular amoxicillin), another received the antibiotic along with a decongestant-antihistamine, and the third received a placebo. When the study was terminated at four weeks, no significant differences were found between the groups. Hearing in all three groups had improved, but 70 percent of the children still had effusion in at least one ear; and among those who didn't, about half had a recurrence of the condition within the next four months. In fact, most had recurrences within a single month. This was true for all groups, treated or not.[12]

The addition of the decongestant-antihistamine to the treatment regimen provided no advantage. This finding confirmed an earlier study by the same researchers, in which these drugs were found ineffective in the treatment of middle ear infections with effusion.[13]

When you take your child to the pediatrician for treatment of an ear infection, you take another risk—that of acquiring an infection in the doctor's office. The October 13, 1988, *New England Journal of Medicine* reported an epidemic of chronic otorrhea (discharge from the ear) that was traced to the instruments used to look in the patient's ears. The instruments were cleaned in an ultrasonic bath that was changed only once a week. It seems the responsible bacteria were transferred through the water from one patient to another.[14]

Antibiotics for strep throat

Another very popular use of antibiotics is in the treatment of strep throat. The justification for this routine practice is to prevent rheumatic fever, which can develop after a streptococcal infection, and can result in serious heart disease.

Ideally, before initiating drug treatment, your doctor would wait for a positive throat culture establishing your sore throat was caused by strep bacteria. But throat culture results take two or three days, and it's not always practical to wait that long. New kits are now available for rapid diagnosis, but they aren't as reliable as the old cultures. So antibiotics are still prescribed routinely, "just in case."

Again, one problem with this practice is that while the drugs kill the strep bacilli, at the same time they prevent the development of antibodies that defend against the disease. This means you're liable to go through the winter with one sore throat after another. Antibiotic treatment can also result in allergic and toxic reactions, bacterial resistance, and superinfections caused by antibiotic-resistant organisms.

All this would be worth the trouble if it were, in fact, preventing serious heart disease. But while rheumatic fever was once a serious threat, deaths due to the disease are now very rare in this country. By 1970, they had plunged to about one per million.

This decline is generally attributed to the widespread use of penicillin to treat sore throats, but rheumatic fever was well on its way to oblivion before the introduction of penicillin. Deaths due to rheumatic fever had already dropped a full 90 percent by the time antibiotics came on the scene. And they've dropped *another* 90 percent in the last twenty years, although antibiotic use hasn't increased during that time. Other researchers suggest that improved nutrition and living standards are more important reasons for the decline. Rheumatic fever is known to be prevalent in areas where crowded and unsanitary living conditions prevail.[15]

Several recent outbreaks of rheumatic fever have been reported in the United States, but these outbreaks weren't due to lax medical treatment. In patients having a positive throat culture, appropriate antibiotic treatment was initiated. The problem was that two-thirds of the patients didn't seek medical treatment because they weren't aware of having a sore throat. The responsible bacteria were apparently a low-symptom strain.[16]

If you do seek medical treatment for your sore throat, your chances of going through an unnecessary round of antibiotics are about 70 percent. This was the finding of a Rhode Island study reported in the *Journal of the American Medical Association* in 1983. It found that more than 157,000 throat cultures were done in the state in 1980—one for every six people in the population. Of these patients, 87 percent received antibiotics before the results were known. Eighty-three percent of the test results were negative. And almost 40 percent of the patients continued to receive antibiotic therapy, even when the culture results were negative.[17]

The study also found only two definite new cases of rheumatic fever, one recurrent case, and seven possible cases in the state over a five-year period. Even counting the merely possible cases, that's a total of ten in a population of nearly a million over five years; or two per million per year. Further, of these ten cases, *six had actually been treated with antibiotics,* so it's not clear the drugs did much good.

Strep throat is a self-limited disease: it will go away by itself without treatment.[18] The odds that your painfully sore throat is caused by strep are less than one in five, and the odds that you'll

contract rheumatic fever from it are two in a million. But your odds
of getting antibiotics if you see a doctor for this symptom are about
nine out of ten. If you do, it won't hurt to at least wait for the throat
culture results before beginning antibiotic treatment—since once
you start, you should finish the full course (see chapter 3).

Antibiotics and the common cold

The most dubious use of antibiotics is in the treatment of the
common cold. Well over a million prescriptions a year are written
for antibiotics for this endemic condition. Yet *colds are caused by
viruses, and antibiotics have no effect against these marauders.*[19]

Again, the professed justification is prophylactic: to treat any bacterial infection that *might* arise. The problems with this theory are
that if an infection does develop, the bacteria will have had an
opportunity to become resistant to the antibiotic, and the patient
runs the unnecessary risk of developing an allergic reaction to the
drug.

We'll look at over-the-counter drugs for the common cold in the
next chapter.

6

COLD AND COUGH REMEDIES: ONE WEEK WITH THEM, SEVEN DAYS WITHOUT

The medical journals are full of articles on the subject of who shall live and who shall die when expensive procedures are rationed, while the really big money is spent on treating the common cold at emergency rooms across the country. It has been estimated that if half the people with the common cold who seek medical advice were to care for themselves, $25 billion could have been saved each year, and that is probably a conservative estimate.

—Stanley Wohl, M.D.[1]

More progress has been made in the drug treatment of disease in this century than in all the rest of medical history. Yet virtually no progress has been made in the battle against the common cold. We still get two or three colds a year, and they still last a week or two, regardless of the method of treatment.[2]

The problem may be in our perception of this natural bodily process. The coughing and sneezing that characterize the common cold are the body's attempt to get rid of offending irritants. If they are suppressed with drugs, toxins can be driven inward, where they do even greater damage. Some medical authorities now believe any attempt to suppress the symptoms of a cold merely prolongs the disease.

Americans spend over two billion dollars a year for over-the-counter cough and cold remedies, although these drugs have no effect on the length of the disease. Drugs often seem to ease the pain, but this impression can be the result of an acquired addiction to them. When you're in the throes of a cold, it's hard to resist reaching for one of the topical decongestants that instantly opens the nasal passages for a breath of fresh air. The problem is the "rebound congestion" that follows two or three hours later. The nasal passages swell to worse than their original condition, and the sufferer can sleep through the night only with another dose of the drug. If you can refrain from starting on these drugs, the overall course of your congestion will be milder and more manageable.

As with all drugs, cold and cough remedies have side effects, and this problem is compounded in the popular products consisting of a combination of drugs. Most of these remedies include several ingredients in fixed combinations. Typically, you don't need the multiple drugs they contain, but you will experience all of their side effects, which are multiplied in combination.

If you take aspirin or acetaminophen (Tylenol) along with these combination products, you can overdose without knowing it. Two cases reported in the *American Journal of Gastroenterology* in 1989 involved the popular liquid cold remedy Nyquil, which also contains acetaminophen. To self-treat a viral illness, one patient had drunk a 14-ounce bottle of Nyquil during the three days before hospital admission, in addition to taking eight to ten Extra Strength Tylenol tablets daily. The other patient had taken no Tylenol but had drunk a 14-ounce bottle of Nyquil in a 24-hour period to treat a chest cold. Both patients had a history of alcoholism, a factor we'll look at in chapter 20. Both wound up with severe liver injury.[3]

Sometimes the drugs in these combination products actually cancel each other out. An example are the cough remedies that combine an expectorant with a cough suppressant. Expectorants stimulate the cough reflex, while suppressants deaden it. In combination, the effects of both agents are suppressed. Unfortunately, the drugs don't cancel out each others' side effects. You get the side effects of two drugs and the effectiveness of neither.

Many combination products contain ingredients in such minute amounts that they have no therapeutic effect. Manufacturers throw in these ingredients simply as a marketing tactic, to make the product their own "unique" formulation. These throw-in ingredients don't do any good and can do harm, particularly if you happen to be allergic to them.

Before you take any of these products, it's good to find out what's in them and what the ingredients will do to you. If they don't do anything that helps your particular condition, pass up the product for one with fewer ingredients. Better yet, pass up the lot and try hot water with lemon and honey.

The ingredients in popular over-the-counter cold, cough, and allergy remedies are discussed by category here, then summarized for your reference in the accompanying charts.

Antihistamines

As their name implies, antihistamines combat "histamine," a natural chemical found in all body tissues. In the central nervous system, histamine acts as a neurotransmitter, or messenger, between neurons. In other parts of the body, it encourages inflammation and allergic reactions.

Antihistamines suppress inflammation. The problem is, inflammation is an important bodily process. It keeps infection from spreading to surrounding tissues. When tissue is infected or damaged, histamine is released from cells and acts on the surrounding capillaries. The capillaries then release greater amounts of substances essential in the healing process—fluid, protein, white blood cells, and "macrophages" (scavenger cells that eliminate unwanted material). That's the microscopic effect. The macroscopic effect is swelling and congestion.

Antihistamines sabotage this eliminatory process by suppressing the release of histamine. Thus, they effectively dry the protective mucus lining of the respiratory system. They do this at the expense of an increased susceptibility to infection. Unfortunately, they can also make cold congestion worse.[4]

Antihistamines will neither prevent nor cure colds. This was shown in a study reported in the *New England Journal of Medicine* nearly forty years ago. Volunteers who took antihistamines as a preventive measure, before they'd contracted the disease, developed no fewer colds than another group taking no antihistamines. Moreover, the colds in each group were equally long. When other volunteers were injected with an infected person's nasal secretions, *more* colds actually developed in volunteers taking antihistamines than in those not taking them.[5]

Antihistamines do have their place. In some people, the body *overreacts* to foreign substances, like pollen and the poison in bee stings. For these overreactors, antihistamines bring welcome relief. It's still the symptom, not the cause, that's being treated. But until the offending allergen can be tracked down and eliminated, antihistamines are an effective suppressant of natural defenses gone awry. To do much good, however, the drugs should be taken at the first sign of an allergic reaction. They aren't very effective after histamine has already been released and the symptoms are full-blown.

Asthma relievers that contain antihistamines should be avoided. Antihistamines dry the tissues, but at the same time they thicken the mucus in the lungs, making it harder to remove and often causing mucus plugs.

We'll look at asthma and allergies in the next chapter. If you don't have them, you don't need antihistamines. Read the labels, and avoid combination cough and cold remedies that contain antihistamines along with other drugs.

Nasal decongestants

Nasal decongestants also sabotage the mechanisms designed to get rid of offending irritants. They do it, however, by another route. They work by affecting the "catecholamines." These are neurotransmitters, or messengers between neurons, including adrenalin (epinephrine) and dopamine.

Adrenalin is what the body releases in emergencies, when it's preparing for "fight or flight." If a wild animal is about to attack, the body has no time for detoxification. It shuts down everything except its emergency system, which speeds up the heart rate for a quick getaway.

Decongestants work by stimulating this fight-or-flight reaction. They afford relief by shutting down the natural cleansing process. This wouldn't be an ideal result even if there were no other side effects. However, the drugs also affect neurons and nerves throughout the body. They can produce restlessness, sleeplessness, and sweating. If taken by mouth in high doses, they can raise the blood pressure and increase the heart rate. Even if you escape these more serious side effects, decongestants can produce an excess dryness in the nose, mouth, and throat that can be more annoying than the original symptoms.

The active ingredients in nasal decongestants are called "sympathomimetic" drugs, because they stimulate the central nervous system. More simply, they're stimulants, or "uppers." They fall in the same class as amphetamines, or "speed." Phenylpropanolamine (PPA), a popular ingredient in nasal decongestants and diet pills, is also an ingredient in "look-alike" uppers sold on the street—including "pink ladies," "black beauties," and "speckled pups." At high doses, their effects resemble amphetamines. Serious complications have been linked with their use, including severe hypertension, stroke, myocardial injury, cardiac arrhythmias, headaches, psychiatric problems, and even death in previously healthy people.[6] We'll look at PPA again in the chapter on "Uppers."

PPA and other sympathomimetics like pseudoephedrine are common ingredients in combination cold and cough formulas (see tables 3, 6, and 7). These drugs are frequently used to treat upper respiratory and ear infections in children. Yet they've been shown to have no effect on the outcome of these ailments; and they can produce amphetamine-like behavioral changes in children, including irritability, hyperactivity, bad temper (slapping and hitting), extreme agitation, restlessness, aggressiveness, and sleep disturbances.[7]

Common over-the-counter cough, cold, and allergy remedies that contain 25 mg or more of PPA are listed in table 3. The immediate-release forms are the most likely to produce severe hypertensive reactions.

Oral decongestants should be avoided particularly by people with

heart disease, high blood pressure, glaucoma, and thyroid and prostate problems. Since they can affect blood sugar, they should also be
avoided by diabetics.

Nasal sprays and drops are easier on the heart than oral decongestants. The problem with them is that they're prone to cause
"rebound congestion." They work by constricting the blood vessels,
but their repeated use tires the muscles that cause the vessels to
constrict. Eventually, the tired muscles let go completely, and the
nose becomes more congested than ever.

Table 3. *Popular Over-the-Counter Cough, Cold, and Asthma
Remedies Containing 25 Mg or More of PPA*[8]

Tablets, capsules:	*Formulation:*
Contac	slow release
Cold Factor 12	slow release
Triaminic 12	immediate release
Allerest	slow release
Prolamine	slow release
Tussagesic	slow release
Super Ordrinex	slow release
A.R.M. Allergy Relief	slow release
Sucrets	slow release
Coryban D	slow release
Dristan	slow release
Head and Chest	slow release
Triaminic	immediate release
Triaminicin	immediate release
Liquid, syrup:	
Cold Factor	liquid
Comtrex	liquid
Formula 44D	liquid
Cremacoat 3	syrup
Cremacoat 4	syrup

The drugs can also inhibit the movement of the cilia that line the
nose and lungs. The cilia serve to remove foreign particles, and if

they're not functioning properly, these particles can enter and infect the lungs.

Nasal sprays and drops should be avoided particularly in the treatment of allergies. These conditions can last for days. In the end, you can wind up intractably addicted to the drugs.

Cough remedies

A cough is a reflex for eliminating foreign substances that block the airways. Drugs that suppress this protective reflex can do you more harm than good. The FDA recommends cough suppressants only for "dry," "unproductive" coughs that aren't bringing anything up. The drugs aren't recommended for smokers or for people with asthma, emphysema, and other conditions involving overproduction of secretions. Their coughs, while chronic and annoying, are still productive.

This means most coughs are best left alone. Assuming, however, that you want to suppress yours, there are ingredients the FDA says are effective and relatively safe for that purpose. They are codeine, dextromethorphan, and diphenhydramine hydrochloride (Benylin). All three are derivatives of the narcotic morphine. Like morphine, they work by drugging the brain. The main drawbacks of codeine are that it can be addictive and very constipating. Dextromethorphan isn't addictive, but overdoses can produce bizarre behavior. Diphenhydramine hydrochloride can make the user very drowsy. This is a hazard particularly if you're driving a car or operating machinery.

The FDA has found other ingredients to be safe in the recommended doses but not to have proven effectiveness in suppressing coughs. Some of these ingredients can also be quite toxic when overdoses are taken by children. Ingredients that are safe but not proven effective are listed in table 4.

The other type of cough remedy is the expectorant. Unlike suppressants, which deaden the cough reflex, expectorants encourage it. Some do this by stimulating the vomiting reflex, others irritate the stomach, and others act on the bronchial tube nerve endings.

If your cough is already productive, you probably don't need expectorants. However, even if you do need them, there are no ingredients that have yet been approved by the FDA as both safe and effective for that purpose. Expectorants considered relatively safe but not proven effective and those found to be clearly unsafe and not proven effective are listed in table 4.

The FDA recommends that cough remedies, if used at all, be taken as single ingredients rather than in fixed-combination products. Combination products increase the risk of side effects without necessarily increasing the product's effectiveness. You're unlikely to

Table 4. *FDA Effectiveness Ratings for Cough Remedy Ingredients*[9]

Cough suppressants

Safe and effective:	codeine, dextromethorphan, diphenhydramine hydrochloride
Safe but not proven effective:	beechwood creosote, camphor, caramiphen edisylate, carbetapentane citrate, cod-liver oil, elm bark, ethylmorphine hydrochloride, eucalyptol and eucalyptus oil, horehound, menthol and peppermint oil, noscapine, thymol, topical or inhaled turpentine oil
Not proven safe or effective:	hydrocodone bitartrate, turpentine oil taken orally

Cough expectorants

Safe and effective:	none
Safe but not proven effective:	ammonium chloride, beechwood creosote, benzoin preparations, camphor, eucalyptol and eucalyptus oil, guaifenesin, ipecac syrup, menthol and peppermint oil, pine-tar preparations, potassium guaiacolsulfonate, sodium citrate, terpin hydrate preparations, tolu preparations, topical or inhaled turpentine oil
Not proven safe or effective:	turpentine oil taken orally, antimony potassium tartrate, chloroform, iodides, ipecac fluid extract, squill and squill extract

need all their ingredients, and even if you do, they're unlikely to be in the proportions appropriate for your particular condition.

Unfortunately, of the 152 products reviewed by the FDA, only 24 were single-ingredient products, so your choice is limited.[10] The most popular single-ingredient expectorants are Robitussin, Terpin Hydrate, and Potassium Iodide Solution. (Note that Robitussin PE and Robitussin CF are combination products.) Benalyn is another single-ingredient cough remedy, but the ingredient is an antihistamine (benadryl), which works mainly by making you drowsy.

Vitamin/mineral therapy

Vitamin C and zinc are two supplements touted as fighting colds. There is no scientific proof, however, that either does any good. Zinc has been shown to inhibit the activity of cold viruses in the laboratory, but in a University of Virginia study involving humans, it neither reduced symptoms nor altered the course of the disease. Vitamin C not only hasn't been proved to fight colds, but can do harm. If taken in megadoses (over 600 mg/day), it can cause nausea, cramps, diarrhea, and kidney stones. And chewable vitamin C can corrode the enamel on your teeth. High doses of zinc can also do harm, by inducing a deficiency of copper.[11] (See chapter 36.)

Nondrug alternatives

Some physicians favor the use of old-fashioned remedies: mixtures of spirits, honey, and lemon juice; hot milk and honey; or chicken soup. Studies have shown that hot drinks can actually make you feel better, by increasing the flow of nasal secretions.[12]

Health food stores supply good herb teas. Licorice root tea can open the bronchioles of the chest. However, drinking large amounts can cause water retention and increase blood pressure, so limit your intake to about three cups a day.

For a cough, secretions can be loosened by breathing the steam from a vaporizer or hot shower.

You'll probably find that if you give up drugs for the treatment of a cold, the condition will become more tolerable of its own accord.

Table 5. *Antihistamines*

Popular generic varieties:	brompheniramine (BP) chlorpheniramine (CP) doxylamine (DX) methapyrilene (MP) phenindamine (PD) phenyltoloxamine (PT) pyrilamine (PY) triprolidine (TP)
Brand names of popular products:	See Table 7.
Intended effects:	Reduce symptoms of allergy (rash, itching, hay fever), prevent motion sickness, induce sleep
Common side effects:	Drowsiness, dizziness, nausea, dry mouth/nose/throat
Uncommon side effects:	Nightmares, irritability, changes in vision, sore throat, fever, rapid heartbeat, unusual bleeding or bruising, difficult urination, fatigue, weakness
Bad drug combinations:	Excess sedation results when taken with antidepressants, other antihistamines, hypnotics, alcohol, narcotics, mind-altering drugs, sedatives, sleep inducers or tranquilizers. Effects of anticholinergic drugs and MAO inhibitors are magnified.
Avoid or use only on the advice of your doctor if you:	have glaucoma, enlarged prostate, asthma, kidney disease, peptic ulcer; are pregnant or nursing; are working around dangerous machinery or engaged in hazardous work; are scheduled for surgery within the next two months. Not recommended for newborns. Elderly people may experience more serious side effects.

Table 6. *Decongestants (Sympathomimetics)*

Popular generic varieties:	ephedrine (EP) epinephrine (EN) phenylephrine (PE) phenylpropanolamine (PP) pseudoephedrine (PS)
Brand names of popular products:	See Table 7.
Intended effects:	Reduce nasal, sinus, and throat congestion from allergies, colds, infections
Common side effects:	Insomnia, agitation
Uncommon side effects:	Dizziness, headache, trembling, weakness, nausea, sweating, paleness; change in heartbeat (irregular, slow, fast, pounding); difficulty breathing or urinating; hallucinations, seizures
Bad drug combinations:	Can either increase or nullify the effects of antidepressants, antihypertensives, beta-blockers, digitalis, epinephrine, ergot, guanethidine, MAO inhibitors. Can produce nervousness and insomnia in combination with caffeine, overstimulation in combination with cocaine, rapid heartbeat in combination with marijuana.
Avoid or use only on the advice of your doctor if you:	are allergic to any sympathomimetic drug; have high blood pressure, heart disease, diabetes, or an overactive thyroid; are scheduled for surgery within two months; have trouble urinating; are pregnant or nursing. Not recommended for children. Elderly people may experience more severe side effects.

Table 7. *Ingredients in Popular Cold and Allergy Remedies*

Product	Antihistamine[A]	Decongestant[B]	Analgesic[C]	Other Ingredients Comments
Actifed	TP	PS	—	
Alka Seltzer Plus	CP	PP	AS	
Allerest	PY, MP	PP	—	time-released
Bayer Children's Cough Tablets	—	PP	AS	
Bayer Decongestant	CP	PP	AS	
Chlor-Trimeton Decongestant	CP	PS	—	
Comtrex	CP	PP	AC	alcohol, dextromethorphan
Congespirin	—	PE	AS	
Contac	CP	PP	—	belladonna; time-released
Coricidin "D"	CP	PP	AS	
CoTylenol	CP	PE	AC	
CoTylenol for Children	CP	PS	AC	alcohol
Dristan	PD	PE	AS	caffeine, aluminum hydroxide, magnesium carbonate
Dristan Time Released	CP	PE	—	time-released
Dimetapp Extentabs	BP	PP	—	
Drixoral	BP	PS	—	
NeoSynephrine Compound	TD	PE	AC	caffeine
Novafed	—	PS	—	alcohol
Nyquil	DX	PS	AC	alcohol, dextromethorphan
Sine-Off	CP	PP	AS	
Sinutab	PT	PP	AC	
St. Joseph Cold Tablets for Children	—	PP	AS	
Sudafed	—	PS	—	
Triaminic	PR, PY	PP	—	

A Key in Table 5.
B Key in Table 6.
C AS = aspirin; AC = acetaminophen.

7

DRUGS FOR ASTHMA AND ALLERGIES

Death during an attack is unknown. The asthmatic pants into old age.

—Sir William Osler[1]

This observation, made by Dr. Osler at the end of the nineteenth century, is no longer true. Not only do people now die from asthma; the mortality rate has doubled in the last decade. The toll in 1987 was 4,000 deaths.[2]

The reason for the alarming rise in asthma deaths isn't clear. Some researchers blame air pollution. Others blame the drugs used to treat the disease. An earlier epidemic of asthma deaths in England, Wales, and New Zealand in the 1960s hit at about the same time that metered-dose inhalers were catching on as the treatment of choice among asthma patients. The epidemic was apparently caused by the increased sale and use of a high-dose aerosol containing the drug isoproteneronol. Patients were relying on self-treatment with this medication rather than seeking medical care.

Today, this drug is no longer available without a prescription and is infrequently used. But the huge increase in availability and use of other aerosol preparations in metered-dose inhalers for dilating the bronchial tubes may be having the same effect. Between 1972 and 1985, when sales of prescription drugs in general increased by only 7 percent, prescriptions for antiasthma products increased by 200 percent. These products afford a false sense of security in the face of a dangerous condition. All antiasthma medications can produce

life-threatening reactions, and their likelihood is multiplied by the
increased use of the medications.[3] Ironically, the unprecedented rise
in asthma deaths comes at a time when doctors now have safer and
more effective drugs than ever before for controlling the condition.
The phenomenon has been attributed to the failure to use these
drugs properly.

An estimated three to six million Americans have asthma, a disorder of breathing characterized by wheezing, difficulty exhaling,
and often, coughing. Most cases are caused by allergies, but the
reaction can also be triggered by aspirin, exercise, or exposure to
cold weather. Asthma and allergies are the leading reasons for hospitalization in children, and account for one out of every eleven
visits to the doctor. They are also responsible for over $11 billion a
year in U.S. drug sales.[4]

In this chapter, we'll look at the drug possibilities and at what's
new in the field for victims of asthma and an even more common
allergy, hay fever. If you have a serious asthmatic condition, however, it's particularly important that you not rely on your medicine
cabinet but seek the regular care of a physician specializing in the
field.

Antiasthma drugs

Drugs for the treatment of asthma fall into four main groups:

(1) Sympathomimetics

These products are used for acute attacks and contain sympathomimetic drugs (see chapter 6). They stimulate the muscles that open
the bronchial tubes.

Ephedrine (contained in Bronkotabs, Mudrane, Quadrinal,
Quibron, and Tedral) has been used for this purpose for thousands
of years. Its drawbacks are that it can cause the heart to pound and
can have other distressing side effects, including nausea, high blood
pressure, dizziness, and sleepless nights.

Aerosol inhalers containing adrenalin in the form of epinephrine

(Primatene, Bronkaid) or isoproterenol (Isuprel, Mucomyst, Medihaler-Iso, Duo-Medihaler, Norisodrine) are newer. However, they can cause some of the same side effects as ephedrine.

The sympathomimetic drugs used in the new aerosol bronchodilators are less likely to have these effects. They include albuterol (Ventolin, Proventil), terbutaline (Brethine), and metaproterenol sulfate (Alupent).

When properly used, these drugs can be very effective. Their improper use, however, is a suspected villain in the alarming increase in asthma deaths. While the newer bronchodilators aren't as risky as isoproterenol, overuse can still cause them to lose their effectiveness, and it can cause a rebound effect that actually makes the condition worse. If the inhaler doesn't have the desired effect, call your doctor immediately.

(2) Xanthine bronchodilators

For daily maintenance treatment, the most common antiasthma drug is theophylline. It's found in the prescription drugs Theo-Dur, SloPhyllin, and Quibrin, and in nonprescription Bronkaid and Primatene tablets. It's also a stimulant found in tea. Theophylline belongs to a group of drugs called "xanthines" that also includes caffeine (found in coffee) and theobromine (found in cocoa). Other xanthines used to treat asthma include aminophylline, dyphylline, and oxtriphylline (see table 10).

While theophylline has been used for nearly 150 years to clear obstructed air passages, new developments in its use have significantly lessened its side effects.

In some studies, the use of theophylline in asthmatic children has been associated with learning disabilities and behavioral disorders, including hyperactivity, inattentiveness, irritability, and sleeplessness. But like caffeine, theophylline affects different people differently, and many children seem to do well on it.[5]

One thing that's important for successful treatment is to keep blood levels of the drug constant. New tests for measuring blood levels are now available that allow more accurate dosing, significantly lessening side effects. Blood levels of theophylline can be affected by many factors, including high intakes of protein or carbo-hydrate, smoking, flu, or flu vaccines. They can also be affected by caffeine-containing products, including cola drinks and chocolate, which should be studiously avoided. The amounts of caffeine in popular foods and drinks are listed in table 8.[6]

Another new development in theophylline use is the slow-release preparation. The older immediate-release forms were bitter to the taste and had to be taken every four to six hours, day and night. The new slow-release capsules allow twice- or even once-a-day dos-ing, and they can be opened and used as a sprinkle for children who can't swallow capsules whole. It's best to stick to one preparation and to take it in a consistent way, since the drug varies in absorp-tion depending on the formulation and how it's taken. If you're

Table 8.   *Caffeine in Popular Foods and Drinks*[7]

Product	Serving	Mg/caffeine per serving
Coffee (brewed)	5 oz.	100–164
(instant)		50–75
Cocoa	8 oz.	50
Chocolate milk	8 oz.	7.5
Chocolate candy	8 oz.	7.7
Chocolate pudding	4 oz.	5.5
Fudge brownie	1¼ oz.	7.7
Soft drinks	12 oz.	
Coca-Cola		45
Diet Rite		17
Dr. Pepper		39.6
(diet)		39.6
Jolt Cola		71
Mountain Dew		54
Pepsi-Cola		38.4
(diet)		36
Royal Crown Cola		30
(diet)		25
Tab		46.5

using a generic brand, have your pharmacist order from the same manufacturer each time, since dosing may not be consistent between formulations.

Regardless of the preparation, theophylline can have side effects, including nausea, vomiting, abdominal pain, loss of appetite, headache, nervousness, anxiety, increased heart rate, heart palpitations, behavioral changes, and short-term memory loss. These can sometimes be eliminated by lowering the dose. If they can't be eliminated, the treatment plan should be changed rather than putting up with them.

Theophylline isn't recommended for children whose symptoms are only intermittent, whose behavior changes on the drug, or who do better on other drugs. It is also not recommended for pregnant women or nursing mothers. It should be used only with caution by people with liver disease or uncontrolled hyperthyroidism. It can aggravate ulcers, fibrocystic breast disease, and heart disorders.[8]

(3) Corticosteroids (Steroids)

Natural steroids are hormones produced by the adrenal glands. The pharmaceutical varieties are used to treat many disorders. Steroids reduce inflammation, opening the airways of the chest. They suppress much of the immune system's response to allergens. However, the drugs don't cure the problem. They act mainly by inhibiting the body's reaction to it. The trouble with taking extra steroids is that your adrenals quit making their own. This means that when you need the natural steroids to cope with stressful emergencies, they're no longer available. Steroids' serious side effects include cataracts, bone loss, weight gain, easy bruising, and emotional and growth problems in children. They shouldn't be taken by people with ulcers, tuberculosis, or ocular herpes, and should be used only with caution by children, pregnant women, and nursing mothers.

For asthma emergencies, steroids like methylprednisolone (the injectable form) or prednisone (the oral form) can be very effective. However, these systemic steroids shouldn't be used long-term, and they should be used only when all other treatments fail. In children, they can't be used for asthma attacks more than about four times a year without significant adverse effects.

Many of the side effects of oral steroids have been eliminated by steroid inhalers (Asmacort, AeroBid, Beclovent, Vanceril) that are sprayed directly into the lungs. Because they're inhaled and are poorly absorbed, the potential for adrenal suppression is minimized. They are considered safe enough for daily use, even by children. In fact, they must be used regularly to be effective. Steroid inhalers aren't effective if reserved only for acute attacks. Because they can contribute to the development of fungal mouth infections, use of a mouthwash is advised after each dose.[9]

(4) Cromolyn

The newest of the asthma inhalers contains cromolyn sodium (Intal). Cromolyn is actually new only to Western medicine. In the form of ammi seeds, it's been part of Bedouin folk medicine for centuries.[10]

Asthma not only constricts the bronchial tubes but causes inflammation. Cromolyn inhibits both of these responses. It prevents the cells in the lungs that release histamine and other immune-system chemicals from reacting to allergens. Unlike antihistamines, which generally battle histamine only after it's already been released, cromolyn actually prevents histamine release.

Cromolyn has been used for years in Europe as the drug of choice for asthma, and it's now challenging theophylline for that position in the United States. It's the preferred drug for children who don't do well on theophylline or whose condition is characterized more by coughing than wheezing.[11]

Drugs to control hay fever

Government estimates are that one in five Americans suffers from allergies of some sort. Allergies also take credit for one in five visits to the pediatrician. Hay fever, or allergic rhinitis, is an inflammation of the nasal passages caused by an irritant. It strikes an estimated six million children annually. Its treatment includes drugs similar to those for asthma and colds. As with asthma, newer, better versions of these drugs are now available.

One of them is, again, cromolyn sodium. It comes either as a nasal spray (Nasalcrom) or eyedrops (Opticrom). Like the asthma version (Intal), the hay-fever products actually prevent allergies before they start. They do this by preventing white blood cells from releasing histamine and other immune-system chemicals. Their major drawback is that they need to be used three to six times a day, all through hay fever season. They can also have side effects, including headaches, sneezing, nosebleeds, and stinging in the nose. These drawbacks aside, the cromolyn sodium drugs represent a major advance over the antihistamines, which are sleep-inducing and tend to reach histamine only after the allergic response is in full swing.

There are, however, also new developments in the antihistamine line. The antihistamines familiar in treating colds are actually more helpful in the treatment of allergies, since allergies result from the *inappropriate* release of histamine into the blood stream. Antihistamines have been available since the 1940s. However, the older versions (Benadryl, Allerest, Chlor-Trimeton) produce drowsiness, making it unsafe for the user to drive a car or operate machinery, and difficult to work. A newer-model antihistamine called terfenadine (Seldane) has overcome this defect. It costs about ten times as much, but that didn't stop it from becoming the number-one prescription drug by the end of 1985, the year it came out. Its success may also have been due to a new marketing technique. Although it's a prescription drug, advertisements were aimed directly at consumers rather than merely at the doctor/middleman. Two other new nonsedating antihistamines, Histamanal and Claritin, which are longer acting than Seldane, are expected to receive FDA approval in the near future.[12]

As in the treatment of asthma, there are also new steroid-containing nasal sprays for the treatment of hay fever that have reduced the serious side effects of steroids taken by mouth. Like Beclovent and Vanceril inhalers, Beconase and Vancenase sprays contain beclomethasone dipropionate. Nasalide contains a similar agent called flunisolide. The steroid spray hits only the nose, not the whole body, so systemic effects are minimized. This feature can, however, give rise to an annoying side effect—sneezing or stinging in the nose. This effect is less likely with Beconase and Vancenase than with the older Nasalide.

For the treatment of hay fever, decongestants or decongestant/ antihistamine combinations should be avoided. These drugs can cause a rebound effect, and they're potentially addicting if used for more than a few days. Hay fever, unfortunately, tends to last more than a few days.

Allergy shots

Allergy-desensitization injections are also available, but they're generally reserved for people with severe allergies. They are a long and expensive commitment with an uncertain outcome. A typical course can take three to five years, and it may be a full year before you see any improvement. At ten to twenty dollars each, the required once- or twice-weekly office visits have been called annuities for allergists. Whether the shots actually reduce or eliminate allergies has never been proven, since many young people outgrow their allergies even without treatment.[13]

Nondrug alternatives

The first defense against allergies is to avoid the offender. Unfortunately, for serious cases of allergy to airborne substances, this may mean staying indoors all through hay fever season. An air conditioner or air filter on your heating system can help. A humidifier or vaporizer can, too, but it can also aggravate some allergies by producing a moist environment that encourages the growth of allergy-producing molds.

For congestion, you can try hot tea made with natural decongestants, like fenugreek, anise, and sage. Hot and spicy foods and garlic and onions can also thin out mucus.

Another trick is the nasal douche, washing out your nose with saltwater. This can be done with a nose dropper.

Exercise is a natural adrenalin stimulant. It can produce direct nervous stimulation to the nose.[14]

Besides hay fever, allergies account for many less obvious childhood symptoms, including eczema (skin rash), chronic coughs and bronchitis, diarrhea, migraine headaches, colitis, and ear aches.[15] These allergic reactions are often traced to certain foods, notably eggs, milk, nuts, soy, and wheat. Substantial improvement may result from avoiding these offenders. This can be a lot of trouble for the parent, but it's liable to be worth the effort, since children often outgrow their allergies. If the food isn't avoided, the allergy is more likely to remain.[16]

The desensitization process can actually be started before the child is born. If one parent has allergies, the chances are one in three that the child will, too. If both parents have them, the chances are two in three. Mothers who suspect allergies can start by passing up allergy-causing foods while they're pregnant and nursing. Eggs, milk products, nuts, and peanut butter are leading suspects to be avoided.[17]

For asthma, an alternative therapy that may be effective is acupuncture. A Chinese study published in 1989 reported a disappearance or decreased frequency of asthma attacks in 88.9 percent of cases treated by a particular acupuncture method. Biofeedback techniques have also been used clinically to treat asthma.[18]

Table 9. *Sympathomimetic Bronchodilators*[19]

Generic name:
  albuterol
  metaproterenol
  terbutaline
	Brand name:
	  Proventil, Ventolin
	  Alupent
	  Brethine

Uses:	Bronchial tube relaxer to aid breathing in bronchial asthma and emphysema. Terbutaline is also used to treat premature labor.
Side effects:	Nervousness, shaking, dizziness, insomnia, headache, heartburn, nausea, vomiting. Excessive use of metaproterenol has resulted in heart attacks.
Adverse interactions and cautions:	Dangerous in combination with other bronchodilators, decongestants, epinephrine or MAO inhibitors. Effectiveness may be decreased by beta-blockers. Hazardous for pregnant or nursing women, diabetics, children under 12, and people with heart disease or high blood pressure, overactive thyroid, seizures, or sensitivity to sympathomimetic drugs.

Table 10. *Xanthines*

Generic name:
  aminophylline
  dyphylline
  oxtriphylline
  theophylline
	Brand name:
	  Aminophyllin, Somophyllin-DF
	  Lufyllin
	  Choledyl
	  Elixophyllin, Slo-Bid, Slo-Phyllin, Theo-Dur, Theolair

Uses:	Bronchial tube relaxer for the treatment of bronchial asthma, bronchitis, emphysema, and other lung disorders
Side effects:	Restlessness, dizziness, insomnia, convulsions, palpitations, nausea, vomiting, loss of appetite
Adverse interactions and cautions:	Altered drug effects likely in combination with diuretics, beta-blockers, lithium, hexamethonium, erythromycin, chlordiazepoxide, rauwolfia drugs, or other xanthines. Effectiveness reduced by smoking, high-protein diets, or barbecued foods. Risky for people with heart disease or high blood pressure, ulcers, liver disease, lung damage, overactive thyroid, infants or the elderly.

Table 11. *Corticosteroids* *

Generic name:	Brand name:
beclomethasone	Beclovent, Vanceril, Beconase, Vancenase
betamethasone	Celestone
dexamethasone	AeroBid, Decadron
flunisolide	Nasalide
hydrocortisone	Cortef, Solu-Cortef
methylprednisolone	Medrol, Solu-Medrol
prednisone	Deltasone, Orasone
triamcinolone	Azmacort, Aristocort, Kenalog

Uses: Adrenal hormones with anti-inflammatory properties used to control allergic reactions; relieve rheumatic symptoms and breathing problems; supplement natural hormones; and treat certain blood, digestive, and nervous system disorders

Side effects: Ulcers, insomnia, elevated blood sugar levels, low potassium levels, fluid retention, weakness, dizziness, headache, slow growth in children, mood swings, congestive heart failure; serious eye and nerve problems and fungal infections with prolonged use; decreased resistance to infection; may mask symptoms of infection

Adverse interactions and cautions: Altered drug effects in combination with barbiturates, diabetes drugs, anticonvulsants. Serious ulcers may result in combination with aspirin. Effects increased by heavy smoking. Causes birth defects in animals. Passed in mother's milk.

* For topical corticosteroids applied to the skin, see chapter 27.

8

REDUCING FEVER WITH DRUGS

*Humanity has but three great enemies: Fever, Famine,
and War. Of these, by far the greatest, by far the most
terrible, is fever.*

—Sir William Osler

This late-nineteenth-century view of fever has been challenged by
recent research, which supports an even older theory dating back to
Hippocrates. The Father of Medicine thought fever was a beneficial
process designed to "cook out" invaders. Current controversy,
which we'll look at in this chapter, centers on whether fever should
be treated with antibiotics, with aspirin, with acetaminophen (Tylenol), or at all.

Should you reduce a fever with antibiotics?

High fever is one of the most common symptoms prompting parents to bring their young children to the doctor. Most fevers are
caused by viral disorders that will go away by themselves without
treatment. But 3–15 percent are caused by bacteria, including those
with the Latin names *Streptococcus pneumoniae, Haemophilus influenzae, Neisseria meningitidis,* and *Salmonella.* Since infections
from these microbes can be serious, some pediatricians routinely
treat fevers with antibiotics, even before they have laboratory evidence of bacterial infection. A recent study in the *New England
Journal of Medicine,* however, raised doubts about this common
practice.

The study involved 955 children aged 3–36 months with temperatures over 102.2 degrees F but without apparent local infection. The children were randomly assigned to two groups, either antibiotic (amoxicillin) or placebo. Blood cultures established that only 2.8 percent of the children had bacterial infections caused by disease-producing organisms.

There was no evidence that early antibiotic treatment prevented new, serious bacterial infections (meningitis, pneumonia, etc.), which weren't statistically different in the two groups. Moreover, the antibiotics themselves produced side effects, including diarrhea and rash. The researchers concluded that the routine treatment of high fever with standard oral doses of amoxicillin in small children is unwarranted, except when actual laboratory evidence of a bacterial infection justifies it.[1]

Should you reduce a fever with aspirin?

In children, reducing fever not only with anitbiotics but with aspirin should be avoided. The aspirin treatment of viral infections is strongly associated with Reye's syndrome, one of the top ten child-killers. The condition is characterized by vomiting and lethargy, sometimes followed by delirium and coma. Half its victims die, and some who live through it wind up permanently brain damaged.

Reye's syndrome usually develops several days after a virus infection—flu, chicken pox, or a cold. Symptoms to watch for are persistent vomiting, listlessness, drowsiness, personality changes, disorientation, delirium, convulsions, or loss of consciousness.

Reye's syndrome develops with little warning and is often misdiagnosed, as in the case of 9-year-old Cindy Robbins. At first, Cindy just came down with a cold. Four days later she vomited—only once, but since this was unusual for her, her mother telephoned the pediatrician. The pediatrician assured her it was nothing to worry about and suggested she was being overprotective. Cindy was listless and had clammy hands, but she had no fever or other symptoms.

When Cindy vomited a second time, her mother again called the pediatrician, with the same result.

When Cindy vomited a third time the next day, her mother brought her to the pediatrician's office, where she was seen after several hours' wait. The pediatrician said Cindy was badly dehydrated and should be hospitalized. She was later transferred to a major medical center for further testing and treatment.

By the time Reye's syndrome was diagnosed, Cindy had lapsed into a coma. Her brain continued to swell until, three days later, she died.[2]

While the condition was previously thought to be limited to children and teenagers, aspirin-related Reye's syndrome has now been documented in adults.[3] Teenagers have a particularly high incidence of the condition, because they often take aspirin on their own.

If your child is sick, avoid giving her not only plain aspirin but any cough and cold remedy that might contain it.

Should you lower a fever with Tylenol?

Because of the risk of Reye's syndrome, acetaminophen (Tylenol and others) is generally recommended for reducing fever in children. Aspirin, acetaminophen, and ibuprofen are about equally effective in reducing fever; and acetaminophen is the safest.

However, a recent study of children with chicken pox treated with acetaminophen suggests that even this practice is unwise. Sixty-eight children with chicken pox were given either acetaminophen or a placebo four times a day for four days. On the second day of treatment, children in the treated group were more active than those in the placebo group. But on the fourth day, the treated children itched more, and their chicken pox took a day longer to scab over. Children typically aren't allowed to return to school until this happens, so many parents of treated children were forced to miss an extra day of work.

The data suggests the effects of fever were actually beneficial in fighting off the virus, and that fever should be allowed to run its course.[4]

Should you reduce a fever at all?

The study of children with chicken pox is only one of many recent studies supporting Hippocrates' pro-fever approach. Hippocrates' attitude actually prevailed until the 1900s, when aspirin was introduced. By the turn of this century, drug companies were promoting aspirin for its ability to reduce fever as well as pain, which seemed to go together. Ultimately, mass advertising turned public sentiment against fever as a natural cleansing process.

New studies, however, have swung the pendulum back to Hippocrates. They show fever cripples many temperature-sensitive viruses. In laboratory experiments, artificially induced fevers have actually decreased the death rate among infected animals, while lowering temperatures has had the opposite effect.

Fever seems to fight disease by means of a substance called interleukin-1 (IL-1), which is released from white blood cells when a foreign agent invades the blood. It raises the thermostat in the hypothalamus, probably by activating prostaglandins, the substances aspirin suppresses. IL-1 speeds the production of the immune system's T cells, which augment natural killer cell activity. When the temperature rises from 98.6 to 102 degrees F, T-cell production increases by as much as twenty times. Conversely, when aspirin is given to rabbits in doses sufficient to prevent fever, the killing activity of their neutrophils (a type of white blood cell) is inhibited. High temperatures also strengthen the effect of interferon, a natural protein that combats viruses.[5]

In a study testing the effects of various drugs on toxic shock syndrome toxin injected into rabbits, the drugs that reduced fever— including aspirin, indomethacin, and cyclosporine—failed to inhibit the toxin's lethal effects. The only drug that worked (methylprednisone) didn't reduce the rabbits' fever.[6]

Before antibiotics, patients with syphilis were deliberately inoculated with typhoid bacteria to induce fever. This treatment was thought to speed recovery by inhibiting the syphilis bacteria from reproducing. In European hydrotherapies, fever is still intentionally induced for its cleansing effects. Heat treatment, or hyperthermia, is now being used experimentally as a form of cancer therapy, apparently with excellent results.[7]

A famous German cancer specialist reported that in a swampy area in Italy where malaria was rife, cancer was unknown. When the area was dried out, the malaria disappeared, but cancer became a problem. The doctor postulated that the high fevers common in malaria had stimulated the natural defenses of the residents so cancer couldn't develop.[8] If this theory is true, our national tendency to pop an aspirin or an acetaminophen at the first sign of a fever may be contributing to our very high incidence of cancer.

Contrary to popular belief, fever in and of itself isn't dangerous. Several investigators who carefully reviewed the literature failed to find any evidence that fever can cause brain damage. The only possible exceptions were patients with meningitis or encephalitis, but these conditions can cause brain damage themselves, independent of the effects of fever. Fever will not cause brain damage below 108 degrees, and temperatures this high are extremely rare.[9]

Still, fevers can be harmful in certain circumstances. They can pose an unnecessary stress on patients with heart or lung disease; they can cause confusion and delirium, especially in the elderly; they can reactivate fever blisters; and they may be harmful to the fetus during the first three months of pregnancy. They can also provoke seizures in children prone to them. However, drugs aren't usually effective in preventing this type of seizure, since by the time the fever is recognized, the seizure is already in full swing. Fortunately, these seizures are harmless.[10] Mothers of children prone to seizures with fever are generally told to give Tylenol prophylactically whenever a fever develops.

It's good to get a doctor's advice for any fever over 103 degrees or for one above 100 degrees that lasts more than three days, especially if it's accompanied by a very sore throat.

9

VACCINES: BENEFITS AND RISKS

What does not destroy me makes me stronger.
—Friedrich Nietzche

Vaccines have eradicated smallpox, and they've reduced polio in the United States to an obscure disease. But like all drugs, they can be problematic. They don't always work; and you need to weigh the risk that you'll get the disease without the vaccine against the risk that you'll get it from the vaccine. Vaccines work by causing your body to produce antibodies that protect you against repeat bouts of the disease. But to do this, they have to expose you to the antigens that cause the disease.

That vaccines carry risks doesn't mean you shouldn't get them. In fact, immunization against polio, diphtheria, tetanus, pertussis (whooping cough), measles, mumps, and rubella is required by law for children entering school. But it's good to be aware of the downside of these drugs, and to be alert to possible side effects. All states allow exceptions if there are medical reasons to predict the possibility of a severe reaction. There may also be the possibility of deferral based on religious or philosophical beliefs.[1]

Polio

The conquest of polio by immunization is one of the major triumphs claimed by medicine. The triumph has been disputed, since polio actually began its decline before the vaccine came into use. In any case, today more cases of the disease are traced to the vaccine than to spontaneous outbreaks.[2] Polio vaccine can have other serious side effects, including muscle wasting, weakness, fever, and inflammation of the nerves and spinal cord.[3]

A case that made legal history in 1988 involved a 2-month-old boy who, one month after receiving an oral polio vaccine, contracted a severe case of the disease that left him paralyzed from the neck down. In a landmark ruling, the U.S. Supreme Court held that the government could be held liable for negligence in licensing and approving dangerous drugs and vaccines. The manufacturer prudently settled out of court.[4]

The biggest risk from polio vaccine is to unvaccinated parents of children receiving it, since the live polio virus can be transmitted in the baby's diapers. This means if your child is getting the vaccine, you should be sure to get it first.

DPT

Diphtheria, pertussis, and tetanus vaccines come in the combination called "DPT." Tetanus vaccine can produce serious complications, but the most controversial in this trio is the "P," pertussis vaccine. It can cause permanent brain damage, epilepsy, retardation, and death.

The United States is the only Western country in which pertussis immunization is mandatory; and some states no longer require it. In Japan, the vaccine was abandoned following the deaths of two infants within a day of receiving it. One in three hundred immunizations has been reported to produce generalized seizures, and the vaccine has been linked to Sudden Infant Death Syndrome (SIDS). In Tennessee in 1978–79, eleven babies died of SIDS within eight days of pertussis vaccination. Nine of the eleven had been vaccinated with the same lot of the vaccine. In *DPT: A Shot in the Dark,* authors Barbara Fisher and Harris Coulter estimate that as many as 943 deaths and 11,666 cases of long-term neurological damage may be attributable annually to pertussis vaccine.[5]

Against the risk of serious side effects, of course, you have to weigh the risk of getting the disease. We know of one mother who regretted the decision not to have her child vaccinated, after nursing him through a bout of whooping cough that persisted for six months. Whooping cough has been making a comeback, up from 1,895 cases in 1982, to 2,925 cases in 1988.

On the other hand, a child who has this much trouble with the disease could have even more trouble with the vaccine. And vaccination doesn't guarantee immunity. Of 795 cases of pertussis reported in 1988, *49 percent had been fully vaccinated against it.* Whooping coughs comeback isn't because mothers are resisting vaccination for their children. Vaccination rates are as high as they've ever been. Rather, the vaccine seems to be wearing off. Most victims are either adults, or very young infants who can't be protected by the vaccine. You can't be revaccinated after the age of seven because the rate of severe complications is unacceptably high. And vaccines don't help infants since full immunity isn't reached until they've completed the full course of immunization. (Five courses of the vaccine are recommended before school.) Even after you get the full course, the vaccine is only 60–85 percent effective.[6]

When your child gets pertussis vaccine, watch for these symptoms of serious reaction: a fever over 104 degrees F, persistent crying, and convulsions. If he has any of these reactions on Round 1, you should think twice about going for Round 2. It's best not to blunt these reactions with acetaminophen (Tylenol), since you may merely be masking a marker for future serious reactions.[7]

MMR

The other mandatory vaccine combination is the "MMR"—measles, mumps, rubella.

Measles inoculations are innocuous, but they may not be effective. The vaccine has a failure rate as high as 10 percent. In the first half of 1989, more than 7,000 cases were reported to the U.S. Centers for Disease Control, a notable increase over previous years. Many of these cases occurred in young people who had been vaccinated against the disease.[8]

The occurrence of the condition called mumps encephalitis (inflammation of the brain) has fallen overall since the mumps vaccine was introduced. However, cases of the condition caused by the vaccine itself have been reported.[9]

As for the rubella vaccine, it has been linked to rheumatoid arthritis; and a 1988 report in the British journal, *Medical Hypotheses*, linked it to Epstein-Barr virus syndrome.[10]

Smallpox, AIDS, and other vaccine-caused epidemics

Smallpox is another vaccination triumph. Again, the disease has been effectively eradicated, except that which has been contracted from the vaccine itself. In fact, smallpox vaccine was the *only* source of smallpox-related deaths for thirty years after spontaneous cases of the disease had disappeared. Given to pregnant women, the vaccine can also cause birth defects in their children.[11]

Smallpox vaccine isn't given today in this country except to servicemen. The rationale for giving it to recruits is to protect them in the event the virus is used as an agent in biological warfare. This rationale has been questioned, since biological warfare has been outlawed by convention, and even if the convention were ignored, the smallpox virus is one of the least suitable agents for carrying it out.[12]

More important, even in apparently healthy servicemen, the vaccine can be risky. The *New England Journal of Medicine* reported the death of a 19-year-old black athlete who developed smallpox and AIDS after receiving a series of immunizations upon entering military service. The series included a live-virus vaccine for smallpox.[13]

One theory actually traces the AIDS epidemic to the World Health Organization's worldwide smallpox immunization program. The African nations most affected by AIDS were also those receiving the most intensive smallpox immunizations. Zaire, the world leader in AIDS cases, received as many as 36 million smallpox vaccines. The same immunization program could account for the high rates of AIDS in Brazil and Haiti.[14]

Another theory traces the AIDS epidemic to polio vaccine. An AIDS-like virus has been found in African monkeys, leading some researchers to suggest that the spread of the disease to humans originated in the widespread immunization of African natives against polio with a monkey-cultured vaccine. Many people were immunized against polio with a vaccine grown in monkey tissue before it was discovered that the culture medium could be heavily contaminated with a virus of monkey origin. A type of virus has also been found in the vaccine that has been linked to brain tumors, a condition that has increased in the last decade.[15]

Dr. Robert Strecker, a Los Angeles physician who specializes in the treatment of AIDS, supports another theory. He believes the AIDS virus originated, not in monkeys, but in the laboratory. He contends the virus is a composite of two animal viruses: Bovine Leukemia Virus, which causes leukemia in cattle, and Visna, the brain rot virus of sheep. Since cattle and sheep don't mate in nature, it's likely these viruses met in the test tube.

Calculating back to when the first cases appeared and using the rate at which the virus doubles, Dr. Strecker shows the AIDS virus must have appeared in many people at once; i.e., probably by inoculation. In the United States, the virus first appeared in five cities simultaneously. Ominously, it was at the same time, in the same cities, in the same group of people, that the New York City Blood Bank conducted its hepatitis B vaccine study. The study involved white, male homosexuals between the ages of 20 and 40. Without actually stating AIDS was a Communist plot, Dr. Strecker notes the study was headed by a Russian-educated Polish scientist who immigrated to the United States and worked his way up to project head from janitor.[16]

Vaccines have been known to cause other epidemics. A report in the April 16, 1987, *New England Journal of Medicine* traced a 1942 epidemic of hepatitis to yellow fever vaccine. Approximately 50,000 men in the U.S. Army were affected. The vaccine had been stabilized in human blood drawn from medical school students, and several of them were later found to have a history of jaundice.[17]

Live-virus vaccines can cause severe complications when given to people with unrecognized impaired immunity. This impaired immunity can result from AIDS, cancer, or treatment with certain drugs. Live vaccines are given not only for smallpox but for polio, measles, mumps, rubella, and tuberculosis (BCG vaccine). Live vaccines have many advantages, and they're considered particularly useful in developing countries. The problem is that developing countries, especially in some parts of Africa, also have high rates of HIV infection, the forerunner of AIDS. The result could be high rates of serious complications from the vaccines.[18]

Immunization may be related in another way to AIDS and other autoimmune diseases, including cancer and rheumatoid arthritis. An autoimmune disease is one in which the body confuses normal cells with foreign invaders and begins attacking itself. Autoimmune diseases have mushroomed in the years since immunization has been required by law. Some researchers suspect the cells' confusion results because foreign invaders have been in the blood since childhood; and because they got there, not in the ordinary way, through organs equipped to buffer them, but through forcible injection directly into the vein.[19]

Table 12.   *Commonly Recommended Immunizations*[20]

Routinely recommended:	0–7	8–24	Age 25–29	30–64	65+
diphtheria	x	x	x	x	x
Haemophilus influenzae B	x				
influenza					x
measles	x	s	s		
mumps	x	s			
pertussis	x				
pneumococcal					x
polio	x				
rubella	x	s	s		
tetanus	x	x	x	x	x

Recommended for certain people or situations:	health care workers	other occupa-tions	Indication immuno-compro-mised	preg-nancy	travelers	chronic illness
diphtheria			x	x		
Haemophilus influenzae B			x			
influenza	x	s	x		s	x
measles	x	s	/	/	x	
mumps			/	/		
pertussis						
pneumococcal			x			x
polio	s	s	*	s	s	
rubella	x	s	/	/	x	
tetanus		s	x	x	x	
adenovirus		s	/			
anthrax		s				
BCG	s		/	/		
cholera			/		s	
hepatitis B	s	s	s	s	s	
meningococcal		s			s	
plague		s			s	
rabies		s			s	
smallpox		s	/	/		
typhoid		s			s	
yellow fever		s	/	s	s	

x = yes, / = no, s = in selected risk situations.
* = inactivated polio vaccine only.

10

ELECTIVE VACCINES

The superior doctor prevents illness; the mediocre doctor cures imminent illness; the inferior doctor treats illness.

—Chinese proverb

Vaccines and antibiotics have been credited with lower childhood mortality in this century, but the premise isn't universally accepted. The diseases targeted by vaccines disappeared not only in the United States, where immunization is required by law, but in Europe, where mass immunization isn't carried out. Furthermore, the major decline in infectious diseases occurred before vaccines and antibiotics came into existence. Diphtheria mortality, for example, dropped 50 percent before the vaccine for it was developed.

Instead of to vaccines, credit for the decrease in childhood deaths may go to improvements in sanitation, nutrition, and general standards of living. Epidemics of diseases like cholera, smallpox, and polio became a serious problem beginning in about the fifteenth century, when travelers in search of treasure brought back unfamiliar germs. There was no acquired immunity for these infections, and lack of sanitation and adequate nutrition reduced resistance to them. The incidence of infectious disease decreased along with the reversal of these unfavorable living conditions. Advances in agriculture brought better nutrition. Contraception improved the standard of living by reducing the number of people competing for society's services. Water purification, sewage disposal, and milk pasteurization cleaned up the carriers in which germs had thrived.[1]

Travelers to Third World countries today face much the same

problems as travelers did in the fifteenth century. In this chapter, we'll look at elective vaccines for them and for two other high-risk groups, preschool children and the elderly.

Immunization and other preventive measures for travelers

The infectious diseases that have been stamped out in the United States are still available for the catching in developing countries. Travelers to them are advised to take some of the same precautions that reduced these diseases historically: thorough boiling of drinking water, or drinking only bottled beverages; eating only food that has been well cooked, or that can be peeled; and the use of condoms.

Immunization is also recommended. Unlike colds and fever, the diseases travelers are exposed to are ones to which their bodies haven't naturally adapted.

One disease that's a threat to travelers is yellow fever. It is carried by indigenous mosquitos, and when indigenous people contract it, fewer than one in twenty die of it. But among travelers who come from abroad, fatality rates can reach 50 percent. If you're traveling to an area where yellow fever is rife, vaccination is recommended or required, depending on the country. One shot is effective for 30–35 years, although the International Health Regulations still require revaccination every ten years.[2]

Another mosquito-borne disease is malaria. Again, for many African natives born and raised in malaria-infested areas, the disease is no worse than an American flu. Some manage to escape its symptoms altogether. But when Americans get it, the disease is at best a miserable experience, and at worst it can be fatal.

Unfortunately, no vaccine effective against the multiple varieties of malaria has yet been developed, and experts say none is likely in the near future. Travelers are reduced to taking various oral antimalarials, and these drugs are losing their effectiveness against new, resistant strains of the disease. The drugs can also have serious side effects, especially when taken for long periods; so it's good to find out the actual risk of the disease in the area to which you're traveling before dosing up with the drugs.

For low-risk areas, merely wearing protective clothing, sleeping under nets, and using mosquito coils that repel the insects may be sufficient. You can also spray your ankles, wrists, and neck with an insect repellent containing "DEET," and spray your sleeping quarters with a pyrethrum-containing flying insect spray (see chapter 27). These poisons aren't particularly good for you, but if you're on a short "safari," the time you need to be exposed to them is much shorter than for antimalarial drugs. Antimalarials may have to be taken for a period beginning a week before you travel until six weeks after you get home. The spray has to be used only from dusk to dawn (the time when malarial mosquitos are said to attack) on the days you're actually exposed. The spray can be hazardous to children, however. It should be used on them with caution, if at all.

Mosquito repellents and long sleeves are a good idea even if you are taking antimalarials, because the drugs may not work.[3] If you contract the disease despite precautions, you should seek immediate medical care. Symptoms to watch for are fever, chills, sweating, and headaches.

The legal vaccination requirements for getting into the country you're visiting must also be met. These requirements aren't actually for your protection, but to keep diseases out of the country you're entering. What's important for your protection is to get the immunizations before you travel. Otherwise, you face injection at the border, and there's no telling whose arms the needles may have been in before yours. For up-to-date requirements and recommendations, write to the Superintendent of Documents, U.S. Government Printing Office, Washington, D.C. 20402, for the publication "Health Information for International Travel," or check with the Centers for Disease Control.

Polio is still alive and well in many developing countries, so immunizations against it should be complete. If you're traveling where food, water, and sanitation are substandard, other immunizations that may be recommended are those for typhoid and hepatitis. Hepatitis B vaccine is recommended for other high-risk groups besides travelers, including most health care workers, homosexual men, injectable-drug abusers, people with bleeding disorders requiring blood products, prisoners, workers in institutions for the mentally retarded, and intimates of carriers of the disease.[4]

Cholera immunization is also recommended or required for entry into some countries. However, the U.S. Public Health Service and the World Health Organization have questioned its benefits. The injection is relatively ineffective, and it's prone to troublesome side effects. Moreover, if you use standard accommodations, you're at virtually no risk of infection from cholera. Again, your best defense is thorough cleaning and cooking of foods, avoidance of raw fruits and vegetables without peels, and drinking only bottled beverages or thoroughly boiled water.[5]

These sanitary precautions can also help protect you against salmonellosis and other diarrheal conditions that are the bane of travelers. If you get traveler's diarrhea anyway, you're better off not suppressing it with drugs, since your body is attempting to get rid of dangerous bacteria (see chapter 23). If you can't get by without a drug, the best choice is Pepto-Bismol. It contains bismuth salts, which kill bacteria. Some doctors recommend antibiotics (Bactrim or doxycycline) for preventative use before you get sick, but other authorities disagree, because these drugs can lead to resistant strains and prolong the period of communicability. In any case, antibiotics may be indicated for people with lowered resistance, including infants under two months old, the elderly, the debilitated, or people with continued high fever pointing to something more serious than a simple intestinal infection.[6]

Shots for tots: should you vaccinate your preschooler against meningitis?

The very young and the very old are high-risk groups targeted for two popular elective vaccines: those against meningitis and flu.

A new vaccine for meningitis has been recommended by the American Academy of Pediatrics and the Centers for Disease Control for all children 24–59 months of age and for those 18 months and up attending day-care centers. Whether this ambitious immunization program is worth the cost or the risks, however, remains controversial. Meningitis is a serious disease that is potentially fatal, so mass immunization would seem to make good sense. But the plan isn't as simple or straightforward as it seems.

One problem is that meningitis isn't a single disease. It can be caused by different viruses and bacteria, which require different preventative measures. Of the bacterial variety, 70 percent of U.S. cases are caused by the strains called *Neisseria meningitidis, Haemophilus influenzae,* and *Streptococcus pneumonia.*

The most serious kind of meningitis comes from *Neisseria meningitidis.* The disease comes on suddenly, with fever, intense headache, nausea, a stiff neck, and often, vomiting, a pink rash, delirium, and coma. The fatality rate used to be over 50 percent, but modern therapeutic measures have reduced this to under 10 percent if the disease is recognized and treated in time. Vaccines for this type of meningitis vary, depending on the strain of *Neisseria meningitidis* organism involved: Group A (which has caused the major epidemics in this country), or Groups B and C (which are currently responsible for most cases). There are vaccines for Group A and Group C, but none is presently available for Group B.[7]

Pneumococcal meningitis also has a high death rate. It is caused by *Streptococcus pneumonia* bacteria, of which there are eighty-three known types and twenty-three common ones. Prevention requires immunization with a vaccine containing the "capsular polysaccharides"—the capsule or shell of the bacteria—for all twenty-three common types.

The most common bacterial meningitis in American children two months to five years old, however, is the *Haemophilus* variety; and this is the one targeted by the new vaccine. *Haemophilus influenzae* type b (Hib) is the most frequent cause not only of meningitis, but of other serious bacterial infections in American children. Its symptoms are fever, vomiting, lethargy, stiff neck or back, and bulging fontanelle (the soft spot on the skull) in infants.[8]

An investigational capsular polysaccharide vaccine was licensed by the FDA in April of 1985, after a field trial apparently confirmed its efficacy against Hib infections. It was then recommended by the American Academy of Pediatrics for all children 24–59 months of age. The recommended age was later lowered to 18 months, after a second-generation Hib vaccine effective in this lower age group was licensed in 1987. One problem is that *70 percent* of serious Hib infections occur in children under 18 months, and there is still no vaccine effective in this age group.[9]

Another problem is that there is some evidence that the vaccine can cause, or contribute to, the very disease it was designed to prevent. A study in the December 18, 1986, *New England Journal of Medicine* reported 55 cases of invasive Hib disease that developed in children inoculated with the vaccine an average of three months earlier. Meningitis developed in 39 of the 55 cases. Three died. Six had serious neurologic complications, including deafness, blindness, and quadriplegia. Five had shock or cerebral edema (swelling of the brain). These were considered "vaccine failures," because the vaccine didn't prevent the disease. The researchers conceded, however, that the high rate of complications may actually have been caused by the vaccine itself.[10]

Another question is whether the vaccine does much good. A case-control study in Minnesota, where use of the vaccine was widespread, failed to document *any* change in the statewide incidence of Hib disease.[11] And in two studies reported in the *New England Journal of Medicine* in 1987, among children who had been directly exposed to active cases at day-care facilities, the incidence of the disease was as low in unvaccinated as in vaccinated children. In one of these studies, *no* subsequent case was found among 361 exposed children under two years of age, the group at particularly high risk. In the other study, among 8,000 day-care contacts directly exposed to a primary case over a seven-year period, only three children contracted the disease—and one of them had been vaccinated against it.

To vaccinate these 8,000 children would have cost an estimated $750,000. Only two cases of the disease might have been prevented, assuming the vaccine worked on them. And other cases might have arisen or been aggravated as a result of the vaccine itself.[12]

The researchers conducting these studies felt that the Immunization Practices Advisory Committee (IPAC) of the Centers for Disease Control incorrectly interpreted their results in forming public policy recommending Hib vaccination.[13]

Shots for seniors

Another high-risk group for viral and bacterial epidemics is the elderly. The average flu epidemic kills twenty thousand people, and most of them are senior citizens. Flu shots are available, but unfortunately they're only 30–40 percent effective in this age group. They are also good only for a single epidemic, since the virus keeps changing. This means the shots have to be repeated every fall. If you're allergic to eggs, you shouldn't get the vaccines, since they're cultured in eggs. And if you're already sick with a fever, you should wait until you're well.[14]

A vaccine is also available against the pneumococcal bacteria, which causes about forty thousand deaths a year. Unfortunately, this vaccine isn't very effective in high-risk elderly patients either. It also shouldn't be given more than once, since severe allergic reactions can occur the second time around.[15]

A more fundamental problem with vaccinating people who are already in a weakened condition is that the vaccines may further impair their immune systems.

II

Prescription Drugs for the Major Killers

11

DRUGS THAT LOWER RISK FACTORS: REASSESSING THE EVIDENCE

No matter how the data are presented, the simple fact is that many people must be treated to benefit relatively few. . . . [W]hen a large population undergoes a treatment alleged to benefit only 1 or 2 percent of its members, the balance of burdens and benefits requires close scrutiny.

—A. Brett, M.D. (1989)[1]

Coronary heart disease (CHD) is the number one American killer, and stroke is number three. Your chances of succumbing to one of these cardiovascular diseases are better than fifty-fifty, and they go up as certain risk factors go up. For CHD, the three major risk factors are high blood pressure (hypertension), elevated serum cholesterol levels, and smoking. For stroke, the single most important risk factor is high blood pressure.[2]

This helps explain why high blood pressure is the number one target of medicine. More than sixty million Americans have it. About 30–50 percent of people over sixty are treated for it. And more drug money is made on it than on any other condition. Annual sales of $7 billion are divided among some sixty hypertension drugs. Diuretics, the most popular, were the subject of over fifty million prescriptions in 1988. Sales of two newer blood pressure drugs called "ACE inhibitors" passed the billion-dollar mark the same year, a distinction held by only three other brand-name drugs.[3]

Yet 75 percent of the people who make up this lucrative market have only "mild" hypertension—and *drug treatment for people in this category has not been proved to significantly increase survival.* Drug therapy became standard treatment long before there was reliable evidence of its benefits, and the matter still remains in doubt.[4]

"Mild" hypertension is typically defined as a diastolic pressure (the bottom number in the equation) of 90–100 or 90–109 mm Hg (millimeters of mercury). The cutoff was dropped from 95 to 90 by the National Heart, Lung, and Blood Institute (NHLBI) in 1984. When high blood pressure is defined in this way, the condition affects up to a quarter of U.S. adults. Antihypertensive drugs have been prescribed for millions of them, although they felt fine before treatment and had no visible symptoms. Once hypertension is diagnosed, the drugs usually have to be taken two or three times a day for life. The average age at diagnosis is fifty. This means the drugs are typically taken for twenty years or more.[5] Since their side effects can significantly impair the quality of life thereafter, it's important to establish that the drugs clearly increase survival before getting started on them. Unfortunately, this has yet to be proved for the largest treatment category, "mild" hypertension. The same is true for drugs aimed at other cardiovascular risk factors.

In the well-known Framingham Heart Study, 5,209 adults living in Framingham, Massachusetts, were followed for eighteen years beginning in 1949. People with lower blood pressure and serum cholesterol levels were found to live significantly longer than people with higher levels. But the people with the lower levels in these studies didn't typically get them from drugs. They got them from their lifestyles or their genes. Long-term studies of people on low-fat, high-fiber vegetarian diets also consistently show a reduction in serum cholesterol and blood pressure levels, as well as an actual increase in life expectancy.[6] But in studies in which blood pressure and serum cholesterol have been lowered *with drugs,* no increase in survival has resulted. The exceptions involve that limited group of high-risk patients who have already suffered a heart attack or stroke, or who have unusually high blood pressure or serum cholesterol levels.

Since the drugs aimed at reducing cardiovascular risk carry risks themselves, you need to know if their benefits have been clearly established before you start on them. So before we compare the merits of different drugs in these categories, let's examine the evidence concerning their effects on longevity in general. We'll look at four popular drug types: those that lower blood pressure, those that lower serum cholesterol, and aspirin and antiarrhythmics used to lower heart attack risk.

Blood-pressure-lowering drugs: trading strokes for heart attacks

The first major study to look at the drug treatment of mild hypertension was the Veterans Administration Cooperative Study. Its first report, published in 1967, focused on severe hypertension, and its second report, published in 1970, focused on mild hypertension. For severe hypertension, drug treatment was shown to be beneficial. It not only lowered blood pressure, but actually saved lives. For mild hypertension, however, the study failed to establish that drugs significantly improved survival.[7]

A later study, reported by the U.S. Public Health Service in 1977, also failed to show drug treatment reduced the overall death rate.[8] The question was left open for further investigation.

Despite these questions, drugs for mild hypertension became standard treatment. A 1976 survey in New York State showed a prescription rate for mild hypertensives of 78 percent. A 1979 follow-up bumped this figure to 90 percent.[9]

It wasn't until 1979 that the already well-established drug craze was vindicated by research—or so it seemed. The landmark study, published in the *Journal of the American Medical Association* in December of that year, was conducted by the Hypertension Detection and Follow-up Program Cooperative Group (HDFP), sponsored by the NHLBI. It involved nearly eleven thousand people aged 30–69 with high blood pressure.

Drug studies usually include a "placebo" group—a group given fake drugs having no physiological effect. The effectiveness of the real drug is measured against the effect in these "controls." But in the HDFP study, drug treatment was already so widely accepted that the researchers considered it unethical to leave a large group of patients untreated. Those in the control group were simply left to their usual medical care. It was assumed they'd get fewer drugs than the "special treatment" group, since the drugs were still experimental.

As it turned out, there wasn't much difference between the groups. By the fifth year, a full 58 percent of the control group was on drugs, compared to 78 percent of the experimental group. Moreover, treatment in the experimental group wasn't limited to drugs. It included counseling to undertake "holistic" changes in lifestyle: to quit smoking, reduce salt intake, and modify diet to lose weight and lower serum cholesterol. Any improvements in the "treated" group could have resulted from these lifestyle changes rather than from the drugs.

The much-publicized result was that five-year mortality from all causes was 20 percent lower in the special-treatment group than the controls.[10] An enthusiastic editorial in the *New England Journal of Medicine* proclaimed:

> The lesson of the HDFP is clear. There is benefit to be derived from assiduous treatment of patients *with any degree of hypertension.*[11]

True, but is there benefit to be derived from assiduous *drug* treatment? This was the conclusion drawn by commentators, until they later spotted the flaws in the study's design.[12] That wasn't until 1985, when an even larger study was reported that did include a placebo group. It was conducted by the British Medical Research Council (MRC). It found *no* significant difference in the death rates of people on active drugs and placebos.[13]

So what caused the 20 percent drop in mortality in the HDFP "special treatment" group? Arguably, it was the holistic changes in lifestyle rather than the drugs. In fact, the drop may have resulted *in spite of* the drugs. This possibility was strongly suggested by a follow-up study, called "MR. FIT."

Published in September of 1982, the Multiple Risk Factor Intervention Trial (MRFIT) was also sponsored by the NHLBI. The trial involved 12,866 men aged 35–57 considered to be at increased risk for CHD. As in the HDFP study, the participants had no clinical evidence of the disease, but they had the risk factors: high blood pressure, high serum cholesterol, and smoking.

The men were randomly assigned to two groups. Again, those in the control group received their usual health care from normal community sources. Those in the experimental group received special care, involving both antihypertensive drugs and counseling to reduce smoking and alter their diets to reduce serum cholesterol. What distinguished MR. FIT from the HDFP study was that not all the men had high blood pressure at entry. That meant not all of them got the drugs.

The disturbing result from MR. FIT was that deaths were actually *higher* in the *experimental* group. The difference wasn't "statistically significant"; it could have come about by chance. Yet it was there. How could more deaths occur in men who'd *reduced* their smoking and their intakes of fat? The researchers suspected some factor in their multiple-risk-factor intervention was counterproductive. The proposed culprit: the antihypertensive medicine itself.

This deduction followed from the fact that in the men who weren't hypertensive at entry (and thus didn't get the drugs), the holistic changes in lifestyle substantially *reduced* the CHD death rate. The reduction was a significant 21 percent. It was only among the men who *were* hypertensive at entry (and thus got the drugs) that coronary heart disease deaths were greater than among the hypertensive controls. It seems the diuretics used to lower blood pressure also increased serum cholesterol and triglyceride levels. Thus, they countered the effects of dietary change, which reduced these risk factors.

In the guarded language typical of medical research, the researchers concluded:

[T]he possibility that the use of pharmacologic [drug] therapy in these subgroups is associated with an increased CHD mortality warrants further investigation. [14]

A second look at a 1980 Norwegian study revealed similar trends. The Oslo Study involved nearly 800 mildly hypertensive but asymptomatic men aged 40–49 years. Half received drugs, half didn't. The patients were followed for 5½ years. Drug treatment reduced blood pressures an average of 17 mm Hg systolic and 10 mm Hg diastolic. Cerebrovascular events (strokes) occurred only in the control group, which received no drugs.

Drug treatment again looked good—until it was observed that CHD incidence, including sudden death, was *50 percent higher* in the drug group than in the no-drug group. This was particularly disturbing, because *hypertensives are five times as likely to die of a heart attack as of a stroke.* The overall result, as in MR. FIT, was that there were 11 percent more deaths from all causes in the treated than in the untreated group. Again, the difference wasn't statistically significant. But neither was the difference in the death rate from strokes. The drug-treated group simply traded the risk of a stroke for the risk of a heart attack—along with the unpleasant side effects of the drugs themselves.[15]

Two other foreign studies seemed to favor drug treatment for mild hypertension. In both, antihypertensive drugs reduced heart attacks as well as strokes. One was the Australian Therapeutic Trial, reported in 1980.[16] The other was the European Working Party on High Blood Pressure in the Elderly Trial, reported in 1985.[17] Their favorable results, however, were dwarfed by the much larger MRC study, also reported in 1985. It involved a longer trial period and 5–20 times as many patients. In fact, the British Medical Research Council study is considered the largest trial of its kind likely to be done in our time.[18] It involved 17,354 mildly hypertensive patients (90–109 mm Hg diastolic) aged 35–64 years. They were treated either with a beta-blocker (propranolol), a diuretic (bendrofluazide), or a placebo. They were followed for five years.

Strokes were cut nearly in half by active treatment. However, the number of strokes in both groups was so low that this reduction was termed an "infrequent benefit." The risk was cut to one stroke per 850 patient/years with treatment; but it was only two strokes per 850 patient/years without treatment. A much greater reduction in risk was seen in nonsmokers as compared to smokers.

More troubling was the lack of an effect on CHD, the most serious and common complication of high blood pressure. Again, the overall result was that no fewer patients died with drugs than without them.[19]

It would have been a draw, except for the side effects of the drugs themselves. Both drugs caused impotence, lethargy, nausea, dizziness, and headache. The diuretic also caused impaired glucose tolerance (predisposing to diabetes), abnormally low potassium levels (predisposing to neuromuscular, kidney, and stomach disorders), gout, and constipation. The beta-blocker caused numbness and pain in the fingers and toes, rashes, and labored breathing.[20]

Newer drugs like the ACE inhibitors seem to have fewer side effects, but their effects on long-term survival haven't yet been established. We'll look at the relative merits of the various blood-pressure-lowering options in the next two chapters.

Aspirin: trading heart attacks for strokes

The aspirin-a-day craze for heart attack prevention was launched by a study reported in the *New England Journal of Medicine* in January of 1988. Earlier studies showed that in patients who had previously suffered a heart attack, daily doses of aspirin significantly reduced disease and death from cardiovascular causes. The Physicians' Health Study looked at healthy men who had not previously had a heart attack. The subjects were 22,071 male doctors aged 40–84.

The study found that in doctors taking 325 mg (5 grains) of aspirin every other day, heart attacks were reduced by 47 percent more than in doctors not taking the drug. There were 171 nonfatal and 18 fatal heart attacks in the placebo group, versus only 99 nonfatal and 5 fatal heart attacks in the aspirin group.[21]

These results were impressive. But again, there was a problem: aspirin had *no* effect on the death rate. Mortality was the same in both groups. There were 72 fewer nonfatal heart attacks among the aspirin takers, but there were no fewer deaths.

This was explained in part by a threefold increase in the number of fatal strokes. Aspirin, it seems, has the opposite effect of blood-pressure-lowering drugs: it *reduces* the risk of heart attack, but it *increases* the risk of stroke.

Aspirin reduces heart attacks by interfering with blood coagulation. It prevents blood from clotting. Decreased clotting, however, means increased bleeding. And cerebral hemorrhage, or bleeding, is the cause of some strokes. Normally, a small hemorrhage in the brain would be closed off by the blood's clotting factor and made harmless. But aspirin can cause the leak to keep bleeding enough to cause a stroke. This type of stroke isn't the most common, but it is the most likely to be fatal.

In the Physicians' Health Study, the increase in strokes in aspirin-takers wasn't statistically significant. The doctor/subjects, however, were unusually healthy. The risk of stroke is likely to be greater in hypertensives, who are already at high risk for the disease.[22] An example is the man in his sixties complaining of impotence discussed in the preface, who took aspirin to prevent a heart attack and wound up with a stroke.

Further grounds for pause came from a similar British study reported the same week. It confirmed the bad news: strokes among aspirin-taking doctors were increased. But it failed to confirm the good news: heart attacks were not decreased. In 5,000 male British doctors taking 500 mg of aspirin daily, total mortality wasn't significantly lower than in doctors taking no aspirin. Total nonfatal heart attacks weren't reduced, and strokes were again increased, this time by a factor of five.[23]

Why the difference? One reason may have been that in the American study, half the doctors taking aspirin were also taking beta-carotene, a vitamin A precursor occurring naturally in plant foods. The vitamin was included to test its effects on cancer incidence, but it may also have influenced the rate of heart disease.

Another proposed difference is that the aspirin in the American study was in the form of Bufferin, which contains magnesium. Like aspirin itself, magnesium prevents blood coagulation and platelet adhesion.[24]

Whatever the explanation, no study has yet shown that a regular aspirin habit will increase life expectancy, except in that high-risk group of people who have already suffered a heart attack. An aspirin habit can also have unwanted side effects. Doctors taking aspirin were 22 percent more likely to suffer an ulcer than those taking placebos, and they were 71 percent more likely to require a blood transfusion.[25]

We'll look at aspirin, its actions, and its side effects more closely in chapter 18.

Cholesterol-lowering drugs: trading heart attacks for gallstones

In long-term trials, drugs to lower serum cholesterol have met similar fates. Three major drug trials have tested three different cholesterol-lowering drugs. In each of them, heart disease and its mortality were reduced. Yet total deaths remained the same, or actually increased.

The first study, reported in 1980, was conducted by the World Health Organization and tested the drug clofibrate. The drug seems to have killed more people than it saved. Deaths in the treated group were one-third higher than in the controls (163 vs. 127).[26]

The second study, reported in 1984, was the Lipid Research Clinics Coronary Primary Prevention Trial. It tested the drug cholestyramine (Questran). Nonfatal heart attacks were reduced by 20 percent, but total deaths in the treated and control groups weren't significantly different (68 vs. 71).[27]

The third study, the Helsinki Heart Study, was reported in 1987. It tested the drug gemfibrozil (Lopid). CHD was reduced by 34 percent, but again, there were actually more deaths in the treated than in the untreated group (45 vs. 42).[28]

Offsetting the reduction in heart disease deaths in each of these studies was an increased fatality from accidents and violence. This finding could have been passed off to coincidence, except that it happened repeatedly. It seems the drugs may have induced mood changes, precipitating the accidental and violent deaths. In addition, people on cholesterol-lowering drugs were more likely to develop gallstones, which in certain cases led to death. They also had higher incidences of certain types of cancer and of bleeding in the brain.[29]

Again, studies *have* shown you can lengthen your life by lowering serum cholesterol with diet.[30] What they *haven't* shown is that you can do it with drugs. Cholesterol-lowering drugs can also have distressing side effects and taking them can be like swallowing sand. For many people, it's harder to get them down in the required doses than to switch to a low-fat, high-fiber diet (see chapter 14).

Lovastatin (Mevacor) is a newer cholesterol-lowering drug that seems to have fewer side effects than the earlier options. It is also easier to swallow. But it has caused cataracts and birth defects in animals, and whether it actually increases survival hasn't been tested in any long-term study.[31] This means taking it can be risky. What can go wrong is illustrated by the recent experience with the antiarrhythmic drugs flecainide and encainide.

Antiarrhythmics: trading the risk of a heart attack for a heart attack

Arrhythmias (irregular heartbeats) are another risk factor that can foreshadow a heart attack. Flecainide (Tambocor) and encainide (Enkaid) are so effective at suppressing irregular heartbeats, both their manufacturers and medical researchers had high hopes for them. The drugs were approved by the FDA and had already been prescribed for over two hundred thousand patients when the National Institutes of Health abruptly terminated its cardiac arrhythmia study in April of 1989. The reason: the drugs were found to be too dangerous to continue the experiment.

The participants in the study were patients who had recently had a heart attack and who had mild arrhythmias without symptoms. The purpose of the study was to see if the drugs would prevent subsequent heart attacks, for which these patients were at high risk. The unexpected result was that the number of patients who died of heart attacks while taking the drugs was *more than double* that of patients taking placebos.

The FDA, which had earlier approved the drugs, has now banned them for mild arrhythmias, their chief former use.

Complained Enkaid's disappointed producers, "It was a growing product."[32]

Cancer chemotherapy

Chemotherapeutic drugs for cancer are also fraught with risks. We are not going to explore them in this book, because the risks and the alternatives cannot be covered adequately in one or two chapters. We must point out, however, that according to a 1985 study in *Scientific American,* only 2–5 percent of cancer deaths are prevented by these very toxic drugs. That means at least 95 percent of patients who get them suffer their devastating side effects needlessly.[33]

Different cancers have substantially different cure rates. If you're diagnosed as having the disease, before beginning treatment, it's very important to ask your doctor about the side effects and the likelihood of cure from the drugs for your particular condition and to solicit the opinions of any other health care professionals interested in your case (other doctors, nurses, pharmacists, etc.).

12

CONVENTIONAL BLOOD PRESSURE DRUGS: DIURETICS AND BETA-BLOCKERS

*The reality of mild hypertension is that most people will
live a long and happy life if you don't do anything.*
—Michael Alderman, M.D. (1989)[1]

Drugs, like species, evolve by trial and error; and the errors are the stuff of which lawsuits are made. Propranolol, the first and most popular beta-blocker for treating high blood pressure, has the drawback that it precipitates bronchial asthma in susceptible patients. In an effort to avoid this problem, researchers developed the beta-blocker practolol by making slight changes in propranolol's structure. The effort succeeded, but the hybrid had other side effects that proved to be much worse. Practolol was the drug discussed in chapter 1, which produced Mary's systemic lupus erythematosus. The better mousetrap turned out to be a major disaster, but the disaster wasn't recognized until it had taken its toll in seven thousand British casualties. Today, propranolol is still one of the most commonly prescribed beta-blockers, although life-threatening adverse reactions have been reported in 2 percent of patients taking it.[2]

Reserpine was another early blood-pressure-lowering drug that is now considered too dangerous to use except in intractable cases. It can cause depression severe enough to end in suicide, and it has been linked to cancer in laboratory animals. But these warnings took thirty years to emerge.[3]

Even the drugs traditionally considered safest for lowering blood pressure, the diuretics, are now coming under scrutiny. They were the antihypertensives in the MR. FIT and Oslo studies that were found to *raise* serum cholesterol levels, and to *increase* the death rate from coronary heart disease.[4]

Diuretics

Diuretics are the most frequently prescribed class of drugs in the United States. Under the conventional "stepped care" approach to hypertension, treatment of nearly every patient begins with one of them.

Diuretics act on the kidneys to increase the amount of water excreted. They're distinguished by the parts of the kidney they act on. "Thiazide" diuretics act on the kidney tubules. "Loop" diuretics act on the "loop of Henle." "Potassium-sparing" diuretics act on the distal tubules. All of them pull water from the blood, decreasing blood volume and thus, blood pressure.

The main problem with this approach is that valuable minerals are pulled out of the blood at the same time. Potassium is the most critical, since its loss can seriously affect the heart's electrical activity. Recent studies have shown that potassium actually helps prevent strokes. Since strokes are what antihypertensive drugs are supposed to prevent, drugs that deplete this mineral are counterproductive even if they do lower blood pressure.

This fact helps explain the disturbing results of two recent studies comparing diuretics and beta-blockers. In the Stockholm Metoprolol Post-Infarction Trial, reported in 1985, patients who had already suffered a heart attack were significantly more likely to have another one if they were on diuretics rather than on beta-blockers. This was true although both drugs lowered blood pressure to the same degree, and although diuretics have traditionally been considered the safest and most conservative first choice of treatment. In a second 1985 study involving 565 older hypertensive patients, the beta-blocker metoprolol (lopressor) again proved to be significantly safer and more effective than the diuretic hydrochlorothiazide.[5]

Despite these findings, in 1988 hydrochlorothiazide remained the generic antihypertensive most often prescribed.[6]

Dyazide was the most popular brand-name antihypertensive that same year. Dyazide combines the usual thiazide diuretic with triamterene, a "potassium-sparing" diuretic that can cause potassium retention. The idea is to avoid potassium loss, but triamterene doesn't always have this effect. All potassium-sparing diuretics can induce either very low or very high blood potassium levels.[7]

Triamterene can have other side effects, including nausea, diarrhea, headache, rash, and mouth dryness. Its more serious side effects, including kidney failure and retention of too much potassium, can be fatal. When you take Dyazide, you also risk the side effects of the thiazide the triamterene is combined with. Taking products that include multiple drugs in fixed combinations is nearly always a bad idea. You may not need all the ingredients, but you will suffer all their side effects. Even if you need all the ingredients, they're unlikely to be combined in the ratio best suited to your particular chemistry.

The second most popular brand-name diuretic of 1988 was the loop diuretic Lasix (furosemide). Lasix is stronger than either hydrochlorothiazide or Dyazide. It's so strong, in fact, that it is recommended only in cases where less toxic thiazide diuretics have failed. Yet Lasix has held its rank near the top of the prescription drug list for many years. This anomaly is best explained by the sensational ads and promotional material issued by its manufacturers. Lasix's side effects include dizziness, fainting, anemia, and loss of hearing. Taking Lasix can result in serious potassium loss and in an overly rapid loss of water and body salts that can cause collapse.[8]

The potassium loss caused by diuretics is sometimes remedied by adding supplemental potassium. The most popular of these products is the prescription drug Slow-K. Potassium supplements, unfortunately, can irritate the digestive tract and produce ulcers.[9] The safer and more natural alternative is to get extra potassium from foods, especially fresh fruits and vegetables.

In a study reported in the *New England Journal of Medicine* in 1987, *adding only a single serving of fruit or vegetables to the daily diet was found to lower the risk of stroke by a full 40 percent.* That's about the same benefit as a full course of antihypertensive drugs, without the side effects. Stroke deaths varied inversely with potassium intake. As potassium went up, deaths went down. Interestingly, the intake of sodium (salt) wasn't significantly related to stroke deaths. Sodium is the dietary variable most often associated with high blood pressure.[10]

Although the favorable effect of potassium on strokes in this study was independent of its effect on blood pressure, potassium also seems to help keep your blood pressure down. In a study reported in the same journal in May of 1989, blood pressure increased from 90.9 to 95 mm Hg in normal people eating a diet low in potassium.[11] In the Hypertension Detection and Follow-up Program (HDFP), a blood pressure difference of this amount was associated with a 20 percent difference in overall mortality over a five-year period.[12]

Other studies suggest it's the ratio of sodium to potassium that's important. Whole cereals, all fruits, and most vegetables contain 10–100 times as much potassium as sodium; but the modern diet contains more sodium than potassium, mainly because potassium is removed and sodium is added during processing and cooking (see table 13).

Unfortunately, eating a high-potassium diet won't solve the problems of diuretics. For one thing, the drugs deplete not only potassium but magnesium, which is necessary to retain potassium in cells. If blood magnesium is low, cells become more permeable. Potassium leaks out, and sodium and calcium leak in. The cells become electrically unstable, producing irregular rhythms. In the worst case, this can mean sudden death.[13]

In a 1980 Australian study, mortality among hypertensives treated with thiazide diuretics—presumably from heart attacks and sudden death—was *twice* that in any other treatment group. The other treatment protocols included not only (1) the beta-blocker propranolol, and (2) simple salt restriction, but (3) a placebo. This means *twice as many deaths occurred among hypertensives taking diuretics as among those receiving no treatment at all.*[14]

Table 13. *Sodium and Potassium Contents of Some Common Foods—Processed vs. Unprocessed*[15]

	[mg/100g]	
	Sodium	*Potassium*
Flour, wholemeal	3	360
White bread	540	100
Rice, polished	6	110
Rice, boiled	2	38
Beef, uncooked	55	280
Beef, corned	950	140
Haddock, uncooked	120	300
Haddock, smoked	790	190
Cabbage, uncooked	7	390
Cabbage, boiled	4	160
Peas, uncooked	1	340
Peas, canned	230	130
Pears, uncooked	2	130
Pears, canned	1	90

Diuretics are also troubled with side effects, including weakness, dizziness, sexual dysfunction, impotence, gastrointestinal distress, rash, muscle cramps, and hearing impairment. In the HDFP study, one out of three patients had to discontinue drug treatment because of intolerable side effects.[16]

In addition, diuretics can increase blood sugar, uric acid, and serum cholesterol levels. These effects aren't merely transient, but can persist for the duration of treatment. This means the drugs can increase your risk of diabetes, gout, and heart disease. Diabetes frequently develops during treatment with diuretics. In the MRC study, only 60 percent of patients who developed this problem had normal glucose tolerance six months after discontinuing treatment. A Swedish study reported in 1989 also found that hydrochlorothiazide (the most often prescribed diuretic) raised total serum cholesterol by 5 percent and LDL ("bad") cholesterol by 6 percent.[17]

So while diuretics remain the treatment favorites, they may not be the ideal blood-pressure-lowering alternative.

The beta-blockers

Under the traditional "stepped care" approach to lowering blood pressure, if a diuretic alone didn't lower it sufficiently, "Step 2" involved adding one of the "antiadrenergic" drugs. These drugs slow the heart by blocking its stimulation by adrenalin (epinephrine). Various antiadrenergic possibilities include reserpine (Serpasil), clonidine (Catapres), guanabenz (Wytensin), methyldopa (Aldomet), and prazosin (Minipress). The usual choice, however, is a beta-blocker, a drug that works by blocking certain nerve receptor sites called "beta receptors." These sites are stimulated by adrenalin and adrenalin-like chemicals to work the heart. When they're blocked, the brain can't signal the heart to beat faster or the arteries to constrict. Heart function is diminished, less blood is forced through the arteries, and blood pressure is reduced.

The problem with this approach is that by slowing your body's pump, beta-blockers can make you very tired. The brain tells the heart to beat faster and pump harder for a reason. In many people, it's because the arteries have become corroded with deposits of calcium and fat. These deposits narrow the arterial openings, requiring a greater pressure to push enough blood through to keep the body running at normal levels. Any artificial reduction in this pressure will at least make you feel tired. At worst, it can weaken your heartbeat enough to cause heart failure. Like reserpine, beta-blockers can also make you depressed, since they kill the "adrenalin rush" that makes life exciting.

By suppressing epinephrine, beta-blockers can trigger bronchial asthma. Epinephrine is the natural chemical that opens up the bronchi, or breathing tubes. In fact, it is often used to *treat* bronchial asthma.

Serious problems can also result if beta-blockers are withdrawn suddenly. This means once you're on them, it's tricky getting off.

Propranolol (Inderal) led the beta-blocker market for many years. It comes with a long list of side effects, including drowsiness, dizziness, low blood pressure, nausea, weakness, diarrhea, numbness and coldness in fingers and toes, dry mouth and skin, impotence, insomnia, hallucinations, nightmares, headaches, difficult breathing, joint pains, confusion, depression, reduced alertness, and constipation. Propranolol can also be dangerous for diabetics. It's a "nonselective" beta-blocker, which blunts the signs of an acute drop in blood sugar and reduces the release of insulin in response to high blood sugar.

All beta-blockers can affect the central nervous system, but propranolol is one of the worst.[18] The result can be nightmares, bizarre dreams, hallucinations, depression, and insomnia.

An interesting case involved an even-tempered, 21-year-old man who was treated with propranolol to relieve migraine headaches. The treatment worked, but the man was no longer himself. He started seeing spiders, hearing voices, and having vivid nightmares and suicidal impulses. In an uncharacteristic outburst of violence, he pushed a fellow worker out of the cab of an excavator at a quarry. The propranolol was stopped, but two weeks later the man was readmitted to the hospital with depression and suicidal fantasies. He saw himself hanging from the ceiling. He saw bars across his bedroom doorway. It took another week for his symptoms to lift, after which drug treatment for his headaches was judiciously discontinued.[19]

Propranolol's market position has now been usurped by newer beta-blockers with fewer side effects. In 1988, Inderal dropped to third place among beta-blocker favorites, while atenolol (Tenormin) moved into first place, and metoprolol (Lopressor) moved into second. Other beta-blockers that are less often prescribed include labetolol, nadolol, pindolol, and timolol.

Atenolol is safer for diabetics, since it doesn't trigger insulin-induced low blood sugar or delay the recovery of blood glucose to normal levels. Atenolol and metoprolol are less likely than propranolol to impair breathing, although this can still happen. They are also less likely to cause insomnia, nightmares, and depression, or to impair sexual function, a major problem for some people on either propranolol or diuretics.[20] In fact, authorities assert there's no longer any good reason to prefer propranolol over these newer alternatives.[21] This raises the question why propranolol remains one of the most-prescribed drugs.

Concerns about the side effects of diuretics prompted the Joint National Committee on Detection, Evaluation and Treatment of High Blood Pressure in 1984 to propose beta-blockers as the first step in stepped-care treatment.[22] Beta-blockers are usually the first-choice drug for younger hypertensives (20–40 years old), whose condition is likely to be caused by a stress-induced stimulation of adrenalin. But they are not the ideal drug for the elderly, who comprise the majority of hypertensives. In older people, hypertension is more likely to be caused by calcified arteries. Blocking their adrenalin rush isn't going to calm them down. It's just going to slow them down and make them tired. Older people are also more likely to suffer side effects from beta-blockers, since their drug clearance is slower. And the drugs aren't as effective in older as in younger people.

The same Swedish research team that in 1989 reported the cholesterol-raising effects of diuretics found similar effects for beta-blockers.[23] And like diuretics, beta-blockers can adversely affect blood glucose. They can provoke asthma, pulmonary disease, congestive heart failure, and peripheral vascular disease. They may not be effective in smokers or blacks.[24] And they are even more likely to impair the overall quality of life than diuretics.

So while beta-blockers have certain advantages over diuretics, they're still not the ideal drug, at least for the elderly, who comprise the vast majority of hypertensives.

Steps 3 and 4

What drugs are left? Under the "stepped care" approach, if Steps 1 and 2 didn't work, you'd add a "Step 3" drug. This was usually a vasodilator that caused the muscles in the small arteries to relax. Possibilities included hydralazine (Apresoline) and the calcium channel blockers.

If that didn't work, it was desperation time. Step 4 meant adding powerful drugs with serious side effects that were considered appropriate only in the most intractable cases. These drugs included minoxidil (Loniten), guanethidine (Ismelin) and the ACE inhibitors.

As we'll see in the next chapter, some of the drugs formerly reserved for Steps 3 and 4 have now proved, for some patients, to be safer and more effective when used alone than the older "first-line" drugs. Like with the older first choices, however, whether these newer options reduce cardiovascular disease and death has yet to be proved.[25]

Table 14.   *Thiazide Diuretics*[26]

Generic name:	*Popular brand names:*
chlorothiazide	Diuril, Adloclor, Aldoril
chlorthalidone	Hygroton
hydrochlorothiazide	Esidrix, HydroDiuril, Apreszide
hydroflumethiazide	Saluron
indapamide	Lozol
methyclothiazide	Enduron
metolazone	Diulo, Microx, Zaroxolyn
Side Effects:	Dizziness, tingling, weakness, anemia and other blood disorders, stomach and intestinal complaints, lung congestion, difficult breathing, shock, blurred vision, photosensitivity, dehydration, rash, fever, kidney and liver damage; elevated blood sugar, cholesterol, calcium, and uric acid levels; low blood potassium
Potential adverse drug interactions with:	Other antihypertensives, cholestyramine, colestipol, insulin, digitalis, adrenocorticoids, tricyclic antidepressants, pain relievers, barbiturates, lithium
Risky for:	People with kidney or liver damage, allergies or bronchial asthma; pregnant women; nursing mothers

Table 15. *Beta-Blockers (Systemic)*

Generic name:	*Popular brand names:*
acebutolol	Sectral
atenolol	Tenormin
metoprolol	Lopressor
nadolol	Corgard
pindolol	Visken
propranolol	Inderal
timolol	Blocadren, Timolide

Side Effects:	Depression, dizziness, numb or cold extremities, diarrhea, dry mouth, fatigue, nausea, hallucinations, difficult breathing, low blood sugar, rash, fever, congestive heart failure
Potential adverse drug interactions with:	Tranquilizers, antihistamines, antidepressants, sedatives, sleeping pills, alcohol, narcotics, reserpine, phenytoin, anti-inflammatories, antidiabetes drugs, insulin
Risky for:	People with asthma or hay fever, pregnant women, nursing mothers, people about to undergo major surgery. May interfere with treatment of overactive thyroid, low blood sugar, diabetes, kidney or liver disease.

13

NEWER BLOOD PRESSURE ALTERNATIVES

Quality of life is an important issue, especially when
treating a largely asymptomatic condition.
                              —Jonathan Edelson, M.D. (1990)[1]

High blood pressure is now known to have different causes. It may be caused by constricted arteries, or a heart that's pumping too hard, or tired kidneys that are retaining fluid. If you can find the right drug for your particular problem, it can be as effective when used alone as multiple drugs used shotgun-fashion. More important, it will produce significantly fewer side effects. The trick is to find the right drug.

Under the traditional "stepped care" approach to hypertension, new drugs were progressively added, but nothing was ever taken away. Yet every time you add something, you compound the risk of side effects. Not only is the single-drug approach calculated to produce fewer side effects, but for many people the newer drugs have fewer of them to start with.

The side-effect-free antihypertensive, however, remains to be discovered. And for mild hypertensives, none of the newer drugs has yet been shown to prolong life, the acid test for determining whether to risk a drug's side effects. In fact, *no* drug has yet passed that test.

Even if it had, there would remain this question: would you rather be drugged and dragged through a somewhat longer old age, or vibrant and alive for a somewhat shorter one? You could actually be vibrant and alive for a longer old age without drugs, if you could reverse the *cause* of your high blood pressure. We'll look at this possibility at the end of this chapter.

The ACE inhibitors

Ironically, the two most profitable antihypertensives now on the market were once considered too dangerous to use except in desperate cases. Unlike practolol, which was thought to be safe until widespread use revealed its risks, the ACE inhibitors were considered dangerous until later studies revealed their virtues. Now, many doctors use them as the first-choice "Step 1" drug to treat new cases of high blood pressure.[2]

ACE inhibitors block the action of angiotensin-converting enzymes (ACE) that constrict the veins. Their very origin suggested caution. The first substances found to be effective for this purpose were isolated from the venom of a Brazilian pit viper.[3] These substances lowered blood pressure, but they were too expensive to be worth pursuing commercially. That was in the 1960s. The first commercial ACE inhibitor wasn't produced until the 1970s, after systematic synthesis and testing of many compounds. The product was called captopril and was marketed by Squibb as Capoten in 1981.

But the drug was still in the trial-and-error stage, and researchers were off on the dose. Moreover, the FDA had restricted its use to the most serious cases. These patients were already so weak that they suffered some serious side effects. The problem was later corrected by lowering the dose, but too late. The drug had acquired a shady reputation that lingered among doctors.

The FDA didn't approve Capoten for general use until 1985, and a virtually identical ACE inhibitor called enalapril got the same approval only six months later. Marketed by Merck as Vasotec, this tough competitor had the advantage that it had to be taken only once a day, to Capoten's twice, and it hadn't suffered Capoten's bad press. Vasotec thus got the edge despite Capoten's early lead, although Capoten hopes to stay in the running with its own once-a-day formula. Merck later increased its market share with a third ACE inhibitor, called Prinivil.

Rivalries aside, these drugs have been incredibly profitable. Collectively, Capoten and Vasotec have grown to over $2.1 billion in sales worldwide.[4] Yet they're not the most-often prescribed antihypertensives. What's the secret of their commercial success? Simple: they doubled the price.

The manufacturers would argue you get what you pay for. They point to a 1986 study in which captopril ranked significantly higher than the older drugs propranolol and methyldopa in improving patients' "quality of life." Patients taking captopril reported fewer side effects, less sexual dysfunction, and greater improvement in general well-being.[5]

True, the study was sponsored by Squibb. Other authorities complained it was incomplete, since Capoten wasn't pitted against the whole array of older, cheaper drugs. And the researchers failed to factor in the cost of the drugs themselves, which to many retired hypertensives is a significant element of the quality of life. But the study made its point, and sales of both drugs soared.[6]

A controversial study reported in the *Journal of the American Medical Association* in January of 1990 found that the beta-blocker propranolol actually outranked captopril in both effectiveness and cost-effectiveness. The researchers projected that for twenty years of simulated therapy from 1990 through 2010, the cost per year of life saved would be $10,900 for propranolol, $16,400 for the diuretic hydrochlorothiazide, $31,600 for nifedipine, $61,900 for prazosin, and $72,100 for captopril. The researchers reached these results by putting existing data into a computer model that forecast the drugs' relative health and cost benefits. Survival benefits were calculated based on the increase in life expectancy found in the Framingham Study for people with lower blood pressures. But as the researchers observed:

> The potential policy implications of any forecasting model are limited by the confidence that can be placed on the assumptions of the model.[7]

One unproved assumption was that lowering blood pressure with drugs improves life expectancy. The Framingham Study established only that people with lower blood pressures live longer than people with higher ones, not that people with higher blood pressures who lower them *with drugs* will live longer.

Another questionable assumption was the one by which the quality of life was factored in. The researchers assumed that a "quality-adjusted life-year" on antihypertensive drugs was equivalent to 99 percent of a year without drugs. In other words, you'd be willing to put up with the drugs' side effects if you got an extra 1 percent of life out of the trade. Yet few people would exchange 20 years of drug-free existence for 20.2 years of impotence, fatigue, depression, and other side effects—at least, not if they knew those were the terms of the deal.

Other studies have confirmed the ACE inhibitors' virtues—at least as compared to the older drugs—in patients for whom they work. ACE inhibitors have been shown to be as effective as diuretics in lowering blood pressure in the elderly, while producing fewer side effects. They can lower blood pressure when used alone, but they generally work better with a diuretic. Either way, side effects are reduced from those produced by a stronger diuretic used alone.[8] Unlike diuretics, ACE inhibitors don't significantly affect serum potassium, uric acid, or glucose levels.[9] According to the Swedish researchers who found that diuretics raise serum cholesterol and decrease glucose sensitivity, ACE inhibitors actually *increase* glucose sensitivity by as much as diuretics decrease it.[10] And patients are more likely to stay on ACE inhibitors than on the older drugs.

One reported case involved an elderly, senile, hypertensive man who just couldn't stay awake on propranolol. He became alert, talkative, and pleasant when his medication was switched to captopril.[11]

ACE inhibitors lower renin activity. Renin is a hormone excreted by the kidneys that regulates the hormone angiotensin. Angiotensin, in turn, regulates blood pressure. Angiotensin is secreted by the kidneys and moves to the lungs, where angiotensin-converting enzyme (ACE) activates it to signal an increase in blood pressure. This means ACE inhibitors are particularly good for younger hypertensives with high renin levels. It also means, however, that the drugs can impair kidney function and the production of blood cells, and can give rise to a persistent cough. ACE inhibitors are risky for people who already have kidney or blood problems. This includes most elderly patients, who generally have some loss of kidney function.

In addition, ACE inhibitors can cause rash, low blood pressure, and potassium loss. They can also react adversely with other medications. Drugs with which they mix poorly include digoxin, nonsteroidal anti-inflammatory drugs, morphine, lithium, loop diuretics, potassium-sparing diuretics, vasodilators, and prazosin.[12]

A further drawback of ACE inhibitors is that they only work in about 70 percent of cases. For patients whose high blood pressure is caused by excess salt in the blood, calcium channel blockers may be better options.

Calcium channel blockers

While diuretics are the antihypertensives most often prescribed, and ACE inhibitors are the fastest growing category, calcium channel blockers are on top in dollar sales (see table 16). Three of these drugs joined the top ten most-prescribed antihypertensives of 1988: Cardizem (diltiazem) at number three, Procardia (nifedipine) at number six, and Calan (verapamil) at number ten.

Table 16. *Top Antihypertensive Drug Treatments of 1988 in Terms of Sales*[13]

Category	Sales Leaders	1988 Sales	1988 Growth Rate
diuretics	hydrochlorothiazide amiloride hydrochlorothiazide	$1.8 billion	2%
beta-blockers	atenolol propranolol	$2.7 billion	7%
ACE inhibitors	Captopril Enalapril	$2.2 billion	45%
calcium channel blockers	nifedipine diltiazem	$3.1 billion	24%

Calcium channel blockers work by keeping calcium on the outside of the arteries, where it has a relaxing effect, instead of inside, where it hardens and tightens them. Calcium must flow in from the surrounding fluid for arteries to contract.

These drugs are particularly appropriate for people whose blood pressure is high because their small arteries are constricted. They are also good alternatives for diabetics, since unlike thiazides and beta-blockers, they don't affect plasma insulin levels.[14] Studies have shown that calcium channel blockers in combination with low doses of diuretics are as effective for lowering blood pressure as either beta-blockers or higher doses of diuretics, and side effects are fewer.[15]

Whether calcium channel blockers actually prolong life in mild hypertensives hasn't been established, but for people with more serious disease, it has. In a 1988 study of people who had suffered a stroke, twice as many patients died during the following month on placebos as on the calcium channel blocker nimodipine.[16]

Because calcium channel blockers act mainly on the muscles of the arteries, they have little effect on other parts of the body. As a result, they have fewer side effects than most antihypertensives. But like all drugs, they can have side effects. The most common are dizziness, headache, fatigue, flushing, heart palpitations, swollen ankles, and constipation. The most serious is heart failure.

Prazosin

Moving up to number twelve among most-often-prescribed antihypertensives is prazosin (Minipress). Prazosin is an "alpha-1 blocker" that works by causing small veins and arteries to dilate. Less pressure is thus required to move the blood through.

Prazosin is another drug that was formerly reserved for the multiple-drug treatment of severe cases of hypertension. It was considered ineffective as first-line treatment. But studies have now shown that in appropriate cases, it can work as well as the older options when used alone.

An important advantage of prazosin over beta-blockers and diuretics is that it not only doesn't raise serum cholesterol and triglyceride levels but can actually lower them.[17] Furthermore, where diuretics can reduce the body's ability to break down blood sugar, prazosin has a favorable effect on insulin sensitivity. This factor may be important in the regulation of blood pressure not only in diabetics but in obese patients. Plasma insulin concentration is increased in obese people with elevated blood pressures.[18]

A 1989 study found prazosin to be as good at lowering blood pressure as the beta-blocker propranolol and the diuretic hydrochlorothiazide, while impairing motor and cognitive skills less—and without affecting serum cholesterol.[19] In another 1989 study, prazosin outperformed even atenolol, the number one beta-blocker and the number two antihypertensive drug. When given as single-drug therapy, prazosin lowered blood pressure more, and atenolol raised triglyceride levels slightly.[20] A third 1989 study compared prazosin with the ACE inhibitor enalapril as single-drug therapy for older hypertensives. All of the patients responded to one of the two drugs, although only half responded to both. In the patients who responded to both, the drug effectively lowered blood pressure when used alone and side effects were mild.[21]

While prazosin has come up in the drug world, it may get bumped by its sister alpha-1 blockers, terazosin (Hytrin) and doxazosin (soon to be approved). These newer versions have longer half-lives, allowing once-daily dosing. Doctors are inclined to prescribe the drug that requires the fewest doses, since patients are inclined to forget.[22]

Terazosin works well alone or in combination with other drugs, has a favorable effect on cholesterol levels, and produces relatively few side effects.[23]

Doxazosin has been shown to lower blood pressure as much as diuretics, with no greater incidence of side effects.[24] It has been proved safe and effective where both ACE inhibitors and calcium channel blockers have failed.[25] It decreases not only blood pressure but serum cholesterol levels.[26] Unlike beta-blockers, it doesn't significantly affect heart rate; and unlike diuretics, it doesn't affect potassium or uric acid levels.[27] It works well either alone or in combination with beta-blockers, thiazide diuretics, or ACE inhibitors.[28]

But like all drugs, the alpha-blockers have side effects that limit their use. In a study comparing prazosin with the calcium channel blocker nifedipine and the vasodilator hydralazine, the drugs lowered blood pressure equally well. They differed significantly *only* in their side effects. With hydralazine, it was headaches. With the calcium channel blocker, it was headaches, flushing, and edema (swelling). With prazosin, it was tiredness and drowsiness.[29] For other side effects, see tables 17, 18, 19, and 20.

Alpha-2 agonists

Clonidine (Catapres) is another third-line drug that has moved up in the eyes of researchers. It's an "alpha-2 agonist" that acts on the brain's "alpha-2 receptors," which control vascular tone. (An "agonist" is the opposite of an "antagonist.")

Methyldopa is an older antihypertensive in this category. It has been outmoded, however, by its serious side effects, including drowsiness, depression, sexual dysfunction, and excessively low blood pressure. Clonidine was thought to have the same limitations, until recent studies showed it to be effective at lower doses than were formerly prescribed. At these doses, side effects are minimal.[30]

One advantage of clonidine is its dosing schedule. Where doxazosin and enalapril got dosing down to once a day, Catapres got it down to once a week. It's the only antihypertensive that can be absorbed by means of a patch on the skin, and the patch lasts a full week.

In one 1987 study, this "transdermal" clonidine proved to be as safe and effective when used as single-drug therapy for mild hypertension as the beta-blocker propranolol.[31] In another study reported the same year, clonidine produced effective blood pressure control with only minimal side effects over a ten-year period. The dropout rate due to intolerable side effects was a little over 3 percent—not bad, compared to the 30 percent dropout rate reported by the Hypertension Detection and Followup Program for the older drugs.[32]

Still, clonidine can have side effects. The most common are drowsiness, constipation, mouth dryness, and itching from the patch. In some studies, skin reactions have been reported by as many as 50 percent of patch users. On the plus side, rebound hypertension, a potentially life-threatening side effect of clonidine, is rarely reported in patch users.[33]

Nondrug alternatives

Although side effects can be diminished by using the newer options and the mono-therapy approach, no antihypertensive drug is without side effects. More important, in people with only mild hypertension, none of these drugs has yet been shown to significantly prolong life. If you are in that broad treatment category, nondrug alternatives remain your most promising course.

For many people with mild hypertension, blood pressure has returned to normal without *any* treatment.[34] For others, blood pressure has proved to be high only in the doctor's office.[35] For this reason, you should always get several readings, preferably in the security of your own home, before starting any drug regimen.

The holistic answer to diuretics is to change your diet. Many studies have shown that a diet low in fat, salt, and animal protein can reduce blood pressure. Weight loss in general can also have this effect. Studies also suggest that the blood-pressure-raising effects of salt may be blocked by eating vegetables, and that lack of calcium may be as important in raising blood pressure as excess sodium. Consuming more than two alcoholic drinks a day, on the other hand, tends to raise blood pressure.[36]

In a Swedish study, hypertensive patients who were unhappy with the side effects of their drugs switched to a "vegan" diet, without animal products or salt. After one year, most of them had succeeded in abandoning their blood pressure medications entirely, while maintaining blood pressure levels that were lower than with drugs by a full 10 mm Hg diastolic.[37]

If your hypertension is linked to tension, relaxation techniques may be your answer to beta-blockers. The sympathetic nervous system increases blood pressure as part of the fight-or-flight response to stress. Beta-blockers reduce blood pressure by blocking the activities of this regulatory system. But the same effect can be achieved without drugs, by simple techniques for letting go of tension.[38] Yoga, meditation, and biofeedback have all been shown to effectively lower blood pressure.[39]

Transcendental Meditation is a simplified Yoga technique that was popularized by the Beatles in the 1960s. Meditators had a hard time convincing researchers to study its effects. When they did, the technique was found to lower blood pressure from the borderline hypertensive range to normal.[40]

Even better results have been reported for meditation reinforced by biofeedback. Biofeedback is a technique that gives you continuous information about the state of your body. Electronic equipment tells you your blood pressure, your heart rate, your skin temperature, and the state of your brain-wave pattern. Just by knowing how these parameters vary, many people can learn to regulate them.

In one study, 77 patients with high blood pressure were trained in biofeedback techniques for dilating the blood vessels in the hands and feet. Of those patients not on antihypertensive drugs, 70 percent were able to bring their blood pressures down to normal. Of those who were on drugs, over half were able to get off them and still reduce their blood pressures an average of 15/10 mm Hg. An additional 35 percent succeeded in cutting their prescriptions in half, while reducing their blood pressures an average of 18/10 mm Hg.[41]

In an Indian study, patients trained in biofeedback techniques showed average drops in blood pressure from 158 to 141 mm Hg systolic and from 99 to 87 mm Hg diastolic. These reductions were greater than those induced by drugs in other studies, and they were retained after six months of follow-up. The patients also reported they felt better, slept better, and worked better.[42]

What about using drugs to induce relaxation? This doesn't seem to be effective. The artificial relaxation resulting from sedatives and tranquilizers not only hasn't been shown to lower blood pressure but, like the drugs that do lower it, they are troubled with side effects.[43]

A third cause of hypertension can be drugs themselves. Potential culprits include diet pills, many cold remedies, and oral contraceptives. If you're worried about your blood pressure, you should avoid these pills.[44]

Table 17. *ACE inhibitors*[45]

Generic names:
  captropril
  enalapril
  lisinopril
	Brand names:
	  Capoten
	  Vasotec
	  Prinivil, Zestril

Uses:	For the treatment of hypertension and congestive heart failure
Side effects:	Dizziness, fainting, headaches, low blood pressure, angina, increased heart rate, insomnia, swelling, digestive complaints, cough, weakness, blood problems, rash
Captopril only:	Kidney failure, protein in the urine, congestive heart failure, urinary problems, loss of taste and appetite, fever, infections, numbness, photosensitivity (see chapter 30)
Enalapril only:	Sweating, unconsciousness, cramps, impotence, nervousness
Adverse interactions, cautions:	Effects increased by other antihypertensives, including a possible severe drop in blood pressure if combined with diuretics; may react adversely with cough, cold, and allergy drugs, aspirin and indomethacin, nitrates, digoxin, vasodilators, morphine, and lithium

Table 18. *Calcium Channel Blockers*

Generic names:
  diltiazem
  nifedipine
  verapamil
	Brand names:
	  Cardizem
	  Procardia
	  Calan, Isoptin, Isoptin-SR

Uses:	Antihypertensive, antianginal, vasodilator; treatment of Raynaud's syndrome
Side effects:	Dizziness, flushing, headaches, nausea, heartburn, weakness, fluid retention, low blood pressure, nasal congestion, heart palpitations, nervousness, diarrhea, low potassium levels

Adverse interactions, cautions: May cause heart failure in certain people in combination with beta-blockers; causes birth defects in animals

Table 19. *Alpha-1 Blockers*

Generic names:	Brand names:
prazosin	Minipress
terazocrin	Hytrin

Uses: Antihypertensive

Side effects: Dizziness, headache, drowsiness, weakness, depression, pounding heart, digestive and urinary complaints, rash, hives, nervousness, unconsciousness, lack of coordination, depression, hair loss, nasal congestion, visual problems

Adverse interactions, cautions: May increase effects of other antihypertensives; may cause fainting, especially with first dose

Table 20. *Alpha-2 Agonists*

Generic names:	Brand names:
clonidine	Catapres, Catapres TTS (transdermal patch)
methyldopa	Aldomet

Uses: Antihypertensive

Side effects: Drowsiness, dizziness, dry mouth, liver disorders, digestive complaints, headache, tiredness, impotence, weight gain, psychic disturbances, heart problems, rash, low blood pressure

Methyldopa only: Anemia, liver damage, inability to think clearly, nasal stuffiness, fever, fluid retention, chest pain

Clonidine only: Severe rebound hypertension, nervousness, anxiety, hair loss, urinary problems, blood sugar problems, sore eyes

TTS only: Sensitization, inflammation, blisters, swelling of skin

Adverse interactions, cautions: May increase sedative effects of alcohol and
                                    drugs that induce drowsiness; may react
                                    adversely with antihypertensives and
                                    antidepressants. Methyldopa may cause
                                    serious blood and liver disorders and interacts
                                    with many drugs (ask your doctor). Clonidine
                                    is risky for patients with serious heart or
                                    kidney problems and may cause birth defects.

14

DRUGS THAT LOWER SERUM CHOLESTEROL

I am a heavy eater of beef, and believe it does harm my wit.

—Shakespeare
Twelfth Night

Although high blood pressure is a major risk factor for heart disease, researchers have been unable to prove that for most people with the condition, lowering it with drugs lowers the death rate.[1] Undaunted, intrepid drug men turned to another major risk factor, elevated serum cholesterol levels.

Merck and Co., which brought you Vasotec, also brings you Mevacor, the hottest cholesterol-lowering drug now on the market. Merck is, in fact, the king of the pharmaceutical industry. It has a market value of about $28 billion—more than not only any other drug company, but than such giants as the Ford Motor Company, Coca-Cola, Mobil, and American Express. Its secret of success is said to be a skillful blend of science and commercial enterprise.

Merck predicts that drugs to treat elevated cholesterol will become as common in the early 1990s as antihypertensive drugs are today. Market analysts are even more optimistic. They've predicted the drugs will reach heights in five years that antihypertensives took twenty years to achieve.

But Merck's investment isn't without obstacles. Physicians are hesitant to prescribe a new class of drugs, particularly if they need to be taken indefinitely. Lowering serum cholesterol with drugs hasn't proved to be any more effective at reducing the overall death rate than lowering blood pressure with them. And Mevacor may carry long-term risks.[2]

Merck plans to overcome these obstacles by aggressively promoting the dangers of high serum cholesterol levels. The cholesterol issue is hot, and Merck is fanning the flames. Its marketing tactics include seminars, symposiums, and personal meetings with key heart specialists and internists, along with the usual relentless visits by its drug salesmen to physicians everywhere.

Merck's sales tactics also include a direct appeal to consumers with ads on the cholesterol issue. Merck isn't the only company that has taken to advertising prescription drugs in consumer magazines. Although prescription drug sales nearly tripled between 1980 and 1988—from $10 billion to $27 billion—competition is getting tougher. Advertising executives are looking to prescription drug ads as a new growth category.

Critics, including many doctors, argue these ads mislead the public. They make drugs look like magic potions that will cure users' ills without a change in lifestyle.[3]

Lowering cholesterol to safe levels is one of those goals that can't be achieved by drugs alone. According to Drs. Michael Brown and Joseph Goldstein, whose Nobel Prize-winning research led to Mevacor's development, people who need cholesterol-lowering drugs also need a cholesterol-lowering diet. If they backslide on their diets, their cholesterol levels are liable to creep back up.[4]

In fact, most people can lower their serum cholesterol by changing their diets, without taking drugs. Research has shown average drops in serum cholesterol of 25–40 percent in people who switched to a very low-fat, low-cholesterol diet, high in fiber. From the more moderate changes advocated by the American Heart Association, drops of about half that amount have resulted.[5] The dietary approach not only can be as effective as drugs; it is without unwanted side effects. What's more important, when cholesterol is lowered in this way, life expectancy is actually increased.[6] This isn't the case with cholesterol-lowering drugs.

Blood fats come in several varieties, including high-density lipoprotein (HDL, the "good" kind), low-density lipoprotein (LDL, the "bad" kind), and very-low-density lipoprotein (VLDL, whose risk-factor status is uncertain). Cholesterol is contained in all of them. In most cases, however, treatment is aimed at lowering elevated levels only of LDL, the bad cholesterol.

Various conditions can cause LDL elevation, but the most common in the United States is excess dietary intake of cholesterol and saturated fat. Cholesterol is found only in animal products, and saturated fat is found mainly in them.[7] This means to get a significant lowering of cholesterol, you may have to eliminate meat and most other animal foods from your diet, and concentrate instead on high-fiber fruits, vegetables, and grains. According to Drs. Brown and Goldstein, however, you can't eat steak and eggs with impunity even if you lower your serum cholesterol with drugs. And if you choose the dietary alternative, you can avoid the side effects of the drugs, which can prove more troublesome than changing your diet.

We'll look at the pros and cons of the various drug options in this chapter. Before you dose up with any of them, however, it's important to make sure you're a proper candidate for drug treatment.

First, you need to know if the laboratory your doctor is using to test your cholesterol is reliable. The Laboratory Standardization Panel of the National Cholesterol Education Program reports that fully *half* the cholesterol measurements made in the United States have been done in laboratories with suboptimal precision and accuracy. Cholesterol reports are frequently 15 percent off in either direction. This can make the difference between 200 mg/dl (considered normal) and 230 mg/dl (considered high).[8]

To get a reliable measurement of lipoprotein levels, you need to fast for 10–12 hours first. You should get at least two readings, and you should get tested only when you're in otherwise good health, at your usual weight, and on your usual diet. Then, if your cholesterol levels test high, try lowering them with diet before turning to drugs. Dietary change should be tried for at least six months.[9] Getting regular exercise and cutting out smoking can also help. Drugs should be resorted to only when these causal approaches fail, since no cholesterol-lowering drug is an ideal remedy.

Here is a rundown of the available options.

Fibric acid derivatives

The drugs first promoted in the anticholesterol campaign were the "fibric acid derivatives." They act by affecting certain enzymes and preventing the formation of cholesterol.

The first of these drugs thought to be sufficiently safe and effective to test in long-term trials was clofibrate (Atromid-S). However, its long-term use has now been associated with severe complications. In a five-year study involving over 15,000 men, clofibrate not only did not reduce the number of deaths; the drug actually increased the death rate by a third (77 in the clofibrate group vs. 47 in the control group). The excess deaths were mainly related to the liver, intestines, and gallbladder.[10]

Another option in this category, gemfibrozil (Lopid), has fewer serious side effects than clofibrate and has done better in long-term trials—better, but not good enough, since more deaths still resulted in people taking gemfibrozil than in those not taking it (45 vs. 42). More also wound up with gallstones.[11]

Besides gallbladder problems, these drugs can cause nausea, abdominal pain, decreased sex drive, weight gain, inflammation and degeneration of the muscles, arrhythmias, and drowsiness. In people with high triglyceride levels, the drugs can also cause LDL (bad cholesterol) to rise.[12]

Probucol

Probucol (Lorelco) lowers serum cholesterol by increasing the breakdown of cholesterol to bile salts. However, it can lower HDL, the good cholesterol, more than total cholesterol. It also hasn't been shown to prevent CHD in humans, and its long-term safety is unknown. Side effects experienced by 10 percent of patients include diarrhea, stomach pain, gas, and nausea.[13]

Bile-acid resins

The current first-choice drugs in most cases are the bile-acid resins and niacin. They have the longest track records for safety and effectiveness in lowering serum cholesterol. However, your particular blood fat profile may determine which drug your doctor prescribes, since different cholesterol-lowering drugs affect different blood fat components. Bile-acid resins lower LDL but have only minimal effects on VLDL and HDL, while gemfibrozil not only lowers LDL but elevates HDL, and lowers VLDL.

The bile-acid resins include cholestyramine (Questran) and colestipol (Colestid). They work by forcing the liver to produce more bile acid, the digestive juice that breaks down dietary fats. Cholesterol is thus used up in the blood. The drugs can lower serum cholesterol by 15–20 percent. Unfortunately, they have to be taken in large amounts to be effective; and this can be a challenging proposition, because they're insoluble powders with the consistency of sand.

Bile-acid resins aren't absorbed, so they have no systemic (whole-body) side effects. They do, however, have side effects. The most common is constipation, experienced by nearly a third of patients. Others are heartburn (17 percent of patients), belching (9 percent), and nausea (8 percent). The drugs work by interfering with the absorption of fat, but they can also interfere with the absorption of other nutrients and fat-soluble vitamins (especially A and D), and of other drugs.[14]

Niacin

Only one medical remedy for lowering cholesterol has clearly been shown to decrease the overall death rate, and this showing wasn't in asymptomatic people who merely had high serum cholesterol levels. It was in men who had already had a heart attack.[15] Furthermore, the remedy isn't exactly a drug. It's niacin, a B vitamin (also called nicotinic acid).

That doesn't make niacin a natural remedy. What takes it out of the natural category is that, to be effective, it has to be ingested at doses that are about one hundred times the recommended daily requirement. At these huge, unnatural doses, niacin can cause very annoying side effects. Skin flushing occurs in nearly everyone taking it. Flushing and itching may go away in a few weeks, but liver damage and jaundice can show up later. Other side effects include upset stomach, peptic ulcers, gastritis, hepatitis, glucose intolerance, high uric acid levels, and cardiac arrhythmias. Hepatitis and upset stomach are particularly common with sustained-release preparations. These side effects can be so distressing that many patients refuse to take the remedy despite its favorable effects on cholesterol levels.[16]

Lovastatin

Merck's answer to these problems was lovastatin (Mevacor). Lovastatin can reduce serum cholesterol as much as 30 percent. It's easier to swallow than the bile-acid resins, and it doesn't produce the annoying side effects of niacin. While it has side effects, they tend to be relatively mild ones, most commonly, gas, diarrhea, and sleep disorders.[17]

Lovastatin may offer advantages for diabetics, who are considered a high-risk group. Coronary heart disease is about twice as prevalent in diabetics as in the general population. Other cholesterol-lowering drugs, such as gemfibrozil and nicotinic acid, can raise glucose levels. Lovastatin is effective without this side effect.

Unfortunately, lovastatin poses other risks for diabetics. The primary one is cataracts, for which diabetics are already at higher risk than other people. Cataracts have developed in beagle dogs given high doses of lovastatin; and in a clinical study of humans, the drug increased the opacity of the eyes in 13 of 101 patients after 18 weeks of use.[18]

The main problem with lovastatin is that its long-term effects are unknown. Besides the risk of cataracts, some people taking it develop liver problems and pain and inflammation in the muscles.[19]

Your doctor is therefore likely to prescribe one of the older, more tested remedies, even if it does mean suffering greater side effects than with this hot new item.

Fish oil capsules

Another popular cholesterol-lowering option is fish oil. When megadoses of the omega-3 fatty acids found in fish oil are substituted in the diet for other fats, they can lower certain blood fat components. What keeps these capsules from qualifying as a natural remedy is, again, the high concentrations you need to take to get the effect. In these concentrated doses, fish oil can interfere with platelet function and cause bleeding. It can also result in toxic doses of vitamin A.

There are other problems with this alternative. No studies are available comparing the safety and effectiveness of fish oil capsules with other lipid-lowering drugs, or showing they cause atherosclerotic lesions to regress.[20] The capsules effectively lower VLDL and triglycerides, but the role of these blood components in most heart disease is uncertain. The components that play a more certain role are LDL and HDL, and fish oils have unfavorable effects on these components. They tend to *raise* LDL levels, and often, to depress HDL levels.[21]

The side effects of fish oil capsules can be avoided simply by eating fish three times a week, a habit that has been shown to significantly reduce heart disease risk. If you're not into fish, you can get about the same effect by substituting dietary polyunsaturated vegetable oils (which come from plants) for saturated fats (which come mainly from animals). Essentially, this means switching to a plant-foods diet.[22]

Psyllium

A cholesterol-lowering tactic that's more natural than either fish oil capsules or niacin capsules is a diet high in plant fiber. The type that lowers serum cholesterol most is the soluble fiber in fruits, vegetables, and oat bran. Unlike the insoluble fibers, which remain coarse and gritty in water, the soluble fibers dissolve to form a gel.

All plant foods are rich in both types of fiber, but some contain more of one than the other. Both are useful, but in different ways. Insoluble fiber, the kind in wheat bran, increases stool bulk and promotes bowel function. Soluble fiber, the kind in oat bran, forms a gel that traps cholesterol-rich bile acids. These bile acids would otherwise be recycled. When they're trapped and eliminated, the body has to use up other cholesterol to make more bile acids, and serum cholesterol is reduced.[23]

Soluble fiber is also the kind found in bulk laxatives containing psyllium, including Metamucil, Konsyl, and Modane Bulk. In a 1988 study, volunteers with an average serum cholesterol level of 250 mg/dl were given a teaspoonful of Metamucil three times a day. After eight weeks, their cholesterol levels had dropped an average of 35 mg/dl, or 14 percent. This result was about as good as with the bile-acid resins Questran and Colestin.

In fact, psyllium works in much the same way as these drugs. It binds bile acids in the intestines and prevents them from being reabsorbed. The advantages of psyllium are that it's easier to swallow, and its side effects are limited to occasional mild stomach cramps and gas.[24]

Psyllium comes from the seed of a common weed you probably wouldn't eat except in processed form. If you're into the truly natural, you can get its effects from common edible plant fibers, including the pectin found in apples and other fruits and vegetables. The mechanism is the same as with the bile-acid resins. In combination with calcium, pectin binds readily to bile acids, rendering them useless as digestive enzymes. The liver senses there is a shortage of bile acid and compensates by extracting cholesterol molecules from the blood. These molecules are then modified into bile molecules. The result is a drop in serum cholesterol.[25]

A high-fiber diet is particularly good for diabetics. Soluble fibers reduce serum cholesterol and triglyceride levels without the drug side effects that are especially hazardous to diabetics. They also reduce blood sugar levels and aid in their control, and reduce insulin requirements. Fiber of both types also helps regulate the metabolism of glucose, by slowing its absorption from the intestines.[26] For a list of foods high in these fibers, see table 24 in chapter 16.

Thyroid hormone

Thyroid hormone is sometimes used to treat high serum cholesterol in elderly patients. At one time, this drug was also an accepted treatment for obesity, infertility, and fatigue. However, doctors writing in the *Journal of the American Medical Association* in 1989 noted that these indications are no longer valid; and that in the elderly particularly, the drug can contribute to the risk of cardiovascular disease. They stressed that thyroid hormone is appropriate only to treat hypothyroidism, goiter, and certain other thyroid diseases.[27]

Serum cholesterol and other drugs

In some cases, the cause of elevated serum cholesterol may be other drugs. Medications that can raise LDL levels include the antihypertensives thiazide and furosemide, isotretinoin, and anabolic steroids. (These are the steroids taken illicitly by athletes; see chapter 33.) If drugs are the cause of your elevated cholesterol levels, it's best not to try to reduce them with other drugs. It's better to abandon the suspect pills.[28]

Table 21.   *Cholesterol-Lowering Drugs*[29]

Category:	bile acid resins
Generic and brand names:	cholestyramine (Questran), colestipol (Colestid)
Action:	combines with bile acid to form an insoluble compound that is excreted
Effects:	lowers LDL, slightly increases HDL
Side effects:	constipation, abdominal pain, nausea, bloating
Adverse interactions:	can interfere with the action of other drugs
Category:	3-Hydroxy-3-methylglutaryl coenzyme A reductase inhibitors
Generic and brand names:	lovastatin (Mevacor), pravastatin, fluvastatin
Action:	inhibits an early step in the synthesis of cholesterol
Effects:	lowers LDL
Side effects:	hepatitis, myositis (degeneration and inflammation of the muscles), birth defects, headache, dizziness, constipation, diarrhea, nausea
Adverse interactions:	increased risk of myositis if taken with gemfibrozil
Category:	fibric acid derivatives
Generic and brand names:	clofibrate (Atromid-S, Claripex), gemfibrozil (Lopid), fenofibrate
Action:	inhibits the breakdown of fats to fatty acids, reduces triglyceride synthesis
Effects:	lowers VLDL, raises HDL, may raise or lower LDL
Side effects:	gallstones, hepatitis, high LDL, decreased sex drive, myositis, arrhythmia, increased appetite, abdominal pain, nausea
Adverse interactions:	effect antagonized or increased by oral contraceptives, rifampin, probenecid
Category:	probucol
Generic and brand names:	Lorelco (Probucol)
Action:	unknown, but seems to inhibit cholesterol transport to the intestines and may decrease cholesterol synthesis
Effects:	lowers LDL and HDL
Side effects:	low HDL, diarrhea, bloating, nausea, abdominal pain
Adverse interactions:	none significant

Category:	niacin (vitamin B3, nicotinic acid)
Generic and brand names:	Niacin, also called Vitamin B3 or Nicotinic Acid, (Nico-400, Nicobid, Nicolar, Nico-Span)
Action:	possibly inhibits the breakdown of fats to fatty acids, and triglyceride production
Effects:	lowers LDL and VLDL, raises HDL
Side effects:	hepatitis, gout, insomnia, flushing, arrhythmias, nausea, vomiting, diarrhea
Adverse interactions:	can cause very low blood pressure if taken with beta-blockers and other sympathetic-blocking antihypertensive drugs

Category:	dextrothyroxine
Generic and brand names:	dextrothyroxine (Choloxin)
Action:	stimulates metabolism of cholesterol
Effects:	lowers LDL and HDL
Side effects:	insomnia, weight loss, sweating, increased risk of heart attack
Adverse interactions:	none significant

15

BEFORE AND AFTER YOUR HEART ATTACK

Extreme remedies are very appropriate for extreme diseases.

—Hippocrates

Heart attacks strike more than 1.5 million Americans a year. Not long ago, doctors couldn't do much to stop them once they were occurring. Now, however, there are drugs that actually dissolve the clots that bring heart attacks on. Studies suggest that if these clot-dissolving drugs are used within hours of the first symptoms of a heart attack, deaths can be reduced as much as 50 percent. This is a good argument for getting to the hospital at the first sign of symptoms.[1]

Heart attacks are typically caused by the rapid formation of a blood clot, or "thrombus," which blocks the flow of blood in one of the coronary arteries. The role of clots in causing heart attacks has been suspected since the 1940s. Clinical trials with the available anticoagulant drugs, heparin and warfarin (Coumadin), however, failed to increase patient survival. Apparently, these drugs, while preventing new clots from forming, didn't affect clots that were already there.

A substance that does dissolve existing clots, a bacterial protein called "streptokinase," was isolated in 1933. Early studies failed to show it helped after a heart attack, apparently because the studies were poorly designed and dosing was inadequate. Researchers back then weren't sure of the link between heart attacks and clots, and interest waned. It was revived in 1980, when an important study established that 90 percent of heart attacks are caused by a fresh blood clot in a coronary artery.

High-tech genetic engineering soon produced another clot-dissolving substance from human cells, called "tissue plasminogen activator" or TPA. TPA dissolves clots at a higher rate than streptokinase, and it has the theoretical (though not yet proven) advantage that its clot-dissolving action may be more containable in the heart. Streptokinase promotes bleeding throughout the body, so that patients taking it run the risk of bleeding to death from ordinary tissue damage.[2]

TPA (Activase) generates half the revenues of its producer, Genentech, Inc. That helps explain why Genentech has used bold and aggressive lobbying and sales tactics to slow the introduction of a competitor drug, SmithKline's Eminase. Ironically, the competitor that may actually wipe out Genentech's investment is the older, natural enzyme streptokinase, which has the consummate advantage of price. TPA costs around $2,200 for a single course of therapy, compared to streptokinase's $200.[3] Health-care financing officials have declined to reimburse hospitals at a higher rate for TPA treatment of Medicare patients until studies demonstrate its superiority over the older drug.

A surprise blow to the new technology came with a New Zealand study published in the *New England Journal of Medicine* in the spring of 1989, which found that TPA and streptokinase were equally effective in preserving the pumping power of the heart. The drugs were also equally effective in reopening clogged arteries. These findings were confirmed in a larger Italian study, released in March of 1990. Apparently, the higher rate at which TPA dissolves clots doesn't correspond to a better outcome for heart attack patients.[4]

Atherosclerosis and angina

Unfortunately, neither drug affects the underlying problem in most heart attacks, atherosclerotic plaque that promotes the formation of clots. Atherosclerosis is the hardening of the arteries that generally precedes a heart attack. It's been called a "silent killer," because for one out of four victims, the first sign of trouble is sudden death.[5]

Lesions in which function has been impaired by atherosclerotic growths develop in Western men at an average age of twenty. These lesions spread so that they cover about 2 percent more of the surface of the coronary arteries every year. By the time 60 percent of this surface has been covered with coronary lesions, the opening through which blood passes is narrowed enough to set the stage for trouble. Until they reach this critical threshold, these lesions cause no symptoms; but then they can take only minutes to manifest as a fatal heart attack.[6]

For the luckier 75 percent of victims, trouble is signaled by "angina pectoris," or chest pain on exertion. Chest pain results when the supply of blood fails to meet demand, and the heart muscle cells can't get enough oxygen to pump at required levels. Insufficient oxygen delivery usually results from fatty plaque build-up in the arteries, which diminishes blood flow.

Angina drugs

Drug treatment for angina generally involves beta-blockers, calcium channel blockers, nitrates, or some combination of them.

We've already looked at the first two options. Beta-blockers reduce angina pain by preventing the nervous system from stimulating the heart to work harder. Calcium channel blockers do it by dilating the blood vessels, making more room for blood to flow through. Both can have side effects, ranging from annoying to life-threatening.

A combination of low doses of these two drug types has become popular in angina treatment, on the theory that the combination will cover more bases with fewer side effects. But recent data suggest that in most patients, combination therapy actually increases side effects, without increasing benefits.[7]

Nitrates include nitroglycerin, isosorbide dinitrate, and pentaerythritol tetranitrate. They work by dilating the blood vessels in the heart. They don't affect peripheral blood vessels, but they do dilate blood vessels in the head. This leads to their most troublesome side effect, painful headaches. Up to 50 percent of users suffer from headaches at one time or another.

Nitroglycerin tablets that can be dissolved under the tongue are used either to relieve angina attacks that are in progress, or to prevent anticipated attacks from exertion. They work for about thirty minutes.

The newest in drug delivery systems is the transdermal patch, a device that lets controlled doses of the drug enter the bloodstream continuously through the skin. It can't be used for acute attacks, since maximum concentrations don't reach the blood until an hour or two after application; but for maintenance therapy it has several advantages over the pills, including convenience and constant bioavailability (see chapter 27).

The major drawback of the transdermal nitroglycerin patch is that continuous doses can cause the body to develop a tolerance to the drug. This means not only that it won't work, but that serious problems can result on withdrawal.

The hazards of nitrate withdrawal were first recognized in workers in the explosives industry. When first exposed to the nitrate used in the munitions, workers experienced severe headaches. These headaches would clear after several days, but on Monday morning or other times after being away from the shop, the headaches would recur. The workers learned to avoid them by putting a pinch of nitrate in their hatbands when they were away. If they didn't, coronary pain and sometimes even death would result.[8]

Some physicians counsel their patients to avoid habituation by a brief interval without the patch in the morning or during sleep; but whether this solves the problem is hard to tell from the published studies. Two 1987 studies found that in patients using the patch, exercise ability was increased, anginal attacks were reduced, and side effects, though common, were tolerable.[9] A 1989 study, on the other hand, found that even intermittently applied nitroglycerin patches failed to prolong the ability to exercise on a treadmill, and 25 of the 36 patients in the study suffered from headaches. The researchers concluded that in most patients with stable angina, side effects of the patch outweighed its benefits.[10]

Another problem with the transdermal patch is that it can irritate the skin. In one study, this effect was found in 75 percent of nitroglycerin-patch users. Other studies have found lower rates of irritation, suggesting the sensitization may be caused by patch components other than the drug itself. If you have this problem, before giving up the patch you might try another brand.[11]

Antiarrhythmics

Cardiac arrhythmias (irregular heartbeats) are another potential risk factor that can warn of an impending heart attack. Arrythmias can be caused not only by heart disease but by infections, hypertension, and emotional stress. They can also be caused by drugs, including nicotine, caffeine, diet pills, and other stimulants. They may be accompanied by symptoms like weakness, fainting, or shortness of breath; but sometimes they're the only symptom.

Whether or not arrhythmias foreshadow a heart attack, recent studies question the wisdom of treating them routinely with drugs. Cardiac arrhythmia is a known risk factor for subsequent sudden death in people who have already had a heart attack. However, in a major recent study that we looked at in chapter 11, the popular antiarrhythmics flecainide (Tambocor) and encainide (Enkaid) not only did not forestall a second heart attack in these patients, the drugs actually doubled the chances of having one.[12]

Atrial fibrillation, or dysrhythmia in the atrium of the heart, is also considered a risk factor for stroke, since it occurs twelve times as often in stroke patients as in other adults. For this reason, anticoagulant drugs have routinely been prescribed to treat the symptom. But a study reported in the *New England Journal of Medicine* in 1987 found that atrial fibrillation unaccompanied by other symptoms is associated with a very low risk of stroke, at least in patients under sixty. Again, the researchers concluded that routine medication is probably unwarranted.[13]

Anticoagulants

Anticoagulants are also used to treat people who have a tendency to form blood clots. The tendency can be the result of atherosclerosis, heart-valve disease, inflammation, poor circulation, or extended bed rest. Warfarin (Coumadin) is the most commonly used of these drugs. It and other anticoagulants are effective, but they are also hazardous. They must be taken exactly as prescribed, and they shouldn't be mixed with other drugs of any sort, prescription or nonprescription, without your doctor's knowledge and approval.[14]

Aspirin and warfarin are a particularly bad mix, since both thin the blood and increase bleeding. It used to be thought that acetaminophen was a safe alternative, but dire results have been reported even with this combination.[15]

What about daily anticoagulant therapy with aspirin? We've seen that studies have failed to show an increase in overall survival from this regimen in normal middle-aged doctors. However, studies have shown increased survival in patients who have already suffered a heart attack or stroke.[16]

Drugs for congestive heart failure

Drug treatment can also increase survival in patients with congestive heart failure. This condition results when the heart is too weak to pump as hard as it should, and blood backs up into the lungs and veins. This is a case of desperate diseases calling for desperate measures, since even with everything medicine has to offer, the prognosis for patients with congestive heart failure remains very poor. The annual death rate is from 15 percent to 60 percent, and nearly two hundred thousand Americans die from the condition each year.

Treatment begins with rest, diuretics combined with a low-salt diet to reduce fluid retention, and digitalis drugs to strengthen the heart. If that doesn't work, vasodilators may be added. In fact, new studies suggest they should be added even if the patient seems to be improving without them.[17]

Vasodilators

Vasodilator drugs work by redistributing blood volume and by lowering pressure and reducing volume in the failing left ventricle of the heart. Vasodilator possibilities include oral nitrates (isosorbide), nitrates plus hydralazine, ACE inhibitors (captopril and enalapril), prazosin (Minipress), and calcium channel antagonists (Procardia).

Only two of these options, however, have been shown to increase survival in patients with congestive heart failure; and that was only when they were combined with digitalis and diuretics. One of these successful alternatives was enalapril. (Captopril would probably work as well.) In one study, the combination of enalapril, diuretics, and other vasodilators reduced mortality by 31 percent at the end of one year.[18] The other successful combination was isosorbide nitrate with hydralazine. The combination of isosorbide, hydralazine, digitalis, and diuretics decreased mortality when compared with a placebo by 34 percent at the end of two years.[19]

These vasodilators also carry serious risks, and patients must be monitored carefully; but in these extremities, the risks are probably worth hazarding.[20]

Digitalis

Digitalis drugs are obtained from plants and have been around for centuries. They were used historically as rat poisons and arrow poisons. In large doses, they're fatal to humans. Unfortunately, there's not much difference between the dose that speeds up the heart and the dose that stops it altogether, and the overly aggressive use of digitalis can be quite hazardous. In one study, its long-term use after heart attacks was actually found to *increase* mortality in the four to six months following the attacks.

Even if the drugs are expertly administered, your chances of suffering from digitalis toxicity are 5–15 percent. In fact, digitalis intoxication is one of the most common adverse drug reactions. Warning signs include visual disturbances, nausea, vomiting, stomach pain, sleepiness, headache, depression, and irregular heartbeats.[21]

Despite these risks, digoxin (Lanoxin), the most popular of the digitalis drugs, ranked *number two* among bestselling prescription drugs in 1988.

Nondrug alternatives

An alternative that takes more motivation than drug therapy but carries fewer risks is dietary change. New studies show that the arterial blockage reducing blood flow can actually be reversed by this method, and the angina pain accompanying it can be eliminated.

At the annual meeting of the American Heart Association in November of 1989, Dean Ornish and Shirley Brown, researchers at the University of California at San Francisco, confirmed preliminary results reported in 1988 demonstrating actual reductions in arterial blockage in their patients. Their study involved about fifty patients with severe heart disease. Half were counseled (but not required) to lower cholesterol and blood pressure, and to quit smoking. The other half were required to quit smoking, to walk one hour three times a week, to reduce stress by daily yoga and meditation, and to eat a low-fat vegetarian diet. The only animal products allowed were nonfat milk and yogurt. Only 8–10 percent of their total calories came from fat—about a quarter of the usual American intake.

After a year, arterial blockage was significantly reduced in 10 of 12 patients in the vegetarian group. By comparison, 11 of 17 patients in the control group got worse. Cholesterol levels also dropped markedly in the vegetarian group while decreasing only modestly in the other group.[22]

If cutting your fat intake to 8–10 percent of total calories sounds too drastic, you can stop the formation of new lesions simply by cutting fat to about 27 percent of total calories (compared to 36–37 percent in the normal diet). This was the finding of a second study, sponsored by the National Heart, Lung, and Blood Institute, conducted by Dr. David Blankenhorn at the University of Southern California.[23]

A strict vegetarian diet can also help conquer angina pain. In a British study, four out of four patients with severe angina became symptom-free after five to six months on a "vegan" diet that entirely excluded animal products. Their conditions had not responded to medication, but they were able to engage in strenuous activities without pain on the diet. One patient was followed for a full ten years, during which his pain did not return even when mountain climbing.[24]

In an earlier study, when six angina patients were put on a diet consisting of rice, fruits, vegetables, and a specially-prepared mixture of amino acids, their angina pain decreased, their ability to exercise increased, and their serum cholesterol levels dropped nearly 40 percent. Again, drug treatment had failed to improve their conditions.[25]

Exercise is hard for people with angina, but it, too, has been shown to reduce angina pain. A regular exercise routine lowers the pulse rate, which means the heart doesn't have to work so hard or use so much oxygen.

A study reported in the medical journal *Mayo Clinic Proceedings* involved eight men aged 44–50 with mild angina. Half had previously had heart attacks. They were put on an exercise program that involved 45-minute sessions three times a week. After one year, five were completely symptom-free, and three experienced significant reductions in angina pain.[26]

Exercise can also prevent angina from developing. An Israeli study of more than ten thousand middle-aged men and women found that the risk of developing angina was more than twice as great for men with sedentary lifestyles as for those who were more active. For sedentary women, it was more than three times as great.[27]

Table 22.   Nitrates[28]

Generic name:	Brand names:
isosorbide dinitrate	Isordil, Sorbitrate
nitroglycerin (systemic)	Nitrolingual (aerosol spray)
	Nitrostat (tablets)
	Nitro-Bid (tablets)
nitroglycerin (topical)	Nitrol (ointment)
	Nitrodisc (skin pad)
	Nitro-Dur (skin pad)
	Transderm-Nitro (skin pad)
pentaerythritol tetranitrate	Peritrate, Peritrate SA

Intended effects:	Reduce oxygen demand, enlarge blood vessels to increase circulation to the heart; reduce angina pain.
Side effects:	Headache, flushing, dizziness, weakness, nausea, vomiting, blurred vision, dry mouth, skin irritation (patch), burning under tongue (tablets)
Adverse interactions:	May cause a severe drop in blood pressure in combination with alcohol or antihypertensives; may antagonize the action of norepinephrine, acetylcholine, or histamine; effects may be altered in combination with over-the-counter cold and allergy remedies
Risky for:	People with glaucoma, severe anemia, low blood pressure, heart malfunctions or impending heart attack. People allergic to aspirin may be allergic to some nitrates.

Table 23.   Digitalis

Generic name:	Brand name:
digoxin	Lanoxin

Intended effects:	To slow, strengthen, and regulate heartbeat; reduce fluid retention; treat congestive heart failure.
Side effects:	Fatigue, weakness, increased severity of congestive heart failure, arrhythmias, low blood pressure, blurred vision, nausea, vomiting, diarrhea,

headache, hallucinations, dizziness, stupor, agitation. Heart disturbances may be life-threatening.

Adverse interactions: Disturbances in heart rhythm or toxicity may result in combination with antibiotics, steroids, thyroid hormones, diuretics, reserpine, ephedrine, epinephrine, or any drugs affecting the heart. Absorption may be altered by antibiotics, phenytoin, antacids, laxatives, kaolin-pectin, phenobarbital, phenylbutazone, cholestyramine, colestipol, metoclopramide, diltiazem, nifedipine, verapamil, and other drugs. Increased absorption can cause digoxin toxicity.

Risky for: Elderly people; people with kidney or liver problems, rheumatic heart disease, or any illness causing diarrhea, vomiting, or dehydration; obese people; pregnant women or nursing mothers. If heart rate is less than 60 beats per minute, don't use; contact doctor immediately.

16

DRUGS FOR DIABETICS: ASSESSING THE RISKS

The benefits of various treatment approaches for NIDDM [non-insulin-dependent diabetes mellitus] remain ambiguous. Although hyperglycemia is clearly a risk factor, it has not been clearly established that alternative treatment approaches improve survival and reduce disease complications.

—R. Kaplan, M.D.
T. Ganiats, M.D. (1989)[1]

Diabetes develops when the body fails to regulate the amount of sugar circulating in the blood and blood sugar rises to abnormal levels. It affects fourteen million people in the United States and Canada. At the beginning of this century, serious cases of diabetes inevitably led to severe dehydration, coma, and death. Then Canadian researchers discovered the disease could be treated with extracts of the pancreas. The pancreas is the organ that releases insulin, the hormone that helps sugar get into the tissues.

Although their prognosis is much better at the end of this century than it was at the beginning, diabetics still have serious long-term health problems. Prolonged hyperglycemia (elevated blood sugar) is a risk factor for the development of such chronic complications as visual loss, kidney failure, high blood pressure, cardiovascular disease, and neurological disorders. These complications result from adverse reactions between glucose and various body tissues. Among U.S. adults aged 20–74, diabetes is the leading cause of noncongenital blindness, which results when blood vessels in the retina multiply and then explode. Diabetes is also the leading cause of kidney failure, which results from circulatory problems in the blood vessels of the kidney. It's a leading cause of amputation caused by gangrene in the feet and toes, resulting from poor circulation. Worst of all, diabetics have twice the risk of heart disease as other people.

Diabetes that begins in childhood, called Type I or insulin-dependent diabetes mellitus (IDDM), is nearly always due to severe insulin deficiency. Its victims produce little or no insulin, so they must obtain the hormone by artificial means. Recent research suggests IDDM is actually an autoimmune disease. It results when confused antibodies mistake the beta cells in the pancreas for foreign invaders and destroy them. In Canada and Europe, immunotherapy to suppress this immune response has resulted in the remission of diabetes, at least so long as the patient is taking the immunosuppressive drug. The problems with this therapy to date are that it requires suppression of the entire immune system, which is very dangerous, and the drug (cyclosporine) is very toxic. Cyclosporine eventually damages the kidneys, perhaps irreversibly; and complete immunosuppression leaves the patient vulnerable to any infection he is exposed to. At present, the cure is worse than the disease.[2]

Fortunately, child-onset diabetes constitutes only 7–10 percent of all diabetes cases.[3] The remainder are Type II, adult-onset, noninsulin dependent diabetes mellitus (NIDDM). People with NIDDM may actually have normal or even elevated levels of insulin. The hormone just isn't working properly. Why isn't certain, but the number one predisposing risk factor is obesity.

Other cases of adult-onset diabetes are actually induced by drugs. Known offenders include steroids, birth control pills, and diuretics. Diabetes, or impaired glucose tolerance, frequently develops during antihypertensive therapy with diuretics, and often, the condition doesn't go away when treatment is discontinued.[4]

Most patients with NIDDM don't need daily insulin injections to control their condition. Many can do it simply by changing their diets and losing weight or by giving up the precipitating drugs. Even many insulin-dependent diabetics can reduce or eliminate the need for insulin by changing their diets.[5]

Dietary modification does more than allow diabetics to control their blood sugar without drugs. Recent research suggests dietary and other lifestyle changes may be the *only* way to reduce or prevent long-term diabetic complications. In this chapter, we'll look at studies questioning the benefits of drugs for prolonging survival in diabetics, and at the dietary alternative. In the next chapter, we'll look at the drugs themselves, and at what's new in diabetes treatment.

Blood-sugar-lowering drugs and long-term survival

Just as for high blood pressure, studies *have* established that prolonged elevated blood sugar is a risk factor for long-term complications; but they *haven't* established that that risk is reduced by lowering blood sugar *with drugs.* Coronary heart disease is the main cause of premature death in diabetics. This increased CHD mortality, however, doesn't seem to be closely linked to blood sugar control. In fact, there is some evidence that oral sugar-lowering drugs actually *increase* the diabetic's risk of death from CHD.[6]

Oral sugar-lowering drugs

For many years, the long-term benefits of lowering the blood sugar were simply assumed, and adult-onset diabetics were routinely treated with oral drugs that brought their blood sugar down. Called "sulfonylureas," these drugs are modified versions of the sulfonamide antibiotics. The discovery that they could lower blood sugar came about by accident when the properties of the modified antibiotics were being investigated during World War II. By the 1950s, the sulfonylureas were standard treatment for NIDDM.[7]

Doubts weren't cast until 1970, when the preliminary results were reported of a large multicentered study known as the University Group Diabetes Program (UGDP). Over eight hundred patients with NIDDM were randomly assigned to one of five groups. Two got insulin injections, on different dosing schedules. The third got a sulfonylurea drug called tolbutamide (Orinase). The fourth group got a drug that produced complications so early in the study that its use was discontinued. The fifth group got a placebo. The patients were followed for eight years.

When mortality rates were compared, the two insulin groups fared no better than the placebo group. Worse, for the tolbutamide group, the probability of death from cardiovascular disease was actually significantly *greater* than for the placebo group.

Three other studies reported in the 1970s also suggested a link between sulfonylurea drugs and heart attack incidence and mortality in diabetics. In all three, diabetics taking the tablets were about *twice* as likely to suffer a heart attack as those treated with diet alone.[8]

Later studies failed to confirm this increased risk, and some commentators concluded the earlier findings were flawed. But the later studies also failed to show long-term benefits from oral hypoglycemic treatment.

Sales of sulfonylurea drugs plunged after the UGDP results were announced, but they've now climbed back up. Recent prescriptions tend to be for the "second generation" sulfonylureas. Conveniently, they weren't tested in the UGDP trial, so there is no evidence they increase cardiovascular risk. However, they also haven't been shown to decrease it; and whether they're more effective or safer than the first generation agents is still under debate.

Based on the evidence to date, oral hypoglycemics may be worth taking only if they improve the quality of the patient's life by relieving symptoms. But this hasn't been established either. In fact, it hasn't been studied.[9]

Oral drugs are more convenient than insulin, which has to be injected, sometimes several times a day. All attempts at oral administration of insulin have failed, because stomach acid quickly destroys the drug. Insulin can also cause allergic reactions, pitting or thickening of the skin at the site of injection, increased appetite leading to weight gain, and too-low drops in blood sugar.

But oral hypoglycemics, too, can have side effects. They can cause skin reactions, gastrointestinal upset, and an improper secretion of antidiuretic hormone that results in headaches, tiredness, stupor, and seizures. On top of this is the "nuisance factor" associated with regular drug use.[10]

Insulin: standard vs. intensive therapy

Because prolonged elevated blood sugar has been linked to chronic diabetic complications, diabetes specialists are focusing on stricter control to keep blood sugar at near-normal levels. Its effects on long-term survival, however, are still under debate.

The issue is whether the progression of late diabetic complications can be decreased or prevented by aggressive insulin therapy to keep blood sugar at near-normal levels. The first study suggesting it could was the Oslo Study, reported in the *British Medical Journal* in 1986. Norwegian researchers found that after two years on the conventional two-shot-a-day insulin treatment, retinal microaneurysms and hemorrhages (minute swellings and bleedings in the capillaries of the retina) significantly increased. Patients who were treated either by continuous subcutaneous insulin infusion (the "insulin pump") or by multiple injections (five or six daily) had significantly fewer of these complications.[11]

But later analysis showed that after forty months of therapy, no important differences in retinal disorders were apparent among the three groups. In fact, according to commentators writing in the *New England Journal of Medicine* in 1988, the most consistent finding of this and similar studies was the short-term *worsening* of retinal disorders with intensive therapy. They cautioned:

The recommendation to proceed with intensive therapy on the basis of such scant data might be countenanced if such therapy were widely accepted by patients with insulin-dependent diabetes mellitus and if it were without added risk as compared with conventional therapy. Such is not the case. The documentation of increased frequency of mild and severe hypoglycemia and ketoacidosis in subjects treated intensively mandates that the benefit-risk ratio for such therapy be evaluated.[12]

These researchers are currently conducting the Diabetes Control and Complications Trial (DCCT). It has been in progress since 1982 and involves over a thousand patients. Its purpose is to definitively determine the benefits and risks of intensive therapy for insulin-dependent diabetics.

The risk of hypoglycemia, with the possibility of coma, is the major complication of insulin therapy. It had been hoped that advances in techniques for insulin delivery and home blood glucose monitoring would improve glucose control in IDDM patients without substantially increasing this risk. But preliminary data from the DCCT show that severe hypoglycemia and coma are two to three times more common in patients treated intensively. Apparently, strict metabolic control of blood sugar blunts the diabetic's already impaired counterregulatory responses to hypoglycemia.[13]

This hazard would be worth putting up with, if aggressive insulin therapy actually delayed the onset of diabetic complications. But until the DCCT results are published, the question mark remains.

Nondrug alternatives

For diabetics without symptoms or with only mild disease, non-drug therapies involving diet and exercise are the preferable first-choice options. NIDDM is more likely to occur in people who are overweight. Simply shedding excess weight can drop elevated blood sugar to near-normal levels.[14]

Even in diabetics who need insulin, dietary change has reduced and, in some cases, even eliminated insulin requirements. In a landmark study, the carbohydrate intake of diabetics was nearly doubled by substituting high-fiber complex carbohydrates for animal foods. The result: diabetics on low doses of insulin managed to give up the drug altogether, and those on high doses substantially reduced their prescriptions.[15]

The high-carbohydrate, high-fiber diet represents a dramatic reversal in diabetic dietary theory. Since carbohydrate is what sugar is made of, eating carbohydrate was assumed to raise blood sugar. Thus, early recommendations involved *reducing* carbohydrate and increasing fat and protein. But this diet wasn't calculated to produce weight loss, and its excess fat increased the risk of hardening of the arteries. This, in turn, increased the risk of heart disease, to which diabetics are already dangerously prone. Accordingly, in 1979, the Food and Nutrition Committee of the American Diabetes Association made a dramatic about-face. It recommended that insulin-dependent diabetics *increase* their carbohydrate intake to 50–60 percent of total calories.[16]

The new diabetic diet stresses complex carbohydrates (whole grains and beans) and fiber. Complex carbohydrates are digested more slowly than simple carbohydrates, and they actually help regulate blood sugar levels. Further, both kinds of fiber—the soluble kind in oats and beans and the insoluble kind in wheat bran—help to regulate glucose metabolism by delaying glucose absorption from the intestines. A high-fiber diet takes longer to digest, and sugar from the food is absorbed over a longer period. Soluble fibers are particularly effective at regulating blood sugar. They improve glycemic control, reduce fasting plasma glucose levels, reduce insulin requirements, and lower cholesterol and triglyceride levels. Fiber also helps keep your weight down. It fills you up with fewer calories and gives you more opportunity to chew.[17]

Beans and other legumes that are slowly digested and absorbed are particularly good foods for diabetics. Studies show that diets based on legumes improve diabetic glucose and insulin profiles, and that slow-release carbohydrates can help relieve the symptoms of the disease.

Legumes remain the traditional staple in parts of the world like Africa and India, where diabetes is uncommon. Legumes were also the staple foods of traditional societies like the Australian Aboriginal and Pacific Island populations. Urbanization has resulted in a dramatic rise in NIDDM in these people during this century. Between 10 percent and 35 percent of them develop the disease when they move to the city, compared to only 3 percent of Caucasians of European descent. The condition in diabetic Aborigines has shown dramatic improvement when they return to their traditional diet—for as few as seven weeks.[18]

Table 24. *Fiber Content of Selected Foods*[19]

Food	Serving size	Insoluble fiber (g)	Soluble fiber (g)	Calories
Grains				
Bread, whole wheat	1 slice	1.2	0.3	61
Barley, pearled, dry	2 tbsp	1.0	1.5	97
Cornmeal, whole grain	2 tbsp	0.8	0.2	54
Oat bran, dry	1/3 cup	2.2	2.0	90
Oats, regular, dry	1/3 cup	1.5	1.3	100
Rice, brown, cooked	1/2 cup	2.2	0.2	97
Fruits				
Apple, raw, with skin	1 fruit	2.1	0.9	80
Banana	1 medium	1.5	0.6	105
Dates, dried	2 fruits	1.2	0.4	50
Figs, dried	1 medium	2.9	3.7	55
Prunes, dried	3 fruits	2.6	1.1	60
Orange, raw	1 medium	1.6	1.6	65
Vegetables				
Broccoli, cooked	1/2 cup	1.1	0.9	28
Brussels sprouts, cooked	1/2 cup	2.3	1.6	30
Cabbage, Chinese, raw	1/2 cup	1.2	1.1	06
Carrots, cooked	1/2 cup	1.2	1.1	21
Cauliflower, cooked	1/2 cup	1.1	0.5	14
Corn, cooked	1/2 cup	2.7	0.2	70
Kale, cooked	1/2 cup	1.4	1.4	20
Peas, green, young, cooked	1/2 cup	3.0	1.1	57
Onion, cooked	1/2 cup	1.4	0.8	32
Potato, white, baked	1/2 medium	1.0	0.9	73
Tomato, raw	1 medium	0.6	0.2	22
Yam, cooked	1/2 medium	1.4	1.5	80
Beans				
Kidney, cooked	1/2 cup	3.3	2.5	109
Lima, cooked	1/2 cup	3.2	1.2	94
Pinto, cooked	1/2 cup	3.3	2.0	114
Lentils, cooked	1/2 cup	1.1	1.0	64
Peas, black-eyed, cooked	1/2 cup	6.8	4.5	100
Peas, split, cooked	1/2 cup	3.4	1.7	71

The diabetic diet now recommended is not only high in complex carbohydrates, but low in fat. Fat, especially the saturated variety, can impair insulin activity.[20] It also contributes to excess pounds. Two-thirds of the fat in the American diet comes from animal foods, while all of its fiber comes from plant foods.[21] Studies have shown a positive association between the consumption of meat, which is high in saturated fat, and blood glucose levels. This may explain why diabetes is more prevalent in beef-eating countries.[22]

A study reported in the *American Journal of Clinical Nutrition* in 1988 involved twenty years of follow-up on twenty-seven thousand Seventh Day Adventists, a religious group that discourages its members from eating meat. The study found that for men who ate meat daily, the risk of developing diabetes was four times as great as for those who ate it once a week or less. Interestingly, no such association was found with the consumption of eggs, milk, or cheese, although those foods are also high in saturated fat.[23]

Exercise can also aid in the control of diabetes. It not only promotes weight loss by burning up excess calories, but improves cardiovascular performance and glucose use. Apparently, exercise blunts the rise in blood glucose that follows carbohydrate consumption, and it increases the sensitivity to insulin.

Major changes in activity levels may, however, require a change in drug dosage, since increased exercise can trigger hypoglycemic episodes. Diabetics who exercise should also pay special attention to their feet, which can lose sensation; and to their eyes, which can be damaged by the increased blood pressure resulting from straining and breath-holding, as in weight lifting. Aerobic activities like walking and swimming are better exercise choices.[24]

17

NEW TREATMENT OPTIONS FOR DIABETICS

While researchers are weighing the long-term benefits and risks of various therapies, dramatic changes are occurring in the treatment options available for diabetics.

The devices

Diabetes specialists are focusing on stricter control of blood sugar to keep it at near-normal levels. This requires close monitoring, which has been facilitated by a variety of home blood glucose monitoring devices (described more fully in chapter 35). Older urine glucose monitoring methods were estimates at best. Home glucose monitoring from pinpricked blood provides immediate, accurate feedback that helps the patient fine tune his treatment program.[1]

Multiple dose schedules have also been made easier by improvements in insulin syringes. Standard syringes have finer needles, and there are a range of automatic syringe options available. There are spring-loaded devices, pen-size devices, and "jet injectors" that blow insulin through the skin.

External insulin infusion pumps are another option. These are worn on the belt or under the clothing. They pump insulin continuously through a catheter to a needle placed under the skin in the abdomen. The syringe and needle are changed every two to three days. These devices allow the pattern of insulin release to be easily adjusted to the anticipated needs of the patient.

Still in the experimental stage is the implanted insulin infusion pump. The ideal is a "closed-loop feedback" system that continuously measures blood sugar levels and then releases appropriate amounts of insulin, just as the pancreas does. But this system is several years away.

What is now at the testing stage is an "open-loop" system. It isn't designed to sense ongoing blood sugar levels but responds to an external transmitter controlled by the patient. The Programmable Implantable Medication System (PIMS), developed at Johns Hopkins, involves an implanted unit that is surgically placed beneath the skin in the left side of the abdomen. In response to commands from the patient, the unit delivers pulses of insulin through a catheter deep in the peritoneal space at variable rates. The PIMS is refilled with insulin every two or three months by injection.[2]

Preliminary tests of the device were reported in the *New England Journal of Medicine* in August of 1989. Eighteen patients received PIMS-delivered insulin for 4–25 months. The system still had a few bugs: one pump broke down because of a manufacturing defect, four wound up with blocked catheters, and two required repair. But the PIMS worked much better than previous attempts, and the patients suffered no surgical, skin, or other serious complications. The study showed that insulin-dependent diabetics can be treated for at least two years without daily injections, with insulin doses programmed to mimic physiologic secretion.[3] These innovations may one day make possible a mechanical system of blood sugar regulation that mimics the body's own.

New insulins

The human system has also been more closely mirrored by the development of human insulin. Earlier varieties were derived from pork or beef. Humulin, marketed by Eli Lilly and Company, is synthesized by a strain of bacteria. It dominates the U.S. human insulin market. Novolin brands are semisynthetic human insulins made from converted pork insulin.[4]

The main advantage of human insulin is that it's less likely to provoke an allergic response than the pork form. Pork insulin, in turn, is less likely to provoke one than insulin derived from beef.

Human insulin costs no more than pork-derived insulin, and may cost less. It is now considered the insulin of first choice for newly-diagnosed diabetics, for diabetics who need insulin only intermittently, and for patients with an allergy or local reaction to animal insulin. Even human insulin, however, provokes an allergic response in 2–3 percent of diabetics during the first year of treatment.[5]

Experts say there is no compelling reason for diabetics presently doing well on pork insulin to change. Many patients seem to be switching on their own, but this can be dangerous. It should be done only under a doctor's supervision.[6]

One problem with human insulin is that it may suppress the symptoms of hypoglycemia, which can kill diabetics. In October of 1989, the British press reported seventeen sudden, unexplained deaths in diabetics, compared to only two in 1985. At least six of the deaths occurred among relatively young diabetics who had switched to human insulin within the past year. Dr. Patrick Toseland, a toxicologist, suggested the deaths may have occurred after human insulin blunted the critical warning signs of hypoglycemia, which usually include sweating, anxiety, and cramps. Diabetics who experience these warnings in time can easily correct hypoglycemia by eating sugary food. But blood sugar drops earlier and faster on human insulin than it does on animal insulin, giving diabetics less time to correct the drop.

The American Diabetic Association issued a statement urging diabetics not to overreact to the report, which to date lacks hard scientific evidence. The British victims were using a Danish product, not Lilly's Humulin. The FDA already requires human insulin products to carry warnings that symptoms of hypoglycemia are less pronounced than with animal-based products.[7]

New oral blood-sugar-lowering drugs

For patients with non-insulin-dependent diabetes, blood sugar may be controlled by oral sulfonylurea drugs; and these, too, have been improved.

The newer-model "second generation" sulfonylureas include

glyburide (DiaBeta, Micronase) and glipizide (Glucotrol). The second generation drugs are more potent than the first, act more quickly, and require fewer daily doses.

Their major drawback is, again, an increased risk of hypoglycemia, especially in elderly people with poor eating habits and a decreased ability to clear drugs from their systems. Whether the second generation sulfonylureas are more effective at increasing long-term survival also remains a matter of debate. Further, the drugs may not work. In up to 20 percent of patients, they don't work at all; and after ten years of treatment, they fail to control blood sugar adequately in 50–70 percent of the rest. If not combined with diet regulation, sulfonylurea therapy is likely to fail at any stage of the disease.[8]

Table 25.   *Insulins Available in the United States*[9]

Source	Brand name	Onset/duration of action
improved pork	Regular Insulin	rapid
improved beef	Semilente Insulin	rapid
	NPH Insulin	intermediate
	Lente Insulin	intermediate
	Ultralente Insulin	long
improved beef-pork	Regular Iletin I	rapid
	Semilente Iletin I	rapid
	Pork NPH Iletin I	intermediate
	Lente Iletin I	intermediate
	Protamine, Zinc & Iletin I	long
	Ultralente Iletin I	long
purified pork	Regular Purified Pork Insulin	rapid
	Semilente Purified Pork	rapid
	Velosulin	rapid
	NPH Purified Pork	intermediate
	NPH Iletin II	intermediate
	Insulatard NPH	intermediate
	Lente Iletin II	intermediate
	Lente Purified Pork Insulin	intermediate
	Protamine, Zinc & Iletin II	long
purified beef	Beef Regular Iletin II	rapid
	Beef NPH Iletin II	intermediate

Source	Brand name	Onset/duration of action
	Lente Iletin II	intermediate
	Protamine, Zinc & Iletin II	long
	Ultralente Purified Beef	long
human (recombinant DNA)	Humulin R	rapid
	Humulin N	intermediate
human (semisynthetic)	Novolin R	rapid
	Novolin N	intermediate
	Novolin L	intermediate

Table 26.   *Sulfonylureas Available in the United States*[10]

Generic name	Brand name	Risky for:	
		elderly/ poor eaters	people with kidney problems
tolbutamide	Orinase	no	no
acetohexamide	Dymelor	no	yes
tolazamide	Tolinase	no	yes
chlorpropamide	Diabinese	yes	yes
glipizide	Glucotrol	maybe	no
glyburide	DiaBeta, Micronase	maybe	maybe

While oral sugar-lowering drugs are more convenient than insulin, insulin has one advantage: it raises HDL ("good") cholesterol more. In a double-blind study conducted at Massachusetts General Hospital in 1988, insulin and glyburide were equally effective at controlling blood sugar in Type-2 diabetics, and both lowered cholesterol by about 5 percent. But after nine months of treatment with insulin, HDL rose by 25 percent, putting it in the recommended range. With glyburide, HDL rose only 10 percent, putting it merely in the borderline range.[11]

Drugs diabetics should avoid

There are other drugs you need to know about if you're diabetic: the ones you should avoid. Many drugs can either increase blood glucose levels or decrease them, thus increasing the risk of hypoglycemia in combination with sugar-lowering drugs. Leading offenders are listed in table 27.

Table 27.   *Drugs that Can Affect Blood Sugar Levels*[12]

Blood glucose levels are decreased by:
  aspirin and other salicylates
  phenylbutazone (a nonsteroidal anti-inflammatory agent)
  coumarin anticoagulants
  ethanol (in alcoholic beverages)
  sulfonamide antibiotics
  trimethoprim (for urinary tract infections)

Blood glucose levels are increased by:
  caffeine (in large quantities)
  corticosteroids
  diazoxide
  ephedrine
  estrogen
  furosemide and thiazide diuretics
  lithium
  nicotinic acid (in large doses)
  phenobarbital
  phenytoin
  rifampin (for the treatment of tuberculosis)
  sugar-containing medications
  thyroid preparations

Beta-blockers should also be avoided, because they can mask the symptoms of hypoglycemia in insulin-dependent diabetics.[13] For diabetics who need antihypertensives, the best alternative may be captopril (Capoten) combined with a thiazide diuretic. Preliminary research suggests this combination can actually halt the progress of kidney failure, the most feared complication of diabetes. This discovery, if confirmed, might prevent thousands of diabetic deaths annually.[14] However, thiazide diuretics can alter insulin requirements and raise sugar levels in the blood and urine.[15] If you're considering this option, consult your doctor first.

Not only prescription but nonprescription drugs can pose a threat to diabetics. Aspirin, the most commonly purchased nonprescription drug, can be dangerous at high doses, since its salicylates can alter urine glucose tests and induce hypoglycemia. High doses of vitamin C can also alter urine test readings. Acetaminophen and ibuprofen, aspirin's leading competitors, aren't ideal choices either, since they can have undesirable effects on the kidneys.

Diabetics who need foot care products should avoid those containing salicylic acid and other irritating chemicals. They should also consult a podiatrist at the first sign of foot problems.

Laxatives can adversely affect blood sugar, either by their high glucose content or by altering intestinal transit time.

Many other over-the-counter drugs contain either sugar or alcohol. Diabetics should avoid both. One clue is to look for ingredients ending in "-ose" or "-ol." However, eliminating these Latin endings won't necessarily hit all the offenders. More than 350,000 drugs are now marketed over the counter, and many of them lack proper labeling. Some, like antacids, are also high in sodium, which is contraindicated for diabetics who have accompanying cardiovascular disease.[16] Your best bet is to take a conservative approach, and cut over-the-counter drug use to the bare bones. When in doubt, ask your pharmacist!

III

Analgesics and Anti-Inflammatory Drugs

18

ASPIRIN: FROM HEADACHES TO HEART ATTACKS

"I'm very brave generally," he went on in a low voice;
"only to-day I happen to have a headache."
— Lewis Carroll
The Walrus and the Carpenter

Analgesics (painkillers) are the most commonly used drugs worldwide. This is probably because pain is the most common symptom of disease. In the United States in 1987, annual sales of over-the-counter analgesics came to $2.1 billion and accounted for one-fourth of the over-the-counter drug market. This lucrative business is divided among aspirin, acetaminophen, and ibuprofen; but aspirin, the oldest analgesic, continues to hold the lead. Aspirin has been around in pill form since 1899, and a naturally occurring form of the drug in willow bark was known to Hippocrates millennia before that. Americans now take about 80 million aspirin tablets a day, not to mention what's contained in many combination drugs.[1]

Aspirin's most popular use is in the relief of simple tension headaches. It not only relieves pain but reduces inflammation, making it the leading drug recommended for arthritis, in which pain comes from the movement and stress of inflamed joints. Aspirin also retards blood clotting and "thins the blood," a property underlying the latest use touted for it, as a preventative for heart attacks.

Aspirin and prostaglandins

The mechanism of aspirin's effects has only recently been pin-pointed. It has to do with certain natural substances called pros-taglandins. There are many prostaglandins, with many biological functions. One targeted by aspirin, called PGE 2, increases the awareness of pain. Apparently, its purpose is to alert the body to disturbances in normal function. Other prostaglandins contribute to the heat and swelling of inflammation, and others promote the co-agulation of blood. Aspirin interferes with the body's biosynthesis of these prostaglandins and thus suppresses inflammation and the awareness of pain.

Other drugs in the aspirin group work by the same mechanism. They're called "nonsteroidal anti-inflammatory drugs" (NSAIDs) —as opposed to the steroids, which also reduce inflammation but have more serious side effects (see chapter 7). In addition to other salicylates in the aspirin family, NSAIDs include ibuprofen (Mo-trin, Advil), indomethacin (Indocin), naproxen (Naprosyn), piroxi-cam (Feldene), sulindac (Clinoril), and other anti-inflammatories. They are described more fully in the next chapter.

All NSAIDs work by suppressing prostaglandin synthesis. The drawback of this approach is that prostaglandins have normal body functions that are inhibited at the same time.

Some prostaglandins help to regulate the flow of blood through the kidneys and the filtration and excretion of sodium and toxins. When aspirin and other NSAIDs inhibit these functions, the result can be fluid retention and the buildup of nitrogenous wastes in the blood.[2]

Other prostaglandins have a direct action on stomach cells. They inhibit acid production and prevent acid damage to the lining of the stomach. When these prostaglandins are suppressed, acid can eat holes in your stomach and intestines. This unwanted effect is, in fact, the largest single cause of disease and death due to aspirin and other NSAIDs.

Aspirin as an anticoagulant

Aspirin's interference with blood coagulation is the basis for its much-publicized ability to reduce heart attacks. But we've seen that when aspirin has been used experimentally for this purpose, the overall death rate in normal middle-aged men hasn't been reduced.[3] One reason is that while the drug reduces heart attacks, it also increases a certain type of stroke. When blood clotting is prevented, bleeding times are extended, sometimes to dangerous lengths. As a result, the risk of stroke from cerebral hemorrhage, or bleeding, goes up. Fish oils, which have also been touted as lowering heart disease risk, work the same way. The fish-eating Eskimos have a low incidence of heart disease, but they also have unusually long bleeding times and a high incidence of strokes.[4]

Aspirin has a tendency to increase bleeding not only in the brain but in the stomach, where its irritating effects contribute to ulcers. Peptic ulcers are very common in this country, affecting some 10 percent of the population. Even if your stomach doesn't actually hemorrhage, you can wind up with iron-deficiency anemia from the daily loss of imperceptible amounts of blood in the stool. This effect is particularly insidious because it may produce no symptoms. It can be a serious threat to older people who don't get enough iron, and to women who have heavy periods. Besides iron, aspirin increases your need for certain vitamins, notably C, B1, and folic acid.

Aspirin has also been linked to the leading cause of blindness in the United States, macular hemorrhage (bleeding) in the aging eye. This means elderly people who regularly take aspirin are at increased risk not only of stroke, but of blindness.[5]

Aspirin can increase the bleeding resulting from wounds, tooth extraction, surgery, and childbirth. Because it keeps blood platelets from sticking together normally, it should be avoided by pregnant women, newborns, and people with clotting disorders or ulcers.

Other hazards

Aspirin overdose can cause dizziness, ringing in the ears, impaired hearing, nausea, vomiting, diarrhea, and confusion. These symptoms will occur in anyone with a large enough dose. Deafness is usually reversible after drug withdrawal, but permanent symptoms can result from continued use.

Accidental overdose is a problem particularly among rheumatoid arthritis victims. The amount of aspirin needed to reduce inflammation is so high that it already approaches toxic levels, and the agony of the condition may prompt sufferers to exceed recommended dosages. Serious overdose can cause hyperventilation, visual impairment, delirium, hallucinations, convulsions, coma, and even death. One arthritic elderly woman whose aspirin dose was accidentally doubled died after only ten days on this regimen. Aspirin's lethal potential is well known to the suicidal, among whom it is second only to barbiturates as the drug of choice.[6]

Aspirin can also cause allergic reactions: shortness of breath, wheezing, rashes, and hives. About 10 percent of people with asthma react to aspirin with bronchial spasms that leave them gasping for breath. Even if you didn't have the condition to start with, you can actually develop bronchial asthma from an intolerance to analgesics. This syndrome, which used to be rare, is being seen more and more often.[7]

Another risk of extended aspirin use is a twofold increase in the likelihood of contracting kidney cancer. We'll look at the risk of kidney disease from analgesics in chapter 20.[8]

Choosing among aspirin products

Major analgesics manufacturers have spent years and fortunes litigating the allegedly false claims of their competitors. However, courts have generally concluded that the litigating manufacturers were about equally guilty of misleading the public, and that all brands of over-the-counter painkillers are about the same.[9]

Buffered aspirin claims to minimize the stomach irritation of regular aspirin, but the Panel on Drugs for Relief of Pain of the National Academy of Sciences/National Research Council asserts there's no convincing support for this claim. Even manufacturer-sponsored studies have failed to prove that regular buffered aspirin is gentler on the stomach than plain aspirin; and highly buffered aspirin, which may be gentler, has the drawback of being very high in sodium. Ironically, this can predispose you to high blood pressure, the major risk factor for the heart disease you may be taking aspirin to prevent.[10]

Enteric-coated aspirin (the kind with the hard candy-like coating) causes considerably less damage to the lining of the stomach than either plain or buffered aspirin.[11] This is because enteric-coated aspirin doesn't dissolve until it gets to the small intestine. But while it bypasses your stomach, it can still eat holes in your duodenum, the portion of the small intestine that attaches to the stomach. It also takes longer than uncoated aspirin to work.

A study reported in 1989 compared the effects of enteric-coated aspirin (Ecotrin) with salsalate, a salicylate in the aspirin family. Salsalate, available as the brand-name drugs Disalcid and Mono-Gesic, was developed as a safer alternative to aspirin. Like enteric-coated aspirin, it doesn't dissolve in the acidic fluids of the stomach. The study compared standard doses (two 325 mg tablets twice daily) of these analgesics taken over a six-day period. It found that coated aspirin was significantly harder on the lining of the stomach and duodenum than salsalate. Only one subject on salsalate had evidence of lining damage, while six of the ten subjects developed pre-ulcerous lesions on Ecotrin, and one developed a duodenal ulcer. Salsalate produced one troublesome side effect in four of the volunteers (ringing in the ears); but five of the ten volunteers experienced side effects while taking Ecotrin (including ringing in the ears, abdominal pain, heartburn, nausea, and nosebleeds).[12]

If you prefer ordinary aspirin, you can also ease stomach irritation by dissolving it in water before you drink it.

Comparing the big three over-the counter-drugs

Some of aspirin's drawbacks are avoided by its competitors, acetaminophen and ibuprofen. However, these analgesics have their own downsides, which we'll look at in the next two chapters. As for their pain-relieving and fever-reducing abilities, they're about the same. Aspirin acts a little quicker. Ibuprofen lasts a little longer. Acetaminophen is easier on the stomach, but it won't reduce the pain associated with inflamed joints. Aspirin is more likely to cause visual disturbances.

Ibuprofen's side effects are similar to aspirin's, but their incidence may be lower. Adverse reactions with other drugs are less likely with ibuprofen, and overdosing is less likely to have serious consequences. According to a recent Vanderbilt University study, however, elderly people who take ibuprofen are four times as likely to die from ulcers and gastrointestinal bleeding as those who don't take it.[13] And like all NSAIDs, ibuprofen tends to cause sodium retention and to inhibit kidney function. It's not recommended for women who are pregnant or nursing, for alcoholics, or for people who have stomach problems or are allergic to aspirin.

Acetaminophen is generally recommended for people who are allergic to aspirin, but there is evidence that people who react to one of these drugs may also react to the other. Acetaminophen has fewer side effects than either aspirin or ibuprofen, but you still don't want to make a daily habit of it, due to its risk of long-term liver and kidney damage.[14]

Table 28. *Comparing the Big Three Over-the-Counter Pain Relievers*[15]

Aspirin

Uses:	Reduce pain, fever, inflammation, blood coagulation
Side effects:	Allergic reactions ranging from itching to asthmatic attacks; stomach bleeding, ulcers, upset stomach, anemia; ringing in the ears, visual disturbances
Risky for:	Pregnant women, nursing mothers; children with chicken pox or flu; people with aspirin allergies, ulcers, or gout; people taking anticoagulants; people who have just had surgery (including oral surgery)
Other factors:	Relatively fast-acting and inexpensive

Acetaminophen

Uses:	Reduce pain, fever
Side effects:	Fewer side effects and allergic reactions than aspirin, but high doses may damage the liver or kidneys
Risky for:	Alcoholics, people with kidney or liver problems, pregnant women or nursing mothers
Other factors:	Somewhat less effective than the other options, but safer for people who react badly to them and for children

Ibuprofen

Uses:	Reduce pain, fever, inflammation, blood coagulation
Side effects:	Similar to, but fewer than, aspirin's. May interfere with diuretic and antihypertensive drugs
Risky for:	Pregnant women, nursing mothers, children under 14; people with gout, ulcers, or aspirin allergies
Other factors:	Longer acting but more expensive; fewer side effects than aspirin but more than acetaminophen

19

ARTHRITIS: CHOOSING AN ANTI-INFLAMMATORY

You can't buy a more potent pain reliever without a prescription.

—Tylenol ad ruled misleading by the
U.S. District Court[1]

Acetaminophen may be easier on the stomach than aspirin and other NSAIDs, but it doesn't reduce inflammation. That means it's not much help in treating toothache, sunburn, sprains, or most forms of arthritis. But for some arthritis sufferers, aspirin isn't the best choice either.

About one in seven Americans suffers from arthritis, and most of them are senior citizens. The most common form of the disease among the elderly is osteoarthritis, the kind that comes from wear and tear on the joints. Osteoarthritis doesn't necessarily involve inflammation. If it doesn't, its pain may respond to acetaminophen.

Rheumatoid arthritis is the most intractable and painful form of the disease. It does involve inflammation, and it is generally treated with anti-inflammatory drugs.

Ankylosing spondylitis is an inflammation of the spine and hip joints. It also generally responds to anti-inflammatory drugs.

Many other conditions involve an element of inflammatory arthritis, including lupus and ulcerative colitis. For these two diseases, however, sufferers shouldn't use aspirin or other NSAIDs, due to their higher risk of kidney or intestinal damage.

Gout, or gouty arthritis, is another arthritic condition on which aspirin won't work. Gout produces an acute pain that's caused by an accumulation of uric acid crystals in the joints. Many kidney stones are also composed of uric acid. Aspirin merely exacerbates these problems, because it causes the *retention* of uric acid. Other NSAIDs don't have this effect.

For most forms of arthritis, however, the most widely recommended anti-inflammatory continues to be aspirin. For many patients with rheumatoid arthritis, aspirin works as well as prescription medications, with fewer side effects. It is also much cheaper.

The non-aspirin NSAIDs

The drugs that are giving aspirin a run for its money are the newer NSAIDs, including ibuprofen (Advil, Motrin, Medipren), naproxen (Naprosyn), piroxicam (Feldene), sulindac (Clinoril), and indomethacin (Indocin).

Of these, only ibuprofen is currently obtainable without a prescription. It, too, was a prescription item until recently. When it was approved in a lower dose for over-the-counter sale, it grabbed nearly 20 percent of the analgesic market. As the blockbuster Advil, ibuprofen took 12 percent of the market in a mere five years. Other popular over-the-counter brands are Genpril, Haltran, Ibuprin, Medipren, Midol 1200, Nuprin, Pamprin IB, and Trendar.

Syntex Corporation, which produces Naprosyn, hopes to duplicate ibuprofen's success by going over-the-counter with its own NSAID, projected to hit the drugstores by 1991.[2] Naprosyn ranked tenth among prescription drug sales in 1988.[3]

Feldene ranked 25th, but that was only in the United States. A 1988 publication by the World Health Organization placed it third worldwide, trailing only the ulcer medications Tagamet and Zantac.[4]

Voltaren (diclofenac sodium) has been promoted as "the number one prescribed antiarthritic in the world." It has been available in other countries for many years but was only recently approved for marketing in the United States. Its sales pitch has been heavy and its initial market performance was good, but sales have recently dropped.[5]

The newer NSAIDs are touted as having the advantages over aspirin of better tolerance, less gastrointestinal distress, once-daily dosing (piroxicam), and general variety of choices. The drugs also cause merely *reversible* blood problems—as opposed to salicylates, which can cause irreversible problems.

Despite these claims, both the FDA and Britain's Committee on Safety of Medicines assert the safety of one NSAID can't be clearly distinguished from any other.[6] In fact, in some cases the newer NSAIDs are actually less safe than aspirin. The authoritative *Medi-*

Table 29.   *Popular Prescription NSAIDs[7]*

Generic name	Brand name	Labeled Indications*						
		RA	OA	JA	AS	APS	AGA	MP
diclofenac sodium	Voltaren	x	x		x			
fenoprofen	Nalfon	x	x					x
flurbiprofen		x	x					
ibuprofen	Motrin, Rufen	x	x					x
indomethacin	Indocin	x	x		x	x	x	
indomethacin (sustained release)	Indocin SR	x	x		x	x		
ketoprofen		x	x					x
meclofenamate	Meclomen	x	x					x
mefanamic acid								x
naproxen	Naprosyn	x	x	x	x	x		x
naproxen sodium	Anaprox	x	x		x	x		x
piroxicam	Feldene	x	x					
sulindac	Clinoril	x	x		x	x	x	
tolmetin	Tolectin, Tolectin DS	x	x	x				

*Key: RA   = rheumatoid arthritis
     OA   = osteoarthritis
     JA   = juvenile arthritis
     AS   = ankylosing spondylitis
     APS = acute painful shoulder
     AGA = acute gouty arthritis
     MP   = mild to moderate pain

cal Letter, an independent, non-drug-industry publication relied on by doctors, warns that all NSAIDs (including aspirin) inhibit the synthesis of prostaglandins that are necessary to regulate kidney blood flow, filtration, and sodium and water excretion. In patients with kidney disease, heart failure, or cirrhosis, kidney toxicity can occur after only a few days of therapy, and the result can be fatal. This can also happen in patients taking diuretics to treat high blood pressure. For this reason, patients taking any NSAIDs should have regular periodic checkups to determine their white blood cell counts and other blood factors.[8]

Non-aspirin NSAIDs: a lower risk of ulcers?

Postmarket surveys suggested the risk of ulcers from non-aspirin NSAIDs wasn't substantial. But a 1986 British study disagreed. It found that people over sixty who took non-aspirin NSAIDs were *three times* as likely as nonusers to be hospitalized with bleeding gastric and duodenal ulcers. About 15 percent of the elderly group studied were current users of these drugs. The researchers projected that in the entire British population of fifty million, about two thousand cases of hemorrhage might be induced each year from this cause, resulting in about two hundred deaths.

Why wasn't this risk detected in postmarket surveys? One reason may have been that the surveys didn't focus on the elderly, who were dwarfed in the broader population covered. Another reason may be that use of the drugs is so widespread. This is a problem with any very popular drug: a risk that looks small in percentage terms can loom large when projected over millions of users. In a sample of ten thousand, a risk of one doesn't look like much; but against a background of twenty million prescriptions annually, the resulting hospitalizations can be counted in the thousands, and the deaths in the hundreds.[9]

Particularly high rates of gastrointestinal bleeding and ulcers have been reported for both indomethacin (Indocin) and piroxicam (Feldene). One reason may be that the powerful pain-killing abilities of NSAIDs can allow peptic ulcers to develop unnoticed. Indomethacin and piroxicam are unusually potent pain-relievers, so they're particularly subject to this effect.[10]

A 1988 Australian study found that the risk of developing a gastric ulcer was more than five times as great in people who used indomethacin daily as in those who used no analgesics. It was also five times as great in daily users of aspirin. It was about three times as great in daily users of ibuprofen and sulindac, and a little over two times as great in daily users of naproxen.[11]

Concerns about these side effects have led the FDA to require new labeling restrictions for NSAIDs. Labels must state, in part:

Serious gastrointestinal toxicity such as bleeding, ulceration, and perforation can occur at any time, with or without warning symptoms, in patients treated chronically with NSAID therapy.

The FDA has also approved a synthetic prostaglandin called misoprostol specifically for use in preventing NSAID-induced ulcers. It works by replacing the prostaglandins NSAIDs inhibit—the ones responsible for producing the mucus that protects the stomach lining from acid. But while misoprostol prevents gastric ulcers caused by NSAIDs, it has no effect on duodenal ulcers or on gastrointestinal pain and discomfort associated with NSAID use. Misoprostol also causes changes in muscle tone, including the muscles of the uterus. Since these changes could lead to miscarriage, the drug isn't prescribed for pregnant women.[12]

For them, and for anyone else who's leery of drugs, there's a more natural alternative. You can eat foods that stimulate the body to make the necessary prostaglandins itself. Foods high in essential fatty acids, found in unsaturated vegetable oils, apparently have this effect.[13]

An even more natural alternative, of course, is to avoid NSAIDs in the first place.

Comparing NSAIDs: effectiveness vs. patient preference

The NSAIDs are all about equally effective, but they differ in their side effects and in patient preference.

In a study comparing the effects of aspirin, ibuprofen, fenoprofen calcium, naproxen, and tolmetin sodium on rheumatoid arthritis, no statistical differences were found in resulting grip strength, walking distance and difficulty, or duration of morning stiffness. But there were significant differences in patient preference, which went in this order: naproxen, ibuprofen, fenoprofen, then aspirin.[14]

In another study comparing naproxen, fenoprofen, ibuprofen, tolmetin, indomethacin, and aspirin, rheumatoid arthritis patients liked all the drugs equally well; but ankylosing spondylitis patients preferred naproxen and indomethacin. This was true although indomethacin had the largest frequency of associated headaches.[15]

Indomethacin also seems to produce a higher incidence of stomach distress and kidney toxicity than other NSAIDs. Sulindac has the lowest incidence of both. Piroxicam and meclofenamate have lower incidences of liver toxicity, while allergic skin rash is most commonly associated with meclofenamate, sulindac, and ibuprofen. Ringing in the ears is most commonly associated with indomethacin.[16]

Feldene: does more expensive mean better?

The NSAID Feldene (piroxicam) has seen a phenomenal rise to success, up to the number three slot worldwide. What does Feldene have that aspirin and other NSAIDs don't? Its only real advantage seems to be that a single capsule will hold you for the day. The cost of this single capsule, however, is over one dollar—many times the cost of an equivalent amount of aspirin. This appears, in fact, to be the source of Feldene's market success. It is so profitable to the manufacturer because it is so expensive to the patient (or his insurance carrier).

Cost, unfortunately, isn't Feldene's only downside. It's the NSAID leader not only in worldwide sales but in the production of gastrointestinal bleeding and ulcers, the largest single cause of side effects and death from NSAIDs.[17] In the elderly, these complications are often fatal. Senior citizens with arthritis are better off taking enteric-coated aspirin. In its generic form, it is not only safer but much cheaper. Even better is salsalate (Disalcid or Mono-Gesic) (see chapter 18). Stomach irritation can also be eased by dissolving aspirin in water before taking it.

When all else fails: steroids and antirheumatic drugs

For some arthritis sufferers, not only acetaminophen but even NSAIDs won't work. For severe rheumatoid arthritis, steroid drugs such as hydrocortisone, prednisone, or dexamethasone used to be given. These drugs are powerful anti-inflammatories. However, starting on them was a major step, because they can have serious side effects, particularly if given inappropriately. One is the risk of ulcers, apparently caused by damage to the lining of the stomach. Other side effects of steroids are listed in chapter 7. Ideally, steroids should be given in small doses on alternate days for only one or two months at a time. Good in theory—but when the drugs are stopped, symptoms can become worse than before you started on them, so in practice you're liable to wind up on them indefinitely. For this reason, steroids are now used only short-term for emergencies.

Like NSAIDs, steroids don't cure arthritis. Joint destruction continues although pain is relieved. Some arthritis specialists believe the progression of rheumatoid arthritis can be slowed if large doses of certain other drugs, called disease-modifying antirheumatic drugs, are given early in the disease. These drugs include gold, taken either by mouth or injection; hydroxychloroquine (Plaquenil), an antimalarial drug; and chemotherapeutic drugs that suppress the immune response, including cyclophosphamide (Cytoxan), methotrexate, and azathioprine (Imuran). Unfortunately, there is little evidence to support these claims.[18] Further, the drugs' side effects can be worse than the disease.

Gold can cause skin rashes, blood disorders, kidney and liver damage. It can also cause acute attacks of arthritis. Gold therapy has to be stopped in about a third of patients due to intolerance. It shouldn't be used by pregnant women, old or very weak people, or patients with high blood pressure, kidney or liver damage, or skin disorders.

Chloroquine must be taken in high doses to be effective, and these doses can cause irreversible damage to the eyes, resulting in blindness.

Immune-suppressing drugs can also have serious side effects. They include damage to the bone marrow, resulting in blood disorders, and deterioration of the muscles.

Another drug often given for severe rheumatoid arthritis is D-penicillamine. How it works isn't certain, but it's a chelating agent that removes excess copper from the blood; and many rheumatoid arthritis patients have abnormally high copper levels. Unfortunately, the drug can also cause serious side effects, including severe blood problems and myasthenia gravis.[19]

If you must resort to any of these drastic therapies, don't mix them but stick to one.

Treating gout

Corticosteroids may also be used for acute attacks of gout that don't respond to NSAIDs. But for long-term treatment, the prescription favorite is allopurinol. It stops the formation of stones and slows kidney damage by reducing the uric acid in the blood. Its drawbacks are that it can trigger acute attacks of gout when first used, and it can produce rash, hives, sleepiness, upset stomach, diarrhea, and headache.

Another alternative is colchicine. A derivative of the meadow saffron plant, colchicine has been used for centuries by gout sufferers. Its short-term side effects include abdominal pain, vomiting, and diarrhea. Its long-term side effects can be much more serious, including bone marrow depression with severe blood abnormalities. Colchicine has also recently been associated with muscular weakness, particularly in people with impaired kidney function.[20] Aged and debilitated patients should use it with great caution, if at all.

Nondrug alternatives

For gout, a side-effect-free alternative is dietary change to reduce uric acid production. Many studies have shown the value of a diet free of meat, the major dietary source of uric acid, in relieving both gout and kidney stones.[21]

For other forms of arthritis, nondrug possibilities include physical and occupational therapy, including warm water swimming and other exercise; heat treatments; acupuncture; homeopathic remedies; and rest. Total bed rest, however, is no longer recommended, since it causes loss of muscle tone. Correcting anatomical problems like unequal leg lengths or abnormal foot positions can also relieve symptoms, and so can exercise that puts the joints through their full range of motion. Trace mineral supplements may also help. Rheumatoid arthritis is often characterized by low iron levels and high copper levels.[22] Some sufferers swear by copper bracelets, obtainable in health food stores.

Like gout, osteoarthritis can be helped by diet, but in this case it's the kind that causes weight loss. Folk remedies include liberal doses of garlic.

Even rheumatoid arthritis may have a dietary component. Recent research traces some forms of the disease to an allergic reaction to certain foods. In a double-blind study, patients were first fed a two-week wash-out diet of foods unlikely to cause allergic reactions. Then they were challenged with capsules of either placebos or known food allergens—dairy products, wheat, corn, citrus, coffee, and chocolate. Although the effect of different foods was a very individual one, about 15 percent improved dramatically and 70 percent showed varying degrees of improvement without their particular offending foods.[23]

Another study linked rheumatoid arthritis to dietary fat. Complete remissions resulted in the six patient/subjects when they changed to a fat-free diet. Symptoms returned within three days of ingesting fat, whether in the form of animal fat or vegetable oils. The researchers concluded that dietary fats in amounts normally eaten in the American diet can cause the inflammatory joint changes seen in rheumatoid arthritis.[24]

20

ACETAMINOPHEN AND OTHER ANALGESIC ALTERNATIVES

The billionaire hermit Howard Hughes consumed 50 to 60 grains of codeine a day. . . . In his final days, he was devouring up to 200 mg of Valium and Librium at one time. He swallowed handfuls of Empirin #4 (codeine, aspirin, caffeine, and phenacetin). The phenacetin killed him, by damaging his kidneys.[1]
—Stanley Siegelman (1989)

Although ibuprofen and other new NSAIDs are giving aspirin a run for its money, its major competitor is still acetaminophen. Acetaminophen is the active ingredient in such analgesics as Tylenol, Datril, Anacin-3, Panadol, and Liquiprin. In 1980, aspirin substitutes accounted for one-fourth of the $1.2 billion Americans spent on analgesics, and most of these substitutes contained acetaminophen. By 1987, analgesics sales had moved up to $1.8 billion and acetaminophen accounted for 37 percent of this market, in hot pursuit of aspirin's 44 percent lead.[2]

A safe aspirin alternative?

The main reason for acetaminophen's rise to fame is that it's easier on your stomach lining than aspirin. The FDA warns, however, that there is no basis for the claim that its all-around safety record is better. While overdoses of aspirin are unlikely to be fatal to adults if treated in time, this isn't true for acetaminophen. Only ten Extra-Strength Tylenol can be fatal to a child, and even small overdoses of either painkiller can be life-threatening to a child. In large doses, acetaminophen can cause death even in adults, by causing irreversible liver damage. Normal doses can also cause liver damage if given daily for long periods.

Liver damage is a problem particularly for the alcoholic who takes acetaminophen to relieve a hangover, since his liver is already impaired. But aspirin isn't any better for this condition, since it can aggravate the upset stomach that typically accompanies a hangover. In fact the mixture of aspirin and alcohol can result in massive bleeding and hemorrhage.[3] For this reason, acetaminophen, which is believed not to cause significant injury to the stomach lining, is often recommended to alcoholics as an aspirin substitute.

Unfortunately, it is not always a safer alternative. What can go wrong is illustrated by the case of a 47-year-old alcoholic who had a bad toothache. He took three 500-mg tablets of Extra-Strength Tylenol every three hours over a twelve-hour period. He wound up with acute hepatitis (inflammation of the liver), followed by acute kidney failure.[4]

Acetaminophen and kidney disease

This case points up a link that has only recently been established: that between acetaminophen and kidney disease. The landmark study, reported in the *New England Journal of Medicine* in May of 1989, found that the risk of disabling kidney disease was more than three times as great for people who took two or more tablets of acetaminophen daily for a year or more, as for infrequent users. The risk was five times greater for daily users of phenacetin, the analgesic that apparently killed Howard Hughes.[5] Phenacetin, acetaminophen's parent, used to be an ingredient in the analgesic Empirin Compound with Codeine, but it has now been removed.

More than $2 billion is spent annually in the United States for the treatment of end-stage kidney disease, in addition to undocumented amounts spent on less serious kidney problems. End-stage kidney disease results when the kidneys shut down entirely and are unable to filter the blood. At this point, the medical alternatives are limited to kidney dialysis or kidney transplantation.

The use of analgesics causes as much as 20 percent of all kidney disease requiring kidney dialysis or transplants. This means 20,000 of the estimated 100,000 Americans who currently require these therapies got that way from analgesics. Few studies have addressed the cause of this serious condition, but enough evidence has now accumulated linking it to these drugs to prompt proposals to limit their easy availability.[6]

Kidney disease resulting from the excessive use of analgesics is called "analgesic-associated nephropathy" (AAN). In some parts of the world, including Australia, it has been shown to be responsible for a third of all kidney dialysis and transplant cases. The condition was first linked to phenacetin. In fact, acetaminophen was introduced in 1963 as a phenacetin alternative, following reports of hardening of the kidneys associated with the parent drug. But it's not clear that the offspring cured the problem. When phenacetin was banned from sale in Australia, no significant decrease in AAN was seen.[7] And when animals are fed phenacetin, it winds up concentrated in their kidneys in the form of acetaminophen. A 1988 Malaysian study documented fifteen cases of AAN directly traceable to acetaminophen. These patients had all overdosed on the drug for many years, in an attempt to relieve migraine headache, gouty arthritis, or joint pain.[8]

Berlin is another place where AAN accounts for a third of all dialysis patients. It's the kidney disease seen most frequently at the dialysis center at the University of Berlin. A 1987 study of these AAN patients found they had taken an average of five analgesic tablets a day over an average of twenty-one years before end-stage renal disease developed. Ninety-three percent took them to treat headaches, although 70 percent gave more than one reason for analgesic use. Most of the patients were women.

The AAN patients had other traits in common. Compared to patients with kidney disease from other causes, they complained more of vague symptoms, complained more about the treatment, smoked more, and were more inclined to reach for the pill bottle to solve their problems. They were more likely to have heart disease, ulcers, diverticulosis, and hemorrhoids. They were also significantly more likely to die of "dialysis dementia," a progressive inflammation of the brain causing the patient to become demented, psychotic, and unable to speak coherently. The increased incidence of this condition was attributed in part to their greater use of antacid medications. Most popular antacids contain aluminum, a metal that has been linked to Alzheimer's disease (see chapter 21). The greater antacid intake by AAN patients was attributed, in turn, to their higher intake of analgesics. The drugs injured the lining of the stomach, necessitating antacid stomach medication.

The AAN patients were also more prone to anemia. This may have been due to their greater intestinal blood loss from ulcers, caused by their excessive analgesic intake. Or it may have been from their higher aluminum intake, which is known to produce anemia.[9]

Aspirin: safer after all?

Does all this tip the balance back in favor of aspirin and other NSAIDs? No, because they seem to be subject to the same hazards.

A multimillion-dollar suit that may make legal history was filed in April of 1989 by all-American defensive back Kenny Easley. In 1985, Easley was earning $650,000 a year playing for the Seattle Seahawks and was regarded as one of the best football players of his generation. His career ended after he took twenty 200-mg ibuprofen pills daily over a five-month period to combat the pain of an injured ankle. He is now saddled to a kidney dialysis machine three times a week.[10]

Kidney specialists report that NSAIDs are second only to the aminoglycoside antibiotics as a cause of acute kidney failure.[11] Although Kenny Easley obviously exceeded the recommended dosage for a long time, the drugs don't have to be taken in large doses long-term to precipitate kidney damage. A 1987 report in the *New England Journal of Medicine* tells of two women who suffered acute kidney failure after taking the NSAID naproxen for a mere seven days each. Only certain patients seem to be candidates for this result, but you can't necessarily tell ahead of time if you're one of them. The two women in this report were later diagnosed as having multiple myeloma (cancer of the bone marrow), but this risk factor wasn't known at the time.[12]

Besides multiple myeloma, other risk factors for kidney failure precipitated by NSAIDs are heart failure, liver disease, underlying kidney disease, and a low blood volume.

Blood volume can be reduced either by disease or by diuretic drugs that stimulate water loss through the urine. The body reacts by bolstering blood pressure with an increase in sympathetic nerve activity. In the kidney, this action makes blood vessels constrict. To counter this effect, kidney prostaglandins dilate the blood vessels. But if NSAIDs are given, prostaglandin synthesis is impaired. Kidney vessel constriction then proceeds unimpaired, and kidney filtration and blood flow decrease. The result can be acute renal failure. This means people on diuretics should studiously avoid NSAIDs.

Phenacetin and acetaminophen, the known causes of AAN, do not inhibit the production of kidney-regulating prostaglandins. In fact, the mechanism of their role in AAN isn't clear. But aspirin and other NSAIDs clearly suppress kidney prostaglandins, and they can have dire consequences for people whose kidney function is already impaired. They can cause water retention (edema), which can exacerbate high blood pressure and heart failure. They can also counter the effects of the diuretics and beta-blockers used to treat high blood pressure. In rabbits and rats, aspirin causes the symptoms of AAN at the same doses as phenacetin, and some 150 reports associate aspirin with AAN in humans.[13]

Treating your aching head

So what do you do if you're suffering from a headache, the most common reason for analgesic pill popping? Acetaminophen may pose long-term risks, but for occasional use it's easier on your stomach than aspirin and other NSAIDs. It is also less likely to provoke an allergic reaction. You should avoid combinations of acetaminophen and aspirin (like Extra-Strength Excedrin and Vanquish), since they expose you to the side effects of both analgesics without affording more pain relief than the same strength dose of either one.

The safest remedy, however, remains simple relaxation. Muscle contraction headaches, including common migraines, may respond to easy neck stretches. Move your head to one side and then the other, resisting against the palm of your hand.[14]

This may not work on serious migraines, but aspirin generally won't work on them either. For the type of migraine attack that lasts from eight hours to two days of unbearable pain, an ergot derivative has now been developed in nasal spray form that's as effective as shots. The drug used, dihydroergotamine mesylate (DHE), is currently approved only for intravenous or intramuscular use. However, in a randomized trial of over one hundred patients, it was shown to give significant pain relief in nasal spray form in 60 percent of patients within about three hours of administration. The drug is good for sufferers whose attacks come on quickly, and who want something fast-acting that doesn't require an injection. It doesn't produce the heavy nausea and vomiting associated with the form of ergotamine administered under the tongue, and it's safe for patients with heart disease who can't use other drugs. In a 1987 study, the nasal spray form of the drug was rated by patients as 52% effective; but they also gave a 41%-effective rating to a placebo that had no pharmacological effect.[15]

Even when this drug works, you're left with a minimum of three hours of excruciating pain. An alternative that reaches the cause would be better yet.

Some migraine sufferers respond to dietary change. Many report relief when they avoid certain foods, including the nitrites found in cured meats like hot dogs, bacon, ham, and salami, and the monosodium glutamate for which Chinese restaurants are notorious. Other suspects include cheese, chocolate, ice cream, alcohol, caffeine, nicotine, and certain drugs.

Migraines have also been blamed on "reactive hypoglycemia." This is the plunge in serum insulin levels that follows a precipitous rise after you overdose on sugar.

A recent British study found that feverfew, a natural herb, was effective against migraines. The herb not only cut the number and severity of headaches but reduced the nausea that goes with them.[16]

It's the fashion to attribute certain headaches to "temporomandibular joint dysfunction," or TMJ. This is a dental condition that results from irritation of the disk connecting the jaw to the skull. If this is your problem, before you succumb to expensive mouth reconstruction, try making a studied effort to relax your jaw. Tension can throw your bite off, which can give you headaches. Your dentist can also fit you with a mouthpiece to wear at night to relieve jaw tension.

Other possibilities are acupuncture and EMG biofeedback, which have been used successfully in the treatment of both tension and migraine headaches.[17]

Another therapy that works for some sufferers is to put your arms in ice water up to the elbows.

Narcotic analgesics

For truly debilitating pain, narcotic analgesics are available by prescription.

The usual option for severe, persistent cancer pain is morphine. New developments in its use include an oral morphine in sustained-release form. It reduces the number of times the medicine must be taken, and allows more even blood levels of the drug. A new technique is also available for injectable morphine: an electronic pump that infuses the drug automatically through a small needle placed under the skin.[18]

Other popular narcotic analgesics related to morphine include codeine (used in cough medicines and for diarrhea), and propoxyphene (Darvon). Both, however, can be addicting; and a virtually universal side effect of narcotic analgesics is constipation. The discomfort of severe constipation from narcotic treatment can rival the pain being treated.

Morphine, codeine, and opium are natural plant derivatives. Structurally related narcotics that are synthetic or semisynthetic include meperidine (Demerol), pentazocine (Talwin), and oxycodone (contained in Percodan with aspirin, and in Percocet with acetaminophen).

Talwin has a particularly high abuse potential. It has been used as a heroin substitute and is the "T" in the street drug "T's and Blues," which combines Talwin with the antihistamine tripelennamine (PBZ). At one time, drug abusers were crushing up Talwin pills and injecting them into their veins. To prevent this, the manufacturer has now added a substance called naloxone, which neutralizes the drug's narcotic effect when it's injected, but not when it's ingested.

Pain and the mind

Recent research suggests the pain-killing abilities of analgesics may be largely in the mind. Pain-killing drugs are particularly subject to the "placebo effect." This is a trick of the mind by which an anticipated effect is produced although the drug contains no active properties known to produce it.

A Mayo clinic study found that for 21 percent of patients tested, as much pain relief resulted from a placebo—a fake pill without active pain-killing properties—as from either aspirin or a stronger drug. The study also found that for pain relief, aspirin was as good as, or better than, any other drug tested, over-the-counter or prescription. The tested drugs included Darvon, the prescription drug favorite.[19]

As noted earlier, up to one-third of prescription drugs, and a much higher percentage of nonprescription drugs, are thought to act primarily as placebos.[20] The patient gets better because he expects to. Placebos apparently work by triggering the release of "endorphins." These substances are the brain's own chemical pain-relievers, which function like opiates in the body.

Pure placebos—pills that have no physiological effect at all—can be effective pain relievers. But drugs that have actual physiological effects work better yet. This is true although their physiological effects are unrelated to the patient's condition. Thus, an anxious patient will feel more relaxed if given a placebo that causes him to be light-headed or dry-mouthed than if given one that does nothing at all. The patient feels the drug is "working" and, having been told it will work to relax him, feels more relaxed.[21]

This effect was illustrated in a study testing different drugs on postherpetic neuralgia, a type of pain that can linger for years after the shingles of herpes have disappeared, and that is frequently unresponsive to treatment. The drugs tested were ibuprofen, codeine, clonidine, and a placebo. The most effective drug proved to be the antihypertensive drug clonidine.

Significantly, clonidine also produced the greatest number of side effects. Several patients remarked to the nurse on noticing its sedative effect, "I feel groggy. I must have gotten the real medicine today." Codeine, which did better than either ibuprofen or the placebo, also produced more side effects than ibuprofen or the placebo.

Even pure placebos can produce side effects. A constant 5–10 percent of patients experience them, including nausea, headache, dizziness, sleepiness, fatigue, depression, numbness, hallucinations, and itching.[22] In this study, the placebo not only produced more side effects than ibuprofen but was more effective in relieving pain. The exceptions were those few patients who reported side effects from ibuprofen. In them, the drug actually resulted in pain relief nearly as great as with clonidine.

This was also true for the placebo, which shouldn't have worked at all. The patients receiving the placebo who *thought* they experienced side effects experienced pain relief nearly as great as from clonidine.[23]

The ideal analgesic would trigger this trick-of-the-mind without pills and their side effects. Christian Scientists do it by faith. Certain biofeedback and meditation techniques are reported to work by triggering the release of natural endorphins. Acupuncture is an effective analgesic that is thought to work the same way. Even the pain of cancer can be reduced by nondrug analgesic therapies, including biofeedback, relaxation training, hypnosis, and behavior modification.[24]

IV

Digestive Remedies

21

OVER-THE-COUNTER STOMACH REMEDIES: ANTACIDS

*It will be interesting to see what happens when the first
American lawyer realizes that Alzheimer's patients may
have been taking aluminium in quite large quantities in
antacid preparations.*

—*Nature* (1987)[1]

After cold remedies and pain-relievers, the bestselling over-the-counter drugs are those for the treatment of digestive complaints. Antacids are alkaline substances that are promoted as relieving a variety of stomach problems, including heartburn, indigestion, bloating, cramps, and gas pains. These ailments are normally traceable to bad eating habits (too much or the wrong types of food), or stress. They can also be caused by other drugs, including birth control pills, antihistamines, and Valium; while ulcers can be caused by drugs like steroids and NSAIDs.[2]

Antacids are advertised as achieving their effects by neutralizing "excess stomach acid." What the advertisers don't tell you is that stomach acid is necessary to the normal digestion of foods. Your digestive enzymes work properly only when the acidity of your stomach is properly balanced, and the amount of stomach acid you secrete is carefully regulated according to the amounts and types of food you eat. The cause of your upset stomach may not be too much acid. It may be too few digestive enzymes to handle an overload, or improper mixture, of foods.

Another thing advertisers fail to mention is that like all drugs, those tasty antacid tablets you get at the candy counter can have unwanted side effects. If the drugs are taken regularly for long periods, these side effects can be quite serious. While different brands of antacids contain different principal ingredients, all of them are subject to negative effects of some kind (see table 30). The major categories are set out below.[3]

Magnesium/aluminum preparations

Magnesium salts (as in Phillips Milk of Magnesia) are effective antacids. Their major drawback is that they tend to cause diarrhea. If used regularly for more than a week or two, the result can be severe. They can also exacerbate kidney problems and cause drowsiness in some people.

Aluminum salts (as in Rolaids) have the opposite drawback. They can obstruct the intestines and cause intractable constipation. The industry solution was to combine these two ingredients, as in Maalox, Mylanta, Gelusil, and Di-Gel Liquid. The theory was that their opposing side effects would cancel each other out. But in practice, these combination products can cause the side effects of either ingredient. In one case, Gelusil became the subject of a lawsuit when a patient on it died of a bowel obstruction that led to peritonitis and gangrene.[4]

Mylanta and Di-Gel also contain simethicone, a drug intended to reduce gas. This is fine if you're troubled with intestinal gas. If you're not, the combination subjects you to unnecessary side effects. One of these, in fact, can be excess gas.

Besides diarrhea and constipation, recent evidence links aluminum antacid preparations to two much more serious side effects: Alzheimer's disease and bone disease. Concerns about these associations prompted the Associated Pharmacists and Toxicologists to petition the FDA in 1982 to restudy the safety of aluminum-containing antacids.[5]

Alzheimer's disease is a form of senility. The link with aluminum has been demonstrated by accumulations of the metal found in the brains of patients who died of the disease. Pathological changes

Table 30. *Active Ingredients in Popular Antacids[6]*

Brand name	Ingredients				
	aluminum hydroxide	magnesium hydroxide	calcium carbonate	sodium bicarbonate	other
Alka-Seltzer Without Aspirin				x	x
Alka-2			x		
Alkets Tablets		x	x		
Almacone II Liquid	x	x			x
Alma-Mag #4 Tablets	x				x
Alternagel	x				
Alu-Cap	x				
Aludrox Suspension	x	x			
Aludrox Tablets	x	x			
Alumid Plus Suspension	x	x			x
Aluminum Hydroxide Gel	x				
Amitone			x		
Amphojel	x				
Arm & Hammer Baking Soda				x	
Basaljel	x				
Bisodol Powder		x		x	
Bisodol Tablets		x	x		
Bromo Seltzer				x	x
Camalox Suspension	x	x	x		
Calcilac Tablets			x		x
Citrocarbonate				x	
Chooz			x		
Delcid Suspension	x	x			
Di-Gel Liquid					
Di-Gel Tablets	x	x			x
Estomul-M Tablets	x	x			x
Gaviscon Tablets	x	x		x	x
Gelusil Tablets	x	x			x
Gustalac Tablets			x		
Kolantyl Tablets	x	x			
Kolantyl Wafers	x	x			

Brand name	Ingredients				
	aluminum hydroxide	magnesium hydroxide	calcium carbonate	sodium bicarbonate	other
Maalox No. 1 Tablets	x	x			
Maalox No. 2 Tablets	x	x			
Maalox Plus Suspension	x	x			x
Maalox Plus Tablets	x	x			
Maalox Suspension	x	x			x
Maalox Therapeutic Concentrate	x	x			
Mag Ox 400		x			
Maox		x			
Mallamint			x		
Milk of Magnesia		x			
Mylanta Liquid	x	x			x
Mylanta Tablets	x	x			x
Mylanta II Tablets	x	x			x
Neosorb Plus Tablets	x	x			x
PAMA #2 Tablets			x		x
Par-Mag		x			
Phillips' Milk of Magnesia		x			
Phosphaljel	x				
Riopan	x	x			
Riopan Plus Chew Tablets	x	x			x
Riopan Plus Suspension	x	x			
Robalate	x				
Rolaids	x			x	
Rolox Suspension	x	x			
Simeco Suspension	x	x			x
Soda Mint				x	
Spastosed Tablets		x	x		
Titralac Liquid			x		x
Titralac Tablets			x		x
Tralmag Suspension	x	x			
Trimagel Tablets	x			x	
Tums			x		
WinGel Liquid	x	x			

similar to those seen in Alzheimer's have also been observed after exposure to aluminum.[7] Earlier observations linking the metal to the disease were confirmed in a 1989 study of 88 county districts in England and Wales. It found a definite connection between the incidence of Alzheimer's and average aluminum levels in the water supply.[8]

Other research has linked the aluminum in common antacids to bone disease. Aluminum displaces calcium from the bones, causing them to be brittle and to break easily—the condition called osteoporosis. Antacids in general also inhibit calcium absorption by neutralizing stomach acid, raising the pH of the stomach. Calcium can be absorbed only in its soluble ionized form, which requires a low pH.

In 1987, the *Annals of Internal Medicine* presented case reports of two 42-year-old women with liver failure requiring liver transplants. Both women had serious bone demineralization which, on x-ray examination, was linked to heavy deposits of aluminum in their bones. Both also had long histories of taking aluminum hydroxide-containing antacids (Amphojel and Mylanta) for the prevention of peptic ulcers.

In one woman, bone pain completely disappeared after the aluminum was removed by chelation therapy. This treatment involves the injection of a solution that chelates, or binds, heavy metals. The metals are then excreted in the urine. (Unfortunately, the solution doesn't cross the blood/brain barrier, so the procedure won't remove metals from the brain.)

The other woman died before a liver donor could be located, but bone staining at autopsy was strongly positive for aluminum.[9]

Aluminum-containing drugs are particularly dangerous when taken with orange juice, with any other citrus fruit or juice, or in drugs containing citrate. This combination increases the absorption of aluminum into the bloodstream by as much as fifty times. The result can be both brain damage and thinning of the bones.

This means you should *at least* avoid combining aluminum and citrus, and some doctors think it's best to avoid aluminum in any form.[10] Aluminum can get into your body not only from antacids, but from aluminum cookware, aluminum cans used for soft drinks and beer, and the aluminum in deodorants.[11]

Calcium carbonate

Calcium carbonate is the chief ingredient in Tums. It used to be the antacid of choice, until prolonged use was found to raise the calcium in the blood. The result can be kidney stones and impaired kidney function. The problem is particularly serious for people whose kidneys are already impaired—or for people who drink a lot of milk, since milk is already high in calcium. Ulcer patients are liable to do just that, since milk has traditionally been recommended for their condition.

Calcium carbonate can also impair iron absorption, can cause constipation, and can produce an "acid rebound" in which its use is followed by significant *increases* in stomach acid. This means you can wind up with more acid in your stomach than before you started on the drug.[12]

Sodium bicarbonate

The major ingredient in Alka Seltzer and Bromo Seltzer is sodium bicarbonate, more commonly known as baking soda. This antacid is relatively harmless for occasional use. But if used repeatedly, it can disturb the body's acid-base balance, especially in people with kidney problems. It can also lead to kidney stones and recurrent urinary tract infections. It is high in sodium, so it's not good for people who have high blood pressure or are in the high risk category for heart disease. Like calcium carbonate, it can also impair iron absorption and can cause an acid rebound.

Alka Seltzer combines sodium bicarbonate with aspirin. If your objective is to relieve a headache, this combination, dissolved in water, can relieve some of the stomach irritation produced by ordinary aspirin tablets. But if your objective is to relieve an upset stomach, the combination is calculated to make it worse, since the aspirin can further irritate your stomach—particularly if your problem is caused by ulcers.

Bromo Seltzer, which combines sodium bicarbonate with acetaminophen instead of aspirin, is easier on the stomach than Alka Seltzer. However, it's harder on the liver. This is a hazard especially to alcoholics (see chapter 20).

Bismuth compounds

Pepto-Bismol is approved by the FDA both as an antacid and as a diarrhea and hangover remedy. It's a "bismuth subsalicylate." That means it contains salicylate, which can have the same adverse effects as aspirin, and bismuth, a potentially lethal nerve poison. Bismuth hasn't been detected in the blood or urine of people taking recommended doses, but overdose can result in kidney failure and liver damage. In France and Australia, bone and joint disorders and encephalopathy (a degenerative disease of the brain) have been reported with the use of bismuth salts even at recommended doses, leading to restriction on their use.[13]

On the plus side, studies show bismuth compounds are actually more effective for preventing ulcer relapses than the prescription ulcer favorites, Tagamet and Zantac. In judging the effectiveness of an ulcer remedy, the relapse rate is considered more important than the healing rate—since nearly every ulcer is eventually followed by another.

On the minus side, bismuth compounds, like other ulcer remedies, are effective only during the first year of treatment. After two years, relapse rates are about 90 percent, no matter what remedy is used.[14]

We'll look at nondrug alternatives in the next chapter, after considering the prescription options.

22

PRESCRIPTION STOMACH REMEDIES: THE H2-BLOCKERS

I am convinced digestion is the great secret of life.
—Rev. Sydney Smith (1859)

According to the World Health Organization, the prescription ulcer medications Tagamet (cimetidine) and Zantac (ranitidine) were the two bestselling drugs worldwide in 1985.[1] Tagamet's rise to stardom was unprecedented. It was the first drug projected to break the billion dollar barrier in annual sales. But by 1986, Zantac had eaten up Tagamet's lead, and by 1989, Zantac had reached the *two* billion dollar mark in annual sales. Tagamet and Zantac are brought to you by rival pharmaceutical companies that are major stock market performers, but Zantac is backed by a more aggressive sales force. It is also a newer drug that hasn't yet suffered the reports of adverse side effects branding 14-year-old Tagamet.[2]

The big question is, where did all the ulcers come from? In 1975, before Tagamet came on the scene, *no* ulcer medicines were among the top ten prescription drugs. Could our increased intake of aspirin and other prostaglandin-suppressing drugs be eating an increasing number of holes in our stomachs? Or could doctors be writing ulcer-drug prescriptions for garden-variety upset stomachs?

Evidence points to the latter. In fact, Tagamet and Zantac are stacking up to be the after-dinner Tums of the 1990s.

Was it their lack of side effects that caused these drugs to take the indigestion market by storm? Or was it because they were more effective than the more established antacids?

The answer seems to be neither. Large doses of aluminum hydroxide and magnesium hydroxide are just as effective as Tagamet and Zantac for treating ulcers; and for minor digestive complaints, there's no evidence that these glamour drugs are effective at all.[3] For forestalling ulcer relapses, bismuth compounds are actually more effective, at least the first year.[4] Further, Tagamet and Zantac have their own side effects, which may be worse in the long run than those of antacids. They're newer drugs, and the evidence isn't all in.

So what's the secret of their success? Like Feldene, the once-a-day NSAID, Tagamet and Zantac seem to have triumphed mainly out of convenience. Instead of sucking all day long on chalk pills, sufferers can take their Tagamet tablets only four times a day. Zantac then got it down to twice a day; and Tagamet, in its new formulation, has followed suit.

There may also be a placebo factor. Tagamet and Zantac are prescription items, while antacids are over-the-counter drugs. If you need a doctor's prescription, it must be a more powerful drug—right? Alas, untrue. Drugs are dispensed by prescription *only* because their side effects are so serious that professional monitoring is required.

A third factor may be addiction. Tagamet and Zantac provide an environment in your stomach that helps your ulcer heal itself, but they don't cure the condition that caused it. After you start on these drugs, you're likely to have a relapse when you go off them. That means another ulcer, unless you make a habit of the drugs. Tagamet and Zantac are officially approved only for "short-term treatment of active ulcer," and a full course of therapy is supposed to be only six to eight weeks.[5] But many patients wind up on the drugs long-term, because they relapse without them.

The FDA is considering over-the-counter status for these drugs. One reason is that they have few apparent side effects. (We'll look at the less apparent long-term effects shortly.) Another is that the need to renew prescriptions for these drugs is a major cause of doctor visits. Many doctors are opposed to over-the-counter approval, perhaps for the same reason.

The H2-blockers

Tagamet and Zantac are the market leaders in a class of drugs known as histamine H2-receptor antagonists, or H2-blockers. Unlike antacids, which neutralize the acid already in your stomach, H2-blockers act by decreasing the amount of acid produced.

Stomach acid is secreted in three ways: (1) by histamine receptors, (2) by the cholinergic nerves in response to stress or stimuli, and (3) by a response of the stomach nerves to food. The H2-blockers act on the first mechanism. It involves the same histamine that is responsible for inflammation and allergic reactions. However, the antihistamines used to suppress hay fever won't work on the histamine in the stomach. The H2-blockers will.

Before the H2-blockers came along, a class of drugs called anticholinergics was used to inhibit stomach acid secretion. Anticholinergic drugs block stomach acid secreted by the second mechanism, through stimulation of the cholinergic nerves. The most popular drug in this class was belladonna. Its use was limited, however, by its unpleasant side effects, including blurred vision, dry mouth, urine retention, constipation, and rapid heartbeat.

When the H2-blockers were developed, the breakthrough was considered revolutionary. The side effects of H2-blockers are much less frequent and annoying than belladonna's, and the drugs are considered unusually safe.

Besides Tagamet and Zantac, other H2-blockers include famotidine (Pepcid) and nizatidine (Axid). Famotidine is the most potent of the group. Ounce for ounce, it's twenty times more potent than cimetidine and 7.5 times more potent than ranitidine. The drug is too new to know its long-term safety record, but it seems to be safer than Tagamet, and as safe as Zantac. However, grand mal seizures and hallucinations have been reported.[6]

Incidentally, the H2-blockers don't always work; and if one doesn't, the others won't either. It won't help to switch from one to another.

Omeprazole (Losec) is another new ulcer drug. It works on stomach acid produced by the third mechanism—that secreted in response to food. Since 90 percent of stomach acid is generated in this way, Losec is the most effective of the available options for suppressing it. But like famotidine, the drug is too new to know its long-term safety record.

The downsides

Although the newer stomach-acid-suppressing drugs represent a major improvement over the anticholinergics, they can still have troubling side effects.

As drugs go, the short-term ones are mild. They are experienced by only 2 percent of patients. Headaches are among the most common. Others include diarrhea, constipation, nausea, skin rash, and dizziness.[7]

Tagamet can also cause a hormonal imbalance that results in breast enlargement and impotence in men. These hormonal effects, fortunately, are reversible when you give up the drug. Other Tagamet side effects include joint and muscle pains, sensitivity to light, and mental confusion. In rare cases, the drug has also depressed the bone marrow, preventing the normal production of blood cells.

Zantac is heavily promoted as giving you the benefits of Tagamet without its adverse effects. The FDA, however, is dubious, since Zantac has now been shown to cause some of the same problems as its competitor.[8] (See table 31.)

Zantac has at least one major advantage over Tagamet: it's less likely to interfere with the absorption of other drugs. Tagamet slows down the metabolism of many drugs, which can build up and produce serious toxic reactions. The list of drugs it can react with is long, and includes the anticoagulant warfarin, some benzodiazepines, lidocaine, theophylline, propranolol, and the anticonvulsant phenytoin. Antacids can also interfere with the absorption of many drugs—and one of them is Tagamet.[9] (See chapter 37.)

If your doctor has prescribed Tagamet, it is important to tell him all the drugs you're taking, and to take no others without advising him first. If you do mix drugs and experience unusual symptoms, you can suspect an adverse drug interaction.

Table 31. *Comparing Side Effects of H2-Blockers[10]*

	Cimetidine	Ranitidine	Famotidine	Nizatidine
Stomach, intestines:	diarrhea, pancreatitis	constipation, nausea, abdominal discomfort	constipation, diarrhea, nausea, loss of appetite, dry mouth	
Liver:	hepatic fibrosis	jaundice, increase in liver enzymes		liver damage
Heart:	arrhythmias	arrthymias	palpitations	increased heart rate
Head:	dizziness, sleepiness, headache, confusion, hallucinations, numbness	dizziness, sleepiness, headache, confusion, hallucinations, insomnia	headache, sleepiness, insomnia, numbness, seizures, depression, anxiety	sleepiness
Hormonal:	male breast enlargement, impotence, decreased sex drive	male breast enlargement, impotence, decreased sex drive	decreased sex drive	male breast enlargement, impotence, decreased sex drive
Muscles, bones:	joint pain, muscle pain	joint pain	joint pain	
Blood:	decreased white blood cells and platelets	decreased white blood cells, red cells, platelets	decreased platelets	decreased platelets

Long-term risks

More ponderous than the immediate and obvious side effects and interactions of the H2-blockers are the subtle and long-term ones. Whenever you tamper with the body's natural secretory mechanisms, you risk upsetting beneficial functions; and this risk holds true for H2-blockers.

Histamine receptors are found not only in the stomach but in the heart and blood vessels. Blockage of these receptors has caused fatal heart attacks in patients receiving H2-blockers by injection.[11]

Not only histamine but stomach acid has beneficial functions that can be suppressed by H2–blockers. One function is to kill bacteria in your stomach and to keep it from being colonized by undesirables. Without the acid, you run the risk of infection by a variety of organisms, including those responsible for typhoid, salmonella, cholera, dysentery, and giardia. The latest research implicates these organisms not only in infections, but as an actual cause of ulcers and ulcer relapses.[12]

A study reported in the *New England Journal of Medicine* in 1987 looked at the risk of infection in 130 patients treated for stress-induced ulcer bleeding. The patients were in intensive care and were breathing by means of endotracheal tubes in their throats. They were chosen for study because their risk of contracting pneumonia was particularly high. Ulcer bleeding was treated either with acid-suppressing drugs (antacids or H2-blockers, or both) or with sucralfate, a drug we'll look at shortly. Sucralfate is as good as the H2-blockers at protecting against bleeding, but it doesn't reduce levels of stomach acid. The study found that patients on acid-suppressing drugs got pneumonia twice as often as those on sucralfate.[13]

Bacteria in the stomach may have a more direct link to ulcers. Recent research suggests many ulcers are actually caused by a certain bacterium, called *Campylobacter pylori*. This germ has definitely been associated with gastritis (inflammation of the stomach), a condition that can also be caused by alcohol, aspirin, and many other drugs. The link between *C. pylori* and ulcers is more tentative, but in some studies the bacterium has been found in 90 percent of duodenal ulcers and 70 percent of stomach ulcers.

Gastritis often heals by itself when patients take Pepto-Bismol or similar bismuth-containing compounds, which are thought to inhibit bacterial growth. Another effective treatment combines a bismuth-containing drug with an antibiotic. The trouble with this alternative is that some antibiotics themselves cause stomach distress. The treatment could turn out to be worse than the disease.[14]

Another necessary function of stomach acid is to aid in the absorption of iron from plant foods. Studies show H2-blockers can block this absorption by 28–65 percent, depending on the dose. This probably isn't a major risk with short-term use; but over the long term, iron deficiency anemia is a real possibility. Vitamin B_{12} absorption can also be impaired, resulting in pernicious anemia.[15]

Another long-term unknown is the risk of cancer. Decreased acidity in the stomach is correlated with increased nitrite and nitrosamine concentrations in the stomach juices. These substances are produced by bacteria from the nitrates in processed meats and other foods, and they are known carcinogens. A clear cause-and-effect relationship between H2-blockers and cancer hasn't been proved and, again, it's probably not a major risk in short-term therapy. But long-term therapy remains an open question.[16]

The problem is that once you get on H2-blockers, your therapy is liable to be long-term, due to the high risk of relapse when you discontinue the drugs. In one study, 85 percent of ulcer patients treated with cimetidine got a second ulcer within a year of treatment. This relapse rate was worse than that found in a second study with no treatment at all. In the second study, only about 50 percent of those treated with placebos relapsed; and less than 40 percent of those treated with colloidal bismuth did.[17]

In a third study, relapse rates after two years weren't significantly different whether ulcers were treated with cimetidine, ranitidine, pirenzepine (an investigational drug), sucralfate, or a placebo. They all varied between 86 percent and 93 percent. After four years, relapse rates varied between 89 percent and 98 percent for all remedies.[18]

There is also a theoretical problem with treating stomach ulcers with acid-suppressing drugs. Unlike duodenal ulcers, stomach ulcers don't heal significantly faster when acid is suppressed. This may be related to the clinical finding that stomach-ulcer patients secrete no more stomach acid than normal people. In fact, sometimes they secrete less.[19]

Sucralfate: coating the hole

All this makes sucralfate (Carafate) look good. Sucralfate doesn't suppress stomach acid. Like the bismuth compounds, it works by forming a coat over the ulcer that actually protects the damaged area while it heals.

Carafate has very few side effects—a little constipation and other mild nonspecific complaints, but nothing much. It does, however, coat your stomach so that the bioavailability of other drugs is decreased. Sucralfate should be taken at least one hour before, or two hours after, other drugs or food. Drugs of particular concern are tetracycline, dilantin, digoxin, coumadin, and Tagamet.

There's another problem with sucralfate. It's an aluminum compound, consisting of aluminum hydroxide and sulfated sucrose. Like aluminum-containing antacids, it causes phosphate depletion that can result in bone loss; and Alzheimer's disease could be a long-term risk. Carafate has been on the market only since 1981, so no one knows for sure.[20]

Nondrug alternatives

For simple stomach complaints, your best bet is to avoid symptom-oriented drugs and look for the cause.

The culprit could be dietary: overeating in general, eating the wrong combinations of foods, or food allergies or intolerances. Common offenders that can provoke upset stomachs in the intolerant are the lactose (milk sugar) in milk, the gluten in wheat, yeast, sugar, coffee, eggs, and soy products.

The theory of "proper food combining" lacks scientific evidence, but sensitive people swear by it. The theory is that different types of food require different digestive enzymes. If you mix your foods improperly, some will sit there and create havoc while others are being processed. If you're prone to indigestion after ordinary-size meals, try separating heavy proteins from heavy starches and fruits, and eating them instead at separate meals.

Specific food sensitivities can also cause the feeling of bloating and distention after eating. Studies show this feeling is *not* caused by "excess gas." Moreover, the FDA has found no over-the-counter drugs that are safe or effective for alleviating it, TV ads notwithstanding.[21]

Excess belching is due mainly to air swallowing rather than to excess intestinal gas production. Stomach gas consists primarily of oxygen and nitrogen, which come from swallowed air. Increased air swallowing can be caused by eating rapidly, gulping, stress, gum chewing, poorly fitting dentures, carbonated soft drinks, thumbsucking, postnasal drip, or dry mouth.

A remedy for intestinal gas that goes back to Hippocrates is charcoal. One quart of charcoal will absorb *eighty* quarts of ammonia gas. Its only downside is that chronic use can interfere with the absorption of nutrients and other drugs.[22]

Other natural remedies for gas, bloating, and overeating are papaya enzyme and peppermint tea.

Ulcer patients can usually eat whatever they want, so long as they don't eat too much, too fast. Small, frequent meals are best. The bland diet heavy in milk fats that used to be recommended for ulcer sufferers is now thought to have done more harm than good. The "sippy diet" consisting of milk products actually increases stomach acid secretion. The latest recommendation is just the reverse: a diet heavy with plant foods that are high in fiber and essential fatty acids (EFAs). Research suggests a high-fiber plant-foods diet may actually help heal ulcers. The vitamin C found in fruits and vegetables is also necessary for healing and tissue repair.[23]

Two important EFAs are linoleic acid and arachidonic acid. Recent research shows they're converted in the stomach and duodenum to prostaglandins. The prostaglandins stimulate the secretion of mucus and bicarbonate, and these protect the stomach lining from injury. Linoleic and arachidonic acids are found particularly in peanut, safflower, soybean, and corn oils.[24]

For alleviating gastric distress, what you don't put into your stomach can be as important as what you do. Aspirin and other NSAIDs can eat holes in it. Other suspects are coffee, alcohol, cigarettes, and spicy foods (if you're not used to them). Smoking is the most certain culprit. In one study of ulcer patients, no matter what form of drug treatment was used, smokers relapsed sooner than nonsmokers.[25]

Ulcers have also responded to EMG biofeedback relaxation techniques, and they show significant placebo healing rates. This means they can go away by themselves if left alone.[26]

If none of these alternatives works, your problem may be something more serious than excess stomach acid. If so, antacids and H2-blockers can mask the symptom while the condition gets worse. Instead of relying on drugs, it's best to get a complete checkup from your doctor.

23

DRUGS FOR DIARRHEA, NAUSEA, CONSTIPATION, AND HEMORRHOIDS

Thousands have found this new miracle ingredient remedies headache, sour stomach, constipation, weak blood, and dizziness . . . Yes, folks! It cures just about anything that ails you . . . .

—1958 TV commercial[1]

A little diarrhea, like a little fever, is actually good for you. Your body is getting rid of things you're better off without. But sometimes the condition can get out of hand. If it's very uncomfortable or socially embarrassing, you may want to suppress it with drugs.

Traveler's diarrhea (locally designated "Montezuma's revenge," "the Aztec two-step," or "Delhi belly") is the kind you don't want to suppress if you can help it. It is always caused by something you ate that your body rejects. If you suppress the eliminatory process, the bacteria will remain inside and can be responsible for serious infectious diseases like typhoid and cholera.

Even if you're not traveling, if your diarrhea is merely the occasional bout, it's likely to be from food poisoning and shouldn't be suppressed. And if it's more than the occasional bout, it may signal a more serious condition that shouldn't be masked with drugs.

Theoretical objections aside, there's another problem with treating diarrhea with drugs: it's hard to find a drug that's really safe and effective for controlling the condition.

Prescription drugs are effective. In fact, they can bring bowel function to a grinding halt, by drugging the nerves that trigger it.

But this result can be hazardous, since bacteria and other toxins remain in the body to create their own havoc; and the drugs contain narcotics that can lead to dependency. Prescription remedies should never be used for mild cases of diarrhea or for more than two or three days. They also shouldn't be used for young children, since the drugs can be very toxic.

Lomotil is a popular prescription remedy that's quite effective. Motofen is a similar product that came on the U.S. market in 1988. However, these drugs are narcotics that can be addicting, and they can actually be fatal if taken in large amounts. They contain diphenoxylate and its metabolite difenoxin, agents that are chemically related to the narcotic meperidine (Demerol). To discourage potential addicts, a bit of atropine is added to give the drugs unpleasant side effects. This means that when you take these drugs, you're going to get some unpleasant side effects. The most common ones are dizziness and sedation. Others include headache, restlessness, depression, nausea, and vomiting.[2]

Paregoric is also a narcotic drug. It's an opium tincture that works very well—so well, it's liable to make you constipated. It can also cause nausea. If used for long periods, it can be addicting. And paregoric can cause diverticular disease by permanently stretching the intestinal wall.

Imodium (loperamide) is a popular prescription item that recently got over-the-counter approval from the FDA. Unlike difenoxin and diphenoxylate, loperamide isn't subject to the Controlled Substances Act. But it, too, commonly causes constipation, by bringing peristaltic activity to a standstill. Other side effects include drowsiness, fatigue, dizziness, dry mouth, and abdominal discomfort.

The FDA says most other over-the-counter antidiarrheal drugs, while safer than prescription remedies, lack evidence of effectiveness.[3]

In animal studies, the active ingredients in Kaopectate—kaolin and pectin—haven't significantly reduced the number of bowel movements, the amount of cramping, or the amount of fluid lost. And Donnagel, which also contains these ingredients, adds several others that haven't been proven effective and have unwanted side effects. These facts aside, kaolin-and-pectin products do seem to ease discomfort, perhaps by firming the stools; and they're considered safe.

Another option that's safe, and that the FDA considers more effective, is polycarbophil (Mitrolan). It's actually a laxative of the bulk-forming variety, but it has the amazing ability to absorb sixty times its weight in water. It eases the discomfort of diarrhea by firming the stools.

Pepto-Bismol, which we looked at under antacids, is also useful for traveler's diarrhea. It is generally considered safe, and travelers report that it works; but the FDA questions the mechanism. The drug provides a protective coat to the gut; but what good is a protective coat against bacteria, after they're already in there causing diarrhea? Another problem with Pepto-Bismol is that the amounts required to be effective are so large, you can wind up with salicylate poisoning. The result can be side effects similar to those from an overdose of aspirin.

If you're taking other medicines, diarrhea remedies can prevent their absorption; so it's best not to take these drugs within an hour of each other.

It may, in fact, be your other medicines that are causing the diarrhea. Known offenders include antibiotics, antacids containing magnesium (including Maalox and Mylanta), laxatives, and medications for high blood pressure and irregular heart beat. Overdosing on vitamin C can also have this effect.

Nausea and vomiting

Like diarrhea, a little vomiting can be good for you. Whether it is or not, you don't have much recourse but to hang on until it goes away, since there are no over-the-counter drugs the FDA considers safe and effective for treating it. There are drugs that work; but they either require a prescription, or the FDA permits their over-the-counter sale only to treat motion sickness. Motion sickness isn't caused by something your body is trying to get rid of, so suppressing it with drugs doesn't mean retaining potential poisons.

Like diarrhea, nausea and vomiting can also be caused by drugs. Offenders include antibiotics, certain heart medications, narcotic painkillers like codeine, birth control pills and other female hormones, and prescription asthma medications. Iron supplements and salt substitutes have also been implicated.

Drugs used to treat cancer are also very toxic and can cause severe nausea. The antinausea drug Reglan (metoclopramide) is generally given before and after chemotherapy. Reglan is good for treating not only nausea but heartburn, persistent feelings of fullness after meals, and a tendency to regurgitate. The drug increases gastric emptying time by stimulating motility of the stomach; but it does this without stimulating secretions, so stomach acid isn't increased. It also has a low incidence of side effects. However, it can cause depression; and 0.2–1.0 percent of patients develop involuntary movements of the limbs and facial grimacing.[4]

Constipation

Constipation is another condition that drugs are more likely to trigger than alleviate. In fact, almost any drug can alter bowel function, causing either constipation or diarrhea. Drugs that commonly slow up the bowels include codeine, antihistamines, diuretics, antispasmodics, narcotics, sleeping pills, antidepressants, tranquilizers, iron supplements, cholesterol-lowering drugs, and antacids containing aluminum or calcium compounds.

Ironically, another major cause of constipation is laxative use. Americans spend more than $400 million a year on these drugs, which include over eight hundred over-the-counter varieties. Laxatives diminish your natural muscle reflexes, so peristalsis occurs only with stronger and stronger stimulation. They can also irritate and inflame the lining of the bowel; cause anal fissures and hemorrhoids; and deplete your body of important substances, including water, calcium, potassium, and magnesium. Water loss causes dehydration, calcium loss weakens the bones, and potassium and magnesium loss weakens the muscles, including the heart.

If you definitely need a laxative, the best are the bulk-forming and stool-softening varieties that encourage normal bowel function. Bulk-formers (Metamucil, Siblin) generally contain psyllium seed. Stool softeners (Doxiden, Colace, Comfolax) generally contain docusate. Bulk-formers should always be taken with eight ounces of water, to prevent blockage of the gastrointestinal tract.

Laxatives to avoid are the stimulant, lubricant, and saline varieties. These laxatives are not only irritating, but, if used for long, can upset the body's mineral balance. Chemical stimulants (Ex-Lax, Dulcolax, Correctol, castor oil) force evacuation by stimulating the nerves controlling the bowel muscles. They are also very irritating to the colon wall; and castor oil, especially, can be very toxic. Lubricant laxatives (mineral oil, liquid paraffin) coat the stools with mineral oil or olive oil. Taken over long periods, they can deplete the body of fat-soluble vitamins (A, D, E, and K) and cause rectal leakage. Saline laxatives (Epsom salts, milk of magnesia, Fleet enemas) pull water into the bowels, often turning the stools liquid. They are not only uncomfortable but can be dangerous for people with heart or kidney failure, or people who should restrict their salt intake.

Laxative use is best limited to a day or two in emergencies; e.g., when you're traveling.[5]

Hemorrhoids

The makers of Preparation H cornered the $100-million-plus hemorrhoid market by aggressive and relentless advertising. Nearly a quarter of their sales proceeds goes to convincing you of their product's efficacy. However, both the FDA and the *Medical Letter* question their advertising claims. These reliable authorities assert there is no acceptable evidence that Preparation H can shrink hemorrhoids, reduce inflammation, or heal injured tissue.[6]

Unfortunately, no other drugs accomplish these feats any better. None of them cures the condition; and most ointments and suppositories can make it worse, by aggravating the trouble and sensitizing the skin.

Hemorrhoids are swollen blood vessels; and the vasoconstrictors touted as shrinking them do work to constrict blood vessels. The problem is that the effect is only temporary; and like the vasoconstrictors used in nasal decongestants, after a few days the drugs can produce a rebound effect. This means the blood vessels become more dilated than before you started treating them. These stimulant drugs are also rapidly absorbed from the lining of the rectum, giving rise to potential systemic side effects including heart palpitations, sleeplessness, and paranoia.

Benzocaine is a local anesthetic found in products like Americaine and Lanacane. It can deaden feeling in the sensitive area; but again, the relief it provides is only temporary, and it doesn't promote healing. In fact, the anesthetic can prolong the healing process, since it tends to be irritating. It can also cause sensitization, rendering you allergic not only to benzocaine but to related anesthetics, including the novocaine used by your dentist.[7]

Hemorrhoidal preparations often include agents for wound-healing, but these too lack evidence of effectiveness; and so do the hydrocortisone products widely marketed for rectal itch. These have the further drawback that if used for long, they can cause skin disorders.[8]

The hemorrhoidal preparation typically used in hospitals is Anusol. However, your best bets may remain old-fashioned petroleum jelly and zinc oxide. They still don't treat the underlying problem, but they can ease anorectal pain and itch without significant side effects; and they're cheaper.

Nondrug remedies

Uncomplicated, external hemorrhoids usually go away by themselves in a couple of weeks. (If they don't, or if you are bleeding from the rectum, you should see your doctor.) Helpful aids while you're waiting include porous underwear that won't trap moisture, sitz baths, moist heat, rest, and cleanliness—though not with a harsh soap or antiseptic, which can also be irritating. More important is to correct the underlying problem, usually constipation.

The dietary solution to constipation is now well known: eat more plant fiber. Wheat bran and psyllium are particularly effective. But relying on pure wheat bran can be dangerous, since it irritates the delicate lining of the intestines and can inhibit mineral absorption. Fortunately, the same laxative effect can be achieved by eating natural foods containing fiber. Raw vegetables, raw and dried fruits, and most beans and whole grains are high in fiber. They create a heavy intestinal mass that travels quickly through the intestines. For a list of common foods that are high in fiber, see chapter 16. Foods to reduce or avoid are those devoid of fiber. This means animal foods, especially cheese; and refined foods, especially sugar. It is also important to drink plenty of water, and to relax, allow time for nature to take its course, and respond when it calls.

Diet is also important for controlling diarrhea. If you're prone to the condition after eating foods that leave your friends unaffected, you may have a food allergy or intolerance. This problem can also underly the "irritable bowel syndrome," a condition characterized by constipation, diarrhea, or both alternately. Try switching to a bland diet, then adding suspicious foods back in, one by one, until you pinpoint the offenders. Avoid dairy products. They contain lactose which is hard to digest and can aggravate diarrhea. Even if you're not allergic to milk in your normal state, milk products can aggravate an active case of diarrhea and should be avoided. You should also avoid caffeinated beverages and any drugs you don't have to take. To replace lost fluids, drink plenty of water or juice diluted with water (but not heavily sugared drinks). Then grin and bear it until it goes away.

This is also the best remedy for nausea and vomiting. However, liquids—especially carbonated drinks—are hard to keep down on an upset stomach. A cracker or other dry food works better. You can drink colas or ginger ales, but they should be flat and at room temperature, taken in small sips. Other good fluids are apple and grape juices at room temperature. Citrus juices aren't so good, because their acidity can be irritating and they often contain solid pulp which is hard to digest.[9]

If diarrhea or nausea and vomiting don't go away by themselves in a couple of days—or if the condition is very serious, or the sufferer is very young or old or debilitated—see a doctor.

Table 32. *Over-the-Counter Remedies Most Recommended by Pharmacists for Digestive Complaints*[10]

Complaint	Brand name	Active agents
Diarrhea	Imodium AD	loperamide
	Donnagel/ Donnagel-PG	kaolin, pectin
	Kaopectate	kaolin, pectin
	Parepectolin	kaolin, pectin
	Pepto-Bismol	bismuth subsalicylate
Constipation	Metamucil	psyllium (bulk-forming)
	Dulcolax	bisacodyl (stimulant)
	Doxidan	docusate calcium (emollient)
	Colace	docusate sodium (emollient)
	Doss	docusate sodium (emollient)
Upset stomach	Pepto-Bismol	bismuth subsalicylate
	Emetrol	levulose, dextrose
	Donnagel/ Donnagel-PG	kaolin, pectin
	Mylanta/ Mylanta II	aluminum, magnesium, magaldrate, simethicone
	Maalox/ Maalox Plus	aluminum, magnesium, magaldrate, simethicone

V

Head Trips

24

DOWNERS: DRUGS FOR INSOMNIA AND ANXIETY

Quick, Watson . . . the needle!
  —Sherlock Holmes ordering an injection
  of cocaine after a hard day[1]

Smith Kline & French, which brought you Tagamet, is also responsible for the major tranquilizers that have cornered the mental illness market, Thorazine (chlorpromazine) and Stelazine (trifluoperazine). In England, Stelazine is one of those "mother's little helpers" sung about by the Rolling Stones, which are prescribed for harassed housewives who find it "difficult to cope."[2]

The major tranquilizers impair attention and diminish aggressiveness. This makes them good alternatives for psychotic patients, who would otherwise be locked up or tied down. They are also good for schizophrenic patients, for whom the alternatives are electroconvulsive therapy or heavy sedation. Since these drugs were introduced in the 1950s, state mental hospital bed occupancy has dropped by more than half (although the fact that state funding has also dropped may take some credit).

The problem with the major tranquilizers is that they have major side effects. They can produce involuntary tremors and jerks, can dangerously lower blood pressure, and can increase the effects of alcohol, sedatives, and anesthetics. They are a major cause of Parkinsonism, a condition characterized by slow and shaky movements and stiff muscles. This means they're not the best options merely for "coping."

Even involuntarily committed patients have contested the enforced use of these drugs. In 1985, a class action lawsuit was filed in San Francisco on behalf of a 45-year-old chronic schizophrenic woman and anyone similarly situated. The principal plaintiff had been committed after engaging in "violent and bizarre acts," and had been forcibly injected with Thorazine. Citing the drug's potential adverse effects, her lawyers argued that involuntarily committed patients should have the same right as other patients to refuse medication. In June of 1989, the California State Supreme Court agreed.[3]

The barbiturates

The barbiturates are a class of sedative/hypnotics that includes phenobarbital, amobarbital, and butabarbital. They produce an intoxication similar to alcohol. Like the major tranquilizers, however, they are dangerous alternatives for merely relieving anxiety. Barbiturates are favorites among the suicidal, since only moderate overdoses can be fatal. They are the drugs that killed Judy Garland, Marilyn Monroe, and Elvis Presley. One gram (about ten capsules) can produce serious poisoning, and two grams or more can produce death. When barbiturates are mixed with alcohol, even smaller doses will do the trick. The drugs induce vomiting and suppress the gag reflex. In many cases, the user actually chokes to death. In extreme overdose, all electrical activity in the brain ceases.

At heavy intake levels, withdrawal from barbiturates can also be fatal; and even if it's not, it can be a nightmare. The barbiturates can produce a host of other side effects, making their use dangerous not only alone but in products that contain them along with other drugs, like antacids and analgesics.

Phenobarbital was the first effective medication available for epilepsy, and it's still in common use for this purpose. In 1938, phenytoin (Dilantin) came on the market; and in the last two decades, other useful anticonvulsants have become available, including carbamazepine (Tegretol), clonazepam (Clonopin), and valproic acid (Depakene). These drugs are generally less sedating than phenobarbital; yet long-term therapy with any of them produces toxic effects. Fortunately, according to a study reported in the *New England Journal of Medicine* in 1988, the majority of epileptics don't need to be on these drugs for life. Approximately two-thirds of epileptic patients who had been free of seizures for two years were safely withdrawn from their medications without relapse.[4]

The minor tranquilizers

The benzodiazepines, or "minor" tranquilizers, were considered a major advance over the barbiturates. Librium (chlordiazepoxide) was the first of these drugs, and Valium (diazepam) was the market leader for many years. In 1980, Valium was among the top five drugs prescribed in the United States; while Dalmane (flurazepam) was the benzodiazepine most often prescribed as a sleep remedy.

When Valium first became popular in the 1960s, it was thought to represent an improvement over the barbiturates in not having addiction potential. Ironically, Valium now heads the list of drugs that cause dependence. Unfortunately, by the time the problem became apparent, thousands of people were already hooked on it. In Britain, where Valium was particularly popular, an estimated 2 percent of the adult population became addicted to it.

The withdrawal problem didn't become obvious until 1980, when enough evidence had accumulated to prompt Britain's Committee on the Review of Medicines to recommend that tranquilizers be used for no more than four months at a time, and sleeping pills for no more than two or three weeks. When thousands of addicts tried to respond to this advisory, they became uncoordinated, experienced muscle-twitching, headaches, vomiting, and insomnia, and felt miserable. Even when withdrawal was done slowly, most people suffered symptoms. Many simply couldn't get off the drugs.[5]

By 1988, when Valium's side effects and addiction potential were well known, it had dropped to 27th among brand-name prescription drugs. Yet its relatives Xanax (alprazolam) and Halcion (triazolam) had climbed to third and sixteenth the same year.[6] Halcion is the world's bestselling sleeping pill, generating $400 million in sales in

1988. These newer benzodiazepines don't actually have fewer side effects than Valium, but they haven't yet suffered its bad press.[7]

At least, they hadn't until recently, when a 58-year-old Utah woman filed suit charging that Halcion made her shoot and kill her 83-year-old mother. The murderess alleged she could remember nothing about the incident.

Other charges have been made linking Halcion to violent behavior, as well as to seizures, amnesia, hallucinations, personality disorders, and other side effects. The only action recommended by an FDA advisory committee reviewing these charges in September of 1989 was a more detailed warning to doctors about an increased risk of amnesia from the drug. Particularly, the committee recommended a warning about "traveling amnesia," an incapacitating condition resulting when a sleeping pill is taken before a flight.[8]

Xanax, Dalmane, and Restoril (temazepam) have also come under scrutiny. Some researchers assert that Xanax is potentially one of the most dangerous drugs on the market. It can cause powerful withdrawal symptoms, including severe convulsions; and it and other benzodiazepines have been linked to everything from highway fatalities to hip fractures caused when elderly patients trip or fall out of bed.[9]

Long-acting versus short-acting benzodiazepines

The benzodiazepines are distinguished mainly by their half-lives. The longer the half-life, the longer the drug lingers in your system. Valium has a long half-life, Xanax's is intermediate, and Halcion's is short. The longer-acting drugs are most often used to treat daytime anxiety, while the shorter-acting drugs are most often used for insomnia (see table 33).

Drugs with longer-lasting effects are better for daytime use, because you're awake two-thirds of the day and asleep only one-third of it. If drugs with long-lasting effects are used to induce sleep at night, you are liable to feel drugged and uncoordinated through the following day. Since the drug isn't entirely cleared from your system when you take the next dose, this dopey feeling and lack of coordination can get worse over time.

The main problem with the newer drugs with shorter half-lives is that they can have more serious side effects when you try to break the habit. Valium stays in your system longer, so withdrawal is more gradual. On shorter-acting benzodiazepines, rebound insomnia and anxiety can occur after only short periods and at only low daily doses. This means you can have *more* trouble sleeping, and feel *more* anxious, than before you started on the drugs. This syndrome can cause you to keep taking them when you'd rather quit. If you're having this problem, try reducing rebound symptoms by gradually tapering the dose.[10]

Table 33. *Benzodiazepines*[11]

Generic Name	Brand Names	Half-Life	Onset of Action
FOR ANXIETY:			
alprazolam	Xanax	intermediate	intermediate
chlordiazepoxide	Librium	long	intermediate
	SK-Lygen		
clorazepate	Tranxene	long	rapid
	Tranxene-SD		
diazepam	Valium	long	rapid
lorazepam	Ativan	intermediate	intermediate
	Loraz		
halazepam	Paxipam	long	intermediate
prazepam	Centrax	long	slow
oxazepam	Serax	intermediate	intermediate
FOR INSOMNIA:			
flurazepam	Dalmane	long	rapid to intermediate
temazepam	Restoril	intermediate	intermediate
	Temaz		
triazolam	Halcion	short	intermediate

After prolonged use, withdrawal reactions on the shorter-acting benzodiazepines are also more frequent, more immediate, and more intense. Severe withdrawal reactions can occur, including seizures and rebound anxiety with psychotic features.[12] Studies also suggest that patients who take Xanax for panic attacks can wind up more anxious than otherwise.[13]

Since rebound insomnia occurs earlier and more intensely on the shorter-acting benzodiazepines, Valium may actually be the safer sleep remedy even though it's not approved by the FDA for this purpose. The tradeoff is that its longer half-life means it stays in your body longer, so you feel drugged the next day.

Buspirone

A new antianxiety drug called buspirone (BuSpar) is touted as avoiding many of the problems of benzodiazepines. It was introduced in the United States in 1987 and soon became Bristol Myers' fastest-selling new drug.

BuSpar produces fewer side effects than benzodiazepines. Drowsiness and psychomotor impairment are less, interactions with alcohol are minimal, and no convulsions result on withdrawal. BuSpar also has a low addiction potential. Unlike benzodiazepines, it is not a controlled substance, and experienced drug abusers show no interest in it. But because it doesn't usually cause sedation, it's not much use as a sleep aid. In fact its side effects can include insomnia and restlessness. Nausea and dysphoria are also more frequent. ("Dysphoria," the opposite of "euphoria," is Greek for excessive pain, anguish, and agitation.)

Studies show that BuSpar is as effective as Valium in patients who have never been on any antianxiety drug. In anxious patients who have been on benzodiazepines long-term, however, it is not effective for suppressing withdrawal symptoms.[14] On the other hand, in patients prone to panic attacks who suffer persistent anxiety on benzodiazepines alone, the addition of BuSpar seems to improve their condition.[15]

The main problem with BuSpar is that many people who use tranquilizers actually *like* their mood-altering, euphoric, mind-obliterating, sedative effects. BuSpar's market is turning out to be limited mainly to first-time tranquilizer users, who don't know what they're missing.[16]

BuSpar may, however, find another use. A Yale study found the drug helped people quit smoking who had previously tried and failed to break the habit.[17]

Prescription vs. over-the-counter sleep aids

For relieving insomnia, prescription drugs have serious drawbacks. They are generally ineffective after about two weeks of continuous use. Users must continually increase the dose, which means increasing the buildup of metabolites (by-products of the drug's active ingredients), along with their hangover-like side effects. Elderly people branded as senile may actually be suffering from the side effects of these drugs. The sleep the drugs induce is drug-like, with insufficient time spent dreaming. Withdrawal can lead to rebound insomnia and other side effects, including anxiety, restlessness, headache, shaking, and visual disturbances. Prescription sleeping pills can be fatal in people with certain health problems, and you can't necessarily tell ahead of time if you're one of them. The drugs can also be fatal if mixed with other drugs, or with narcotics, or alcohol. The benzodiazepines, like the barbiturates, depress brain function; and any drug that does this can be addicting and cause crises on withdrawal.

These concerns have made doctors leery of scribbling prescriptions for sleeping pills. That means inveterate insomniacs are often left to their over-the-counter remedies. In 1979, however, the FDA found that *no* over-the-counter products then on the market were safe or effective for treating insomnia, and it banned the sale of all of them.

Resourceful drug manufacturers then turned to antihistamines, which have the *negative side effect,* officially recognized by the FDA, of inducing drowsiness in some people. Originally marketed for the relief of allergies, antihistamines thus became the main ingredient in over-the-counter insomnia remedies like Nytol and Sominex.

Unfortunately, antihistamines can also expose you to a range of side effects, including nausea and vomiting; dizziness; dryness in the mouth, throat, and nose; ringing in the ears; frequent urination; fatigue; and double vision. Dizziness and confusion are particularly likely in the elderly. In children, the drugs can produce restlessness and insomnia, the very problems they're supposed to prevent. In pregnant women, certain antihistamines can produce birth defects. And breast-fed infants can experience adverse effects from the antihistamines taken by their mothers.

Antihistamines also don't do anything for anxiety. Although artful brand names like Tranquil-Span and Quiet World suggest otherwise, *no* over-the-counter drug is recognized by the FDA as effective for this purpose.[18]

Tryptophan

A remedy that has been touted as a natural sleep inducer is L-tryptophan. It's used to treat not only insomnia, but premenstrual syndrome, depression, stress, and alcohol and drug abuse. Tryptophan is an amino acid rather than a foreign chemical, so it has been considered a safe alternative to drugs. This characterization appeals to the health-conscious patrons of health food stores, where tryptophan has done a brisk business. It's classed as a dietary supplement rather than a drug and has been sold without restriction, making self–medication common. Health food stores, supermarkets, and drug stores together sell an estimated $60 million a year in tryptophan supplements.

But popping processed pills of amino acids, it turns out, may be no safer or more natural than popping other sleeping pills. In 1989, the death of a 58-year-old New York woman was linked to ingestion of tryptophan supplements, and so were some seven hundred cases of a rare disorder characterized by severe pain in muscles and joints, swelling of the arms and legs, skin rash, and sometimes fever. Reports of other deaths followed. In November of 1989, the FDA halted the sale of tryptophan.[19] The problem was traced to a contaminant in the pills rather than to tryptophan itself; but the FDA ban has effectively removed this Japanese-derived product from the market.

Nondrug alternatives

The most active ingredient in over-the-counter sleep aids may actually be the advertising that persuades you they work. Studies have shown four out of ten insomniacs get a good night's sleep on placebos.

For anxiety, relaxation can work as well as drugs. In a study comparing methods for relieving anxiety in patients about to undergo surgery, acupressure (a form of massage) and relaxation/meditation tapes were found to work as well as, or better than, Valium. Biofeedback relaxation methods have also proved effective in relieving both anxiety and insomnia.[20] And some people swear by valerian root, a natural herb relaxant from which the drug Valmid is made.

For inducing sleep, the traditional hot bath, good book, and hot drink remain your most viable course. Giving up drugs of all sorts may also help. Like constipation and diarrhea, insomnia is more likely to be caused by drugs than cured by them. Many drugs contain stimulants—including analgesics like Anacin and Excedrin, which contain caffeine; over-the-counter diet aids, nasal decongestants, and asthma products; and many prescription drugs, including those for asthma, many cough and cold remedies, amphetamines, and thyroid preparations. Beta-blockers, hypnotics, and diuretics taken late in the day can also worsen sleep.[21] Sleeplessness can also result when you try to discontinue the drugs intended to counteract it. This means it's best not to start on them if you can help it.

25

UPPERS: DRUGS FOR LOSING WEIGHT AND SUBDUING HYPERACTIVE CHILDREN

> . . . *Hitler took methamphetamine both orally and intravenously to energize himself; moreover, he took the drug on a daily basis. The fact that amphetamines were dangerous was not recognized at the time. . . . There is little doubt that Hitler's repeated use of amphetamines at high dosages contributed significantly to his violent mood shifts. It is likely, as well, that amphetamines accounted, in part, for his pathological behavior.*[1]
>
> —Stanley Siegelman (1989)

The amphetamines are synthetic stimulants that mimic the effects of adrenalin, the body's own stimulant. Adrenalin is the fight-or-flight hormone produced by emotion, especially fear. Popular synthetic brands include Benzedrine, Dexedrine, and Methedrine.

Amphetamines became popular in the Second World War, when soldiers used them to stay awake. Then students and truck drivers discovered them. By the 1960s, "speed freaks" were injecting them directly into their veins. The initial sensation was usually one of euphoria and brilliance. But severe mood swings were common. Eventually the user could become paranoid, schizophrenic, and pathologically aggressive. Withdrawal produced depression, insomnia, and extreme exhaustion. Addiction led to liver damage, high blood pressure, and cerebral hemorrhage.

Medically, amphetamines have been used to treat depression, obesity, fatigue, hyperactivity in children, and narcolepsy (habitual involuntary sleep). But as the serious side effects and addiction potential of these dangerous drugs became evident, doctors sought other alternatives.

The book *Fatal Vision* is the bestselling true account of Dr. Jeffrey MacDonald, who is now in jail for the brutal murder of his wife and two daughters. A very popular and successful physician, Dr. MacDonald allegedly committed the murders while taking 3–5 capsules daily of Eskatrol, an amphetamine-type diet pill, to help him stay awake while he worked three jobs. Eskatrol has since been taken off the market due to its serious side effects, including paranoid psychosis.[2]

Uppers for weight loss

It used to be that if you wanted to lose a few pounds, you could easily get a prescription for amphetamines. But the psychotic-like side effects and addiction potential of these drugs, as well as their failure to contribute to *long-term* weight loss, have now made doctors very circumspect in their use.

What has stepped in to fill their place are over-the-counter diet pills. Yet these drugs, while not as strong as amphetamines, have the same downsides. They can do the same harm. They just do it more slowly. Like amphetamines, they also don't promote long-term weight loss.

Most over-the-counter antidotes to overeating contain combinations of phenylpropanolamine (PPA), ephedrine derivatives, and caffeine. PPA and ephedrine were originally marketed as cold remedies (see chapter 6). Their chemical structures are very similar to amphetamines, and so are their reactions in the body. They stimulate the sympathetic nervous system, the fight-or-flight emergency system. In high doses, they can produce psychotic-like side effects.

PPA is now the most widely used diet aid; yet no well-controlled study has shown it to be effective in long-term weight control. It can cause high blood pressure, even in healthy young adults who haven't exceeded the recommended dosage. It can also produce potentially fatal heart problems. The drug is particularly hazardous for people who already have high blood pressure, heart disease, diabetes, or thyroid problems. Mixing PPA with other drugs, including MAO inhibitors, certain NSAIDs, and antihypertensive drugs, can precipitate hypertensive crises.[3]

Although amphetamines can be obtained only by prescription, in some ways PPA and ephedrine can do more harm. Because these over-the-counter "uppers" aren't as potent as amphetamines, the user is more likely to take several at a time to get an equivalent effect. Moreover, PPA and ephedrine have much stronger effects on blood pressure than amphetamines, so hypertensive crises and intracerebral hemorrhages are more likely. Some have been reported that ended in death.[4] In one reported case, a 35-year-old woman developed an intracerebral hemorrhage after taking only one tablet of the popular diet aid "Dexatrim, Extra Strength."[5]

Over-the-counter diet aids containing 25 mg or more of PPA are listed in table 34. The immediate-release forms are the most likely to produce severe hypertensive reactions.

Table 34.　*Over-the-Counter Diet Aids Containing 25 Mg or More of PPA*[6]

Brand name:	Formulation:
Acutrim	slow release
Acutrim II	slow release
Dietac	slow release
Dexatrim (caffeine free)	slow release
Dexatrim (plus vitamins)	slow release
Dexatrim (extra strength)	immediate release
Appedrine	slow release

Caffeine is another popular diet-pill ingredient. It isn't particularly harmful in moderate doses—the amount in two or three cups of coffee daily (two cups brewed, three cups instant).[7] But the recommended diet pill dose contains as much caffeine as you'd get in about *five* cups of coffee. This means you're getting too much, particularly if you also drink coffee or cola drinks, or take other medications containing caffeine.

Other dubious diet-pill ingredients include benzocaine (as in Ayds and Slim-Line), and starch blockers. Starch blockers are no longer available, thanks to the FDA; but benzocaine still is. It's an anesthetic that numbs the tongue. The theory is that decreasing the sensation of the taste buds makes food less appealing. At best, however, it works only temporarily; and it doesn't numb the cravings of the stomach. Benzocaine can also produce allergic reactions, sensitizing you not only to it, but to other anesthetics like novocaine.[8]

What about thinning down with fiber pills like Fibre Trim? Many studies have shown that high-fiber foods aid in weight loss. They fill you up with fewer calories, give you the satisfaction of chewing, and slow digestion in your stomach. Fiber pills, unfortunately, don't have the same effect. For one thing, they don't contain much fiber. Five pills provide only 2.5 grams of fiber, a mere tenth of the recommended daily allowance. The pills also don't fill you up or give you the satisfaction of chewing. And their fiber can bind important minerals, making you crave food to fill the lack. Filling up on fiber-rich plant foods doesn't pose this problem, because the foods themselves provide abundant vitamins and minerals. Incidentally, only plant foods contain fiber; and the less refined, the more fiber they have.[9]

The safest, surest and most painless approach to weight loss is dietary substitution. Replace refined foods and fats with whole grains and greens, and cut animal products to a minimum. According to the FDA, animal products are the source of two-thirds of the fat in the American diet; and they contain none of the fiber and complex carbohydrates that quell hunger.[10]

Ritalin: uppers for children

While amphetamines have for the most part been superseded as medical therapies, they remain popular in the treatment of hyperactive children. Between 1985 and 1988, sales of the amphetamine methylphenidate (Ritalin) increased by 97 percent. The drug is now used to treat an estimated one million American children, or some

3–5 percent of the school-age population.[11] Other amphetamines used for this purpose are dextroamphetamine (Dexedrine, Dexampex, Ferndex), and pemoline (Cylert).

Although amphetamines are stimulants, they have the property of calming down hyperactive children. This effect was considered paradoxical, until researchers had a closer look at it. Stimulants, it seems, have the same effect on problem children as on normal adults: they increase the ability to concentrate on a task. The child sits still and gets down to work. Children on Ritalin perform better on certain types of tests, especially those requiring attention and motivation. In one recent study, two-thirds of the hyperactive children tested improved academically, socially, or both, on the drug.[12]

Hyperactive children on Ritalin work faster and make fewer mistakes. This is also true of adults on coffee. Amphetamines are notorious for their illicit use by college students to get through exams. One problem with Ritalin is that high school students are peddling it to their friends for the same purpose.[13]

Another problem is that a significant amount of information learned on Ritalin is forgotten when the child is taken off the drug. This is also a known drawback of studying on "speed." Most reviewers have concluded that Ritalin has neither short-term nor long-term beneficial effects on academic performance.[14]

The main problem with amphetamine treatment is that it doesn't teach the child anything. The ability to concentrate on a task is improved by chemical means, but the drugs don't seem to affect reasoning, problem-solving, or learning, in adults or children. Children on Ritalin who have been followed through high school still have trouble with their families and still have academic and behavior problems at school. Hyperactive boys on Ritalin are no less likely than other hyperactive boys to be arrested and institutionalized for juvenile delinquency. At best, the drug masks the underlying problem, so parents and clinicians can avoid dealing with it.[15]

As any mother knows, coffee is bad for children because it stunts their growth; and Ritalin is also subject to this side effect. Amphetamines affect the release of growth hormone at a time when children are still growing. Most researchers think this doesn't cause an

actual loss of height, since the child catches up on "drug holidays."
But the matter isn't settled.[16]

Ritalin also has other side effects, including sleeplessness, loss of
appetite, irritability, headaches, fatigue, withdrawal, crying for no
apparent reason, abnormal sensitivity to criticism, and depression.
The most serious potential side effect is the development of tics, or
involuntary, darting, purposeless motor movements of the face or
arms. In the worst case, the tics can progress to "Tourette's syndrome," a condition characterized by generalized jerking movements in any part of the body, accompanied by a tendency to use
foul language and to repeat words heard.[17]

These side effects have led to a spate of lawsuits on behalf of
children allegedly harmed by inappropriate use of the drug.

One child/plaintiff was forced by school employees to take
Ritalin to avoid being expelled from school. He took it for about
four years, during which he suffered insomnia, bad dreams, and
slowed growth. He also became violent and suicidal, traits common
to "speed freaks."[18]

Another child is alleged to have suffered from nausea, insomnia,
hallucinations, depression, and suicidal thoughts during his three
years on the drug. His mother reports that on one occasion, he lay
in the street during rush hour because "his mind told him to." On
another occasion, he said he wanted to be dead. He lost weight, was
uncoordinated, and "seemed retarded."[19]

Ritalin is prescribed for children with a condition formally characterized as "attention-deficit hyperactivity disorder," or "minimal
brain dysfunction." The disorder is considered to be a form of brain
damage, but studies have been unable to find consistent, objective
evidence of it. The disorder is also not defined by a consistent clus-
ter of symptoms.[20] In fact, the American Psychiatric Association's
official criteria for its diagnosis could apply to most children. As
comedian Bill Cosby (who has five children) points out:

*All children have brain damage. . . . If you know you're not
supposed to do something and you do it and then people say why
did you do it and you say "I don't know," that's brain damage.*

According to the American Psychiatric Association, a child is
considered to have attention-deficit hyperactivity disorder who

shows eight of the following symptoms for at least six months, beginning before his seventh birthday:

1. Often fidgets his hands or feet or squirms in his seat.
2. Has trouble staying in his seat when required.
3. Is easily distracted.
4. Has trouble waiting his turn.
5. Often blurts out answers before the question is completed.
6. Has trouble doing chores or otherwise following through with instructions.
7. Has trouble sustaining attention to work or play activities.
8. Often shifts from one unfinished task to another.
9. Has trouble playing quietly.
10. Often talks too much.
11. Often interrupts others or butts into other children's games.
12. Doesn't seem to listen to what's being said.
13. Often loses things (toys, pencils, books, assignments).
14. Does dangerous things without considering the consequences, like running into the street without looking.[21]

Most children display some of these symptoms; and it's this vagueness in diagnosis that has led to most of the problems with Ritalin use. Where the only alternative is to institutionalize the child, the drug is obviously the best choice of treatment. But it is often given to children whose problems can be corrected by other means. These problems can include reading or other learning disabilities, problems at home or problems at school (ineffective teaching or boring subject matter). As John Coale, a personal injuries lawyer representing Ritalin victims, observes:

Many of the kids I see [on Ritalin] are highly creative children with high IQs who are obviously just plain bored in school. They're being drugged because they're intelligent.[22]

Other possibilities include nutritional deficiencies, low blood sugar, food allergies, or hay fever and the drugs used to treat it. Hay fever can cause irritability, mood swings, and insomnia; and the drugs

can make victims drowsy and slow. The result can be a short attention span, difficulty learning, and disruptive behavior in school.[23]

Nondrug alternatives

For specific learning disabilities, tutoring or remedial reading
classes are recommended.

If the problem is social or psychological, counseling may help. In
a recent study, boys receiving psychotherapy along with Ritalin
were institutionalized only one-third as often as those receiving the
drug alone, and they were arrested for multiple felonies only half as
often.[24] Another researcher found that difficult childhood behavior
could be modified by bringing the parents together in groups to
discuss ways of handling specific problems. Before they attended the
sessions, the parents read a book on child management.[25]

In some children, hyperactivity has been traced to food allergies.
In a study of over one hundred children reported by pediatrician
and allergist William Crook, hyperactivity was traced to this cause
in about three-fourths of them.

In a study conducted at London's Institute of Child Health and
Hospital for Sick Children, 28 hyperactive children were fed one of
two selected foods, each for one week. The "suspect" food was one
that had been associated with symptoms in the child. The "control"
food was one that hadn't. When the children's behavior was rated
by a psychologist, a pediatric neurologist, and the parents, dramatic
improvement was noted during the week the control food was
eaten.

The late Ben Feingold, M.D., chief of the allergy clinics of the
Kaiser Foundation in California, linked hyperactivity to food addi-
tives and chemicals, including those in Ritalin itself. Other suspect
food allergens are sugar, cow's milk, citrus fruits or juices, wheat,
corn, chocolate, eggs, nuts, fish, and berries.[26]

If you suspect a food allergy in your child, try eliminating possible offenders, then adding them back into his diet one by one. If a
food is definitely implicated by the return of symptoms, eliminate
it from the diet for at least three months. The food can then be

tried cautiously. If no reaction occurs, it can be eaten in moderation.[27]

The drug option

If you elect Ritalin treatment for your child, here are some things you should know:

Generic forms of methylphenidate don't seem to be as effective as the brand-name product. They should be used cautiously, if at all.

Although sustained-release formulations have the advantage of allowing the child to avoid the embarrassment associated with taking his "behavior pills" during the day, the response to these formulations is variable and unpredictable. Once-a-day dosing is more practical with dextroamphetamine, which is twice as strong as methylphenidate and requires only half the dose. Dextroamphetamine may also be effective in children who don't respond to Ritalin.

To lessen insomnia, avoid late-afternoon doses.

To lessen growth problems, give the drug only when school is in, not on weekends or holidays.

Your child should be under the regular supervision of a physician. Prescriptions for refills shouldn't be given over the phone.[28]

26

DRUGS AND DEPRESSION

Grief is itself a med'cine.
—William Cowper (1731–1800)

An estimated fifteen million Americans are clinically depressed. One in five women and one in ten men will experience at least one major episode of depression in their lives; and in a third of them, the condition will become chronic.[1]

Amphetamines have been used for fifty years to give the depressed a "lift." But controlled trials have failed to establish that the drugs relieve depression significantly better than placebos.[2] Amphetamines have now been replaced with other drugs, including the monoamine oxidase (MAO) inhibitors and the tricyclic and other antidepressants. However, for selected cases of major depressive episodes, therapists are showing renewed interest in returning to amphetamines. They are finding that the newer antidepressants can actually pose a greater risk to health than these older alternatives, especially for the elderly and the medically ill.[3]

The latest in antidepressants is fluoxetine (Prozac). It's not an amphetamine, but in some ways it acts like one. Unlike the older antidepressants, it's more likely to wake you up than to put you to sleep, and it's more likely to cause weight loss than weight gain. It can also produce nervousness, sleeplessness, and, in rare cases, suicidal depression. These drawbacks aside, it's considered a major improvement over the older options. Prozac is now the antidepressant most often prescribed, reaping sales in 1989 of $350 million.

That's more than was spent on *all* antidepressants before Prozac hit the market in 1987.[4]

The tricyclic antidepressants

Before Prozac, the treatment favorites were the tricyclic antidepressants, including amitriptyline (Elavil), imipramine (Tofranil), and doxepin (Sinequan). It's not certain how tricyclic antidepressants work, but they may block the re-uptake of certain natural stimulants, increasing their availability at the nerve endings. The tricyclic's antidepressant properties were discovered by accident in the 1950s, when imipramine, the first to be used clinically, failed in its intended use as an antipsychotic for schizophrenic patients—but succeeded in cheering them up.

Though the tricyclic antidepressants lift the mood, they aren't actually stimulants. They are more likely to tranquilize and produce fatigue. They can also have other side effects, including low blood pressure and dizziness (experienced by 18–52 percent of patients, depending on the study), dry mouth (50–74 percent of patients), blurred vision (6–20 percent of patients), and urinary retention (5 percent of patients). More serious potential effects include excessively rapid heart beat, high blood pressure, tremors, and seizures. Since overdoses can be extremely toxic, doctors tend to give the smallest possible dose. The problem is that the drugs have a narrow therapeutic range. This means these small doses are often ineffective.

The tricyclics can also react adversely with other drugs, including tranquilizers, antihistamines, sedatives, sleeping pills, alcohol, narcotics, antihypertensives, levodopa, thyroid hormone, quinidine, MAO inhibitors, and other antidepressants.

Adverse effects and interactions are particularly likely in people over sixty. Yet this age group, constituting less than a seventh of the population, takes a third of all antidepressants prescribed. We'll look at the problem of depression in the elderly in chapter 38. Older people who can't avoid these drugs should at least reduce the dosage.[5]

For younger people, a new use has been found for the tricyclic antidepressant called desipramine. It seems to help curb the desire for cocaine. The drug doesn't cure the addiction, but it eases the craving.[6]

Table 35. *Popular Tricyclic Antidepressants*[7]

Generic Name/ Brand Names	Side Effects			
	sedation	seizures	dizziness on standing	arrhythmias
amitriptyline Amitril Limbitrol Elavil	++++	+++	++	++
amoxapine Asendin	++	+++	+	++
desipramine Norpramin	++	++	+++	+++
doxepin Adapin Sinequan	++++	+++	++	++
imipramine Tofranil	+++	+++	++++	++++
maprotiline Ludiomil	+++	++++	++	+++

++++ = high
+++   = moderate
++   = low
+   = very low

The MAO inhibitors

The first MAO inhibitor, iproniazid, was originally developed as a rocket fuel. Like the tricyclic antidepressants, its uplifting properties were discovered by accident in the 1950s. Iproniazid is no longer commercially available as an antidepressant, but three other MAO inhibitors are: phenelzine (Nardil), isocarboxazid (Marplan), and tranylcypromine (Parnate).

MAO inhibitors work by blocking the breakdown of certain amines in the body, including adrenalin and other chemicals produced in response to emotion. They can also inhibit the breakdown of amines such as tyramine in food. These can collect at the nerve endings and cause high blood pressure, resulting in a stroke or heart attack. Tyramine is found particularly in cheese, which should be strictly avoided by people on these drugs. Other dangerous foods include dairy products in general, pickles, red wine, and beer. In addition, hypertensive crises can occur when MAO inhibitors are mixed with a variety of other drugs, including allergy medications, sympathomimetic amines such as amphetamines, common cold remedies, ephedrine, levodopa, pemoline, narcotic analgesics, reserpine, tricyclic antidepressants, and tryptophan.

Other side effects of MAO inhibitors include tiredness, insomnia, nervousness, convulsions, confusion, dizziness, headaches, impotence, rashes, water retention, and weight gain.

Due to their potential for serious side effects and adverse interactions, MAO inhibitors are now generally limited to intractable cases that don't respond to other treatment.[8]

The newer antidepressants

Some of the MAO inhibitors' adverse effects and interactions are avoided by the newer antidepressants, including trazadone (Desyrel), bupropion (Wellbutrin), and fluoxetine (Prozac).

Trazadone is less likely to affect the heart, produce seizures or result in toxic overdose than other antidepressants. It can, however, cause "orthostatic hypotension," a sudden drop in blood pressure on standing that can be responsible for falls in the elderly. The drug can also be very sedating, interfering with daytime activities.

These problems were avoided by bupropion, which came on the market in 1985. It not only didn't put patients to sleep, but actually woke them up. It lacked significant cardiovascular activity, didn't cause dizziness, and often worked in cases where conventional drugs failed. Moreover where the older antidepressants impaired sexual function, for many patients bupropion actually improved it.

Unfortunately, in one study bupropion was found to be up to four times more likely to induce seizures than the older tricyclics. This downside was responsible for its withdrawal from the market soon after it became available. Other side effects included insomnia, agitation, dry mouth, headache, nausea, vomiting, constipation, and tremor. The drug may be marketed again after more study.

The current favorite is Prozac. It is the preferred alternative for patients with heart abnormalities. Not only bupropion but the tricyclic antidepressants can induce seizures in these patients. Prozac can, too; but the risk is a low 0.2 percent.

Prozac is being used to treat not only depression but anxiety, addiction, and bulimia. It is also good for obsessive-compulsive disorder. The tricyclics are generally ineffective for this condition, with the exception of another new option, clomipramine (Anafril). Prozac isn't sedating, and it has significantly fewer side effects than the older options.

Prozac can, however, have side effects. The most common are sleeplessness, nervousness, nausea, and anxiety. Unlike bupropion, it decreases both sexual interest and the ability to perform. And some 3.5 percent of patients who aren't suicidal before treatment get that way on the drug. Others get jittery and restless or experience tremors—symptoms reminiscent of amphetamines. Prozac works only 60 percent of the time, compared to a potential 80 percent with appropriately-prescribed tricyclics. Further, it's a new drug, whose track record is unknown. Enthusiasm for it rivals the 1960s craze for Valium, which now heads the list of dangerously addictive drugs.[9]

Viloxazine

Viloxazine is a drug marketed as an antidepressant all over the world except in the United States; but it is currently under review by the FDA. It may find a niche in the treatment of narcolepsy, a strange disorder that causes sufferers to fall asleep without warning at any time during the day. Until now, the condition has been treated with amphetamines, other stimulants, and antidepressants.

Viloxazine wakes up narcoleptics as well as the tricyclic antidepressants, but with fewer side effects. The most common side effects experienced by depressed patients using viloxazine are nausea and vomiting; and narcoleptics experience even fewer, since they need less of the drug.[10]

Lithium

Lithium is used to treat manic-depression, a condition characterized by extreme swings in mood, from exaggerated elation to gloomy depression. The drug is generally better for treating the "manic" than the "depressive" phase, since it tends to sedate the patient and make him lethargic.

Unlike most drugs, lithium isn't an organic compound but is a mineral ion. It is in the same family as sodium and potassium, and it competes with these minerals in the body. Lithium can have serious side effects; but for patients who really need it, they're liable to be worth the risk. Older patients should take only one-half to two-thirds the dose of younger adults, since normal therapeutic doses can make them confused and disoriented.[11]

The decision to treat depression with drugs

If antidepressants will prevent a suicide or keep a loved one off the mental wards, they are clearly justified. Suicide accounts for thirty-one thousand deaths a year in this country, and it's the number two cause of death among young adults in the vulnerable years between 15 and 24.

Before resorting to antidepressants, however, it's best to try to locate and eliminate any curable causes of the condition. Drugs may be appropriate in cases that can't be traced to any external, curable source. If your husband hasn't left you, your home life is fine, no one has died, and you're still depressed, you may have a chemical imbalance that can be corrected with drugs. Depression can also be caused by disease, and if the disease itself is incurable, drugs may help alleviate your distress. Diseases in this category are listed in table 36.

Something else to check before you turn to drugs is the ones you're already taking. Drugs themselves can be a major cause of depression. Known offenders include tranquilizers, sleeping pills, barbiturates, the heart drug reserpine, beta-blockers and other antihypertensive drugs, H2-blockers (Tagamet and Zantac), certain antibiotics, corticosteroids, and NSAIDs (see table 37).[12]

Drug-induced depression should not be treated with additional drugs. If you are taking drugs that can have this effect, check with your doctor to see if you can get by without them, or switch to something more uplifting.

If your depression has a recognizable external cause, you are probably better off with counseling than with drugs. If your husband *has* left you, with three kids and no job, drugs are liable to do you more harm than good.

For one thing, unlike the amphetamines that drop weight off, tricyclic antidepressants make you put it on; and what you don't need is to be a heavy divorcée. Your mirror will just make you more depressed. Studies show the weight gain from tricyclics to be linear: the longer you take the drugs, the more you gain. So if you're on them temporarily, get off them as soon as possible. Switching from one tricyclic to another won't do much good, since all of them have similar effects on body weight. The MAO inhibitors are even worse. The only currently available antidepressants not linked to weight gain are trazodone and fluoxetine.[13]

As William Cowper observed in the eighteenth century, grieving in appropriate situations is actually therapeutic. Psychiatrist David Viscott contends that if you repress these normal emotions with drugs, they will build up inside and produce other physical or mental ailments.

Table 36.   *Medical Diseases that Can Cause Depression[14]*

Of the heart and blood:	heart attack, stroke, congestive heart failure
Of the central nervous system:	brain tumors, Parkinson's disease, multiple sclerosis, Alzheimer's disease, Huntington's disease
Of the endocrine system:	diabetes, hypothyroidism, hyperthyroidism, hyperparathyroidism, Cushing's disease, Addison's disease
Miscellaneous:	rheumatoid arthritis, lupus, infectious disease, pernicious anemia, malnutrition, pancreatic disease, carcinoma, metabolic abnormalities

Table 37.   *Drugs that Can Cause Depression*

Mood-altering agents:	alcohol, chloral hydrate, benzodiazepines, barbiturates, meprobamate, major tranquilizers, stimulants (on withdrawal)
Antihypertensive and cardiovascular drugs:	propranolol, metoprolol, prazosin, clonidine, digitalis, procainamide, guanethidine, methyldopa, reserpine, hydralazine
Analgesics and anti-inflammatories:	indomethacin, phenylbutazone, opiates, pentazocine
Steroids:	corticosteroids, oral contraceptives, estrogen (on withdrawal)
Others:	major tranquilizers, stimulants (on withdrawal), cancer chemotherapeutic agents, antiparkinson drugs, ethambutol, certain antibiotics, H2-blockers

Nondrug alternatives

Marshall Mandell, an allergy specialist, estimates that the mood swings of four-fifths of the patients in mental hospitals can be traced to allergies or nutritional deficiencies.[15]

If you're allergic to certain foods, a reaction by the immune system can cause an inflammation in the brain that makes you moody and depressed. In a University of Chicago study, 16 of 23 psychiatric patients who thought their moods were related to food experienced marked irritability, anxiety, and depression when fed capsules of wheat or milk.

Similar effects can result from an inability to metabolize, or break down, certain foods properly. The sugar in milk or the ammonia from meat may be lingering in your system and causing headaches and irritability.

A third possibility is that you're suffering from nutritional deficiencies. Dramatic recoveries have been documented among schizophrenics given doses of certain nutrients.[16]

If you suspect a food allergy or intolerance, try an elimination diet in which you eat only neutral foods for several days—brown rice, sweet potatoes, vegetables, and non-citrus fruits. When your symptoms abate, add a new food you think might be the culprit. If nothing happens, add another. If you react badly, go back to the neutral diet. Try other foods until you've exhausted the likely possibilities.

Studies show exercise can also relieve anxiety and depression. Frequent, noncompetitive aerobic exercise or running seems to alter mood by stimulating endorphins, the brain's own natural "uppers."[17]

VI

Topicals

27

DRUGS TO REPEL BUGS AND RELIEVE ITCHING

We tend to think of drugs applied to the skin as being relatively harmless, since they're not taken into the body like those that are swallowed. This is, however, a misconception. Drugs taken by mouth go through the normal detoxification processes for which the stomach, kidneys, and liver were designed. Although drugs applied to the skin are less well absorbed, they go directly into the bloodstream, without metabolic intervention.

In fact, topical painkillers produce adverse reactions more frequently when applied to the skin than when swallowed. People who are allergic to foods or other substances should be especially careful with them. Babies' skin is particularly absorbent. Topical painkillers should not be used on children under two without a doctor's advice.[1]

The ability of the skin to absorb drugs is the basis for the latest in drug delivery systems, the transdermal patch applied to the skin. There are now transdermal patches for the delivery of motion sickness drugs, estrogen, antihypertensives, and other medications. Patches are the next best thing to continuous intravenous infusion, a delivery method generally limited to hospital patients. Where pills have to be taken according to the clock several times a day, transdermal patches can be left in place for one to three days or, in the case of blood pressure medications, for up to a week. Transdermal patches also have the advantages of constant bioavailability, minimizing fluctuations in blood levels of the drug; and of allowing the drug to bypass the liver, an organ that can render oral drugs inactive and can increase dose requirements.[2]

Itch relief

Of all skin disorders, the most common complaint is pruritis, or itching. It can be caused by insect bites and stings, poison ivy or oak, sunburn, or dry skin. It can also mean something more serious. In an estimated 10–50 percent of cases, generalized itching over a large area of the body that lasts more than a week is a symptom of systemic disease requiring a doctor's attention. Possible underlying causes include diabetes mellitus, hypothyroidism, gout, leukemia, lymphoma (cancer of the lymph nodes), infection by parasites, kidney failure, and liver disease.

Itching of the more mundane variety can be relieved by nonprescription remedies. Nature's remedy is scratching, but this can be overdone, leading to perpetuation rather than relief of symptoms. Over-the-counter anti-itch products may contain local anesthetics, antihistamines, corticosteroids, or counterirritants (see table 38).

Local anesthetics include those with active ingredients ending in "-caine." Their main drawback is that they can cause sensitivity reactions in susceptible people. People who react most severely to poison ivy and poison oak—and thus are in most need of relief—are, unfortunately, also the most likely to have an allergic reaction to local anesthetics. The result can be skin rash, hives, and eruptions, the very symptoms the drugs are intended to relieve.

When large amounts of some local anesthetics are applied to large areas of damaged skin, much of the drug is absorbed; and life-threatening, even lethal, toxic reactions can result. Offenders include lidocaine, dibucaine, and tetracaine. Fortunately, this reaction is rare; and it doesn't happen with the more popular benzocaine, which is insoluble in body fluids.

Antihistamines taken in liquid or chewable tablet form immediately after a sting, bite, or exposure to poison ivy or poison oak can block the histamine receptors before they have time to release their itch-provoking hormone. Antihistamines applied to the skin also seem to relieve itching, but why isn't clear. Relief is too fast for them to work the same way as oral antihistamines.

Methapyrilene was an antihistamine formerly approved for topical use, until studies showed it may cause cancer. It was replaced by the antihistamines phenyltoloxamine dihydrogen citrate and pyrilamine maleate, but their safety and effectiveness haven't yet been assessed by the FDA. Another topical antihistamine that seems to work is diphenhydramine hydrochloride, but it's only good on broken skin. It can't penetrate unbroken skin. It can also lose its effectiveness after several days' use and can eventually cause a skin reaction. The same is true for another topical antihistamine, tripelennamine hydrochloride.

Counterirritants like camphor, menthol, and phenol seem to work by causing a mild irritation at other skin sites, diverting the pain receptors at the site of irritation. Their soothing medicinal odors may also exert a placebo effect. Phenol, however, can cause serious skin burns; and if swallowed, it can cause internal injury,

Table 38. *Active Ingredients in Some Popular Over-the-Counter Products to Relieve Itching*[3]

Product	Active Ingredients
Americaine Anesthetic	benzocaine
Anbesol	benzocaine, phenol
Product	Active Ingredients
Bactine Antiseptic	lidocaine
Benadryl	diphenhydramine
Caladryl	diphenhydramine, calamine, camphor
Dermoplast	benzocaine
Domeboro	aluminum acetate
Ivarest	pyrilamine maleate, benzocaine, calamine
Medi-Quick	lidocaine
Nupercainal	dibucaine
Panthoderm	dexpanthenol
PBZ	tripelennamine
Pontocaine	tetracaine, menthol
Solarcaine	benzocaine, triclosan
Surfadil	diphenhydramine
Tronothane	pramoxine
Xylocaine	lidocaine
Ziradryl	diphenhydramine, zinc oxide

even in very weak concentrations. It should be kept away from children and should never be used to treat diaper rash.

The most effective treatment for itching and excess dryness of the skin (a major cause of itching) is probably the least used: the wet dressing. Wet dressings work because the water evaporating from them cools the skin. They also gently clean the skin.

To apply a wet dressing, soak a layer of gauze or thin cloth in water. (Diluted Burow's solution is sometimes recommended, but it contains high amounts of aluminum that may be absorbed by broken or inflamed skin. See chapter 21.) Apply the wet dressing to the irritated area. Soak and reapply the cloth every two or three minutes for 15–30 minutes. This procedure can be repeated several times a day. If itching covers an area too large for wet dressings, a cool bath can soothe irritation. Cool water constricts blood vessels. Avoid warm baths, which can increase vasodilation and itching.[4]

Topical steroid preparations

Corticosteroids are potent drugs that normally aren't sold without a prescription. However, the FDA has allowed two of them, hydrocortisone and hydrocortisone acetate, to be sold in low dosages over-the-counter for the self-treatment of minor skin irritations. Hydrocortisone is effective at relieving itch, but not pain; and its effects may not be felt for a day or two. Absorption is enhanced as much as fivefold in inflamed skin. Other steroids are sold for topical use by prescription only (see table 39).

A skin rash typically represents the body's attempt to expel irritants, and histamine is released in furtherance of this process (see chapter 6). Steroids are effective because they inhibit this natural elimination. They prevent the release of histamine by stabilizing the membranes of cells. If the irritant itself isn't removed, however, the rash is liable to come back in full force when the drug is stopped. This is another example of the "rebound effect" that plagues many drugs.

When inflammation is reduced, resistance to infection is also lowered. The result can be secondary infection, including boils and thrush. If steroids are used to treat skin disorders caused by infection, much more severe infections can result, which can spread over large areas or produce ugly skin ulcers.

Topical steroids used on children's skin or in large amounts by adults can enter the general circulation and reach the pituitary, where they can have systemic effects like those seen with systemic steroids (see chapter 7). Other potential adverse effects include allergic reactions, irreversible marks on the skin, unwanted hair growth, and acne.[5]

Table 39. *Popular Topical Steroids for Skin and Eyes*[6]

Generic name	Brand name
amcinonide	Cyclocort
betamethasone	Diprosone, Valisone
desonide	Tridesilon
desoximetasone	Topicort
dexamethasone	Decadron
fluocinolone	Synalar
fluocinonide	Lidex
fluorometholone	FML Liquifilm
flurandrenolide	Cordran
halcinonide	Halog
hydrocortisone	Hytone, Westcort
methylprednisolone	Medrol
triamcinolone	Aristocort, Aristocort A, Kenalog
Intended effects:	Relief of symptoms from inflamed or irritated skin or eyes
Adverse effects:	Burning, itching, irritation, dryness, acne, discolored or flattened skin areas, infection, weakening of tissue, unwanted hair growth, allergic reactions

Insect repellents

More people are killed each year by the stinging Hymenoptera—including bees, wasps, hornets, yellow jackets, and fire ants—than by any other poisonous animals, including rattlesnakes. Unfortunately, there are no effective repellents for these attackers. However, most chiggers, ticks, biting flies, mosquitoes, and other insects can be driven off by a topical insect repellent known as "DEET," short for "N,N-diethyl-m-toluamide." DEET is the active ingredient in popular brands of insect repellent like Off. Most brands contain only a little of it, but some, like Muskol, are pure DEET.

In this case, you're better off with the products containing the active ingredient in lower concentrations, since the risk of adverse reactions is highest with the highest-concentration brands. Chemicals that are sprayed on the skin are absorbed into the circulation, and about 10–15 percent of each dose of DEET can be recovered from the urine. Toxic effects are particularly likely in infants and young children, in whom excessive or prolonged use of ordinary insect repellents has caused serious reactions. As for the higher-concentration products, only brief exposure to smaller amounts has caused serious reactions in both children and adults, including anaphylactic shock and grand mal seizures. Swallowing DEET can be fatal.

Other insect repellents include 2-ethyl-1, 3-hexanediol (Rutgers 612) and dimethyl phthalate. They are effective against both mosquitoes and ticks, but not as effective as DEET. Citronella-based repellents (Natrapel and others) probably aren't effective against ticks but may give short-term protection from mosquitoes.

A cult insect repellent that is popular among campers is Avon's Skin-So-Soft. This concentrated bath oil contains di-isopropyl adipate, mineral oil, isopropyl palmitate, dioctyl sodium sulfosuccinate, fragrance, and the sunscreen benzophenone-11. In one study, Skin-So-Soft successfully repelled the mosquito that carries yellow fever. However, its long-term safety and effectiveness are unknown. According to the *Medical Letter,* while products containing DEET are usually effective for one to several hours, Skin-So-Soft may be effective for as little as ten to thirty minutes.[7] Skin-So-Soft has at least one advantage over DEET-based repellents: it smells significantly better.

Another insect repellent possibility is thiamine (a B vitamin). If you take 100 mg/day beginning a week before you're going to need it, it will come out in your skin. Bugs don't seem to like the smell and tend to stay away.

What to do about the stinging Hymenoptera

There are no effective repellents for this class of stinging insects, but there are medications you can use on the bites after you get them.

Normal reactions to insect stings involve pain, redness, swelling, itching, and warmth at the site of the bite. Reactions can be quite painful and annoying; but as long as they're confined to the area of the sting, they are considered normal inflammatory responses. For these normal reactions, ice can help lessen pain and swelling, and itching can be controlled by oral antihistamines or calamine lotion applied to the skin.

The reactions that require emergency treatment are those from multiple bites, which can produce toxic reactions in normal people; and allergic reactions in sensitive people to a single bite, which can be just as serious.

A serious allergic reaction is treated with epinephrine by injection, antihistamines by injection or orally, and adrenal steroids. If you know you're allergic to insect stings, you should keep an emergency insect treatment kit containing these items on hand (available only by prescription).

When determining whether to call a doctor if your child is stung, symptoms to look for are severe pain; redness or itching at the site of the sting; sudden, serious swelling of the lips, tongue, eyes or body; itching all over the body; hives (itchy bumps on the skin); wheezing, sudden coughing, or trouble breathing; dizziness and weakness; serious nausea; or collapse.[8]

Preventive measures include wearing clothes that are close-fitting, that cover as much of the body as possible, and that are boring to insects. Brightly colored clothes may be mistaken for flowers. Dark-colored clothing (brown or black) may also provoke an attack. The least interesting clothes to bees are those made from white or light khaki-colored materials. Scented soaps, perfumes, suntan lotions, and other cosmetics, as well as shiny jewelry or buckles, can also attract stinging insects. Bees won't attack unless you threaten their hives or step on them. If stung, remove the stinger and attached venom sac, since these can continue to inject venom after being torn from the insect.

28

EYE CARE

Drugs dropped into the eyes can reach the general circulation and have systemic effects even faster than those applied to the skin. Since the contact time with the eye is often only a fraction of a minute, eye medications are highly concentrated. They drain rapidly back into the mucus membranes of the nose; and from there, they can enter the bloodstream and reach the heart, lungs, and other organs without being detoxified.[1]

Unfortunately, the eyedrops that can do the worst damage are also the most indispensable: those for the treatment of glaucoma. Yet even over-the-counter eyedrops can be dangerous. If you use eyedrops and have unexplained systemic or psychiatric symptoms, you should report them to your ophthalmologist or physician to determine whether eyedrop absorption may be a possible cause.

Drugs for the treatment of glaucoma

Glaucoma is now estimated to affect nearly two million Americans. Its causes include injury, cataracts, and inflammation in the eye. Glaucoma can also be caused by drugs, including steroids and certain drugs that dilate the pupils.[2]

The condition is characterized by an increase in pressure within the eyeball sufficient to damage the optic nerve that carries images from the eye to the brain. Glaucoma causes visual loss that can lead progressively to blindness, unless the patient adheres to a lifelong daily drug regimen.

The problem is that the most common type, chronic or open-angle glaucoma, is asymptomatic. It causes no pain or immediate disability. On top of that, the drugs used to treat it can have annoying side effects. As a result, it's easy for glaucoma patients to lose interest in taking their medications, a temptation as many as half of them fall into. Failure to take glaucoma medications correctly has been called "a leading cause of glaucoma blindness."

To foster patient compliance, it was particularly important for ophthalmologists to find a drug that was easily administered and that had few side effects. Timolol (Timoptic), a beta-blocker approved for ophthalmologic use in 1978, seemed to be the answer. Its most popular predecessor, pilocarpine, generally had to be administered four times a day and frequently caused annoying side effects, including burning and stinging on application, brow aches, and visual disturbances. Timolol and its companion beta-blockers, betaxolol and levobunolol, had few eye-related side effects, and they had to be administered only once or twice a day.[3]

Timolol soon became the most commonly used antiglaucoma medicine in the world. But by 1987, two thousand cases of systemic toxicity had been reported to the National Registry of Drug-Induced Ocular Side Effects. These side effects were the same as those seen with beta-blockers taken orally. They included severe heart and breathing problems; low blood pressure and slowed heartbeat; acute suicidal depression and major personality disorders requiring hospitalization; and even death, from heart failure or acute asthmatic attack.

Timolol is still the drug of choice for glaucoma, but it is not recommended for patients with asthma or a history of asthma, chronic obstructive pulmonary disease, cardiovascular disease, or those taking oral beta-blocking drugs. If you need to use timolol, side effects can be reduced by proper administration, including pinching the bridge of the nose near the eyes after application. Ask your ophthalmologist for instructions.[4]

Alternative drugs that are now being tested on humans are the renin inhibitors, a class of drug that is also being studied for the treatment of hypertension. In animal studies, one renin inhibitor was found to be more potent and longer lasting than a leading antiglaucoma agent, with few apparent side effects.[5]

Topical eye medications that can cause glaucoma and other serious conditions

One cause of glaucoma can be drugs themselves. Culprits include corticosteroids and corticosteroid/antibiotic combinations. These drugs can have potentially devastating effects if improperly instilled in the eyes. They can not only cause glaucoma and cataracts, but can enhance eye infections. Corticosteroids suppress inflammation, and when inflammation is reduced, resistance is lowered and secondary infections can occur (see chapter 6).

One case involved an 87-year-old nursing home resident with a red eye. The nursing home physician gave her Cortisporin, a combination of corticosteroids and antibiotics. When her condition got worse, she was seen by an ophthalmologist, who diagnosed a herpes infection of the cornea. The condition remained chronic despite appropriate treatment.[6]

A second case involved a 29-year-old man who wore soft contact lenses. His optometrist prescribed Maxitrol, another antibiotic/corticosteroid combination, for an irritation in one of his eyes. His condition, too, got worse. He was subsequently diagnosed as having a herpes simplex keratitis infection, which did not heal. Corneal transplantation was ultimately required.[7]

A third case, described in chapter 4, involved the topical use of Cortisporin over a fifteen-month period to treat a rash around the eyes of a child. He wound up with glaucoma that caused blindness in one eye and partial blindness in the other.[8]

Chloramphenicol (Chloromycetin Ophthalmic) is another antibiotic that is available for topical use in the eyes as an ointment or drops. Oral chloramphenicol, however, is the drug most commonly associated with the potentially fatal blood disorder known as aplastic anemia; and similar blood disorders have been reported following the use of topical chloramphenicol in the eyes. Approximately half of nine such cases reported to the National Registry ended in death.[9]

For these reasons topical ocular chloramphenicol is virtually never indicated, except for conditions in which the infecting organism is resistant to all other antibiotics; and topical corticosteroids are recommended only when the diagnosis is clear and the need is compelling.

Drugs used by ophthalmologists to dilate the pupils have also been associated with glaucoma, as well as with certain rare but serious systemic side effects. One of these drugs is called cyclopentolate hydrochloride. Central nervous system effects, including visual hallucinations and schizophrenic and psychotic reactions, have been reported following its application in the eyes. These reactions were usually in children and involved formulations containing strong concentrations of the drug. A similar drug, called phenylephrine hydrochloride, has also been associated with uncommon but severe cardiovascular and other side effects. Reviewers suggest it should be used with caution, or not at all, for patients with heart conditions or diabetes, and for lightweight children.[10]

Over-the-counter eye medications

The innocuous-looking over-the-counter eye medications that are widely advertised as removing redness can also have dangerous side effects. Cases of blindness have actually been reported from their misuse.[11]

Even if these drops don't ruin your eyesight altogether, their daily use can make your eye problems worse. Like many other drugs, the drops can produce a rebound reaction that makes your eyes redder and more irritated than before you started using them.

Visine is currently the most popular over-the-counter eyedrop preparation. It and similar products contain an agent called tetrahydrozoline HCl, which makes the tiny blood vessels in your eyes constrict. This temporarily clears minor redness due to irritants. However, if you use the medicine repeatedly, your eyes react by dilating. This can lead to a vicious cycle of worsening eye redness and dependency on the drops.

A better option is the Murine formulation which omits the vessel-constricting medication. (There are two Murine formulations, one with tetrahydrozoline HCl, called "Murine Plus," and one without it.) Better yet, omit the drops, rest your eyes, and avoid irritants. If your problem persists, it may indicate something more serious that requires a doctor's attention.[12]

Bacterial eye infections and contact lenses

More than half the people in the United States need corrective lenses, and some twenty-one million of them have chosen to wear contact lenses. In 1987, more than 115,000 people elected to wear contacts just to change the color of their eyes.

Daily cleaning of contact lenses is very important to prevent a severe infection called ulcerative keratitis. This infection can occur when bacteria grow in the space between the contact lens and the cornea. It can result in permanent eye damage and even blindness. Researchers estimate an annual rate of 12,000 cases among contact-lens wearers. Among extended-wear contact-lens users, the risk is especially high. Studies indicate their rate of infection is five times greater than for ordinary lens wearers. If they wear their lenses while sleeping, the risk is ten to fifteen times greater.

There are three basic types of contact lenses—hard, soft, and gas-permeable. For cleaning, each type requires its own contact lens care system. It is particularly important that hard contact lens solutions not be used with soft contact lenses, since this can damage both the lenses and your eyes.[13] Ask your optometrist which products are best for your lenses.

If you are having chronic eye problems, see an ophthalmologist (an M.D. specializing in eye diseases).

29

DRUGS FOR BLEMISHED SKIN

Beauty's but skin deep.

—John Davies (1606)

Given the choice between looking good and feeling good, many people will unflinchingly go for the former.

One woman had such disfiguring acne, she was embarrassed to be seen in public. For her, Accutane was a wonder drug that wiped her mirror clean. Its side effects were a small price to pay for the self-confidence she gained from a normal, clear complexion.

A second woman lived to regret the same choice. A beautiful New York model in her twenties, she had only a few blemishes on otherwise perfect skin; but in her profession, they loomed large. Her dermatologist prescribed Accutane, which she took. Her skin and lips are now permanently dry and chapped, and she can no longer go out much in the sun.

Accutane (isotretinoin) is one of a class of vitamin A derivatives called retinoids. Another drug in this class, etretinate (Tigison), is used mainly in the treatment of psoriasis. These drugs have revolutionized dermatology. In intractable cases, they are indeed wonder drugs; but the price in side effects is very high. A related drug is the "antiwrinkle cream" tretinoin (Retin-A), which we'll look at in the next chapter.

Accutane

In industrialized Western countries, acne in some form affects four out of five teenagers and young adults.[1] Isotretinoin (Accutane) has been called "the greatest single advance thus far" in its treatment. Over a million patients have used it. The drug has produced dramatic clearing of lesions in severe, recalcitrant, cystic acne that is unresponsive to conventional therapy.[2]

Enthusiasm for its beneficial effects, however, has been tempered by concern over its serious side effects and heavy toll in birth defects. In a study of 154 women who took Accutane while pregnant, their odds of having a child with major malformations turned out to be about fifty-fifty. That's if the child was actually born. Spontaneous abortions were also common. In theory, this risk could be eliminated by taking precautions to avoid pregnancy while taking the drug. But among those women for whom contraceptive information was available, a third who bore malformed infants conceived *despite* using contraception.[3]

Not only is it impossible to ensure that young women won't get pregnant while taking Accutane; young users also risk stunted skeletal development. The drug has been linked to premature closure of the bones.[4] These concerns have prompted consumer groups to try to have it removed from the market.

Side effects experienced by Accutane users are similar to those resulting from an overdose of vitamin A. Skin reactions are the most common and annoying. Nearly everyone receiving therapeutic doses of the drug experiences drying and inflammation of the lips. Chapping, itching, inflammation, and dryness of the skin are also frequent. Some patients experience dryness in the eyes and an increased sensitivity to sunlight. These symptoms may not go away after the drug course is completed. Some patients also suffer vague aches and pains in the muscles and bones. Others lose a portion of their hair, or find their skin problems get worse, especially if they're taking tetracycline antibiotics at the same time. Headaches and depression can also result. Liver function can become altered and triglycerides elevated. This means careful monitoring is necessary in patients with a history of coronary artery disease, hepatitis, or inflammation of the pancreas.[5]

For these reasons, specialists recommend that Accutane be used only on patients with deeply seated cystic or pustular acne that is unresponsive to any other form of treatment, and who have been carefully screened for contraindications by physicians who are thoroughly familiar with the drug.[6]

Drugs to avoid if you are taking accutane include vitamin A, tetracycline, micocycline, alcohol, benzoyl peroxide, sulfur, tretinoin, and topical agents that cause drying of the skin.

Topical antibiotics

An older therapy for acne is topical antibiotic treatment. Tetracycline, erythromycin, or clindamycin (Cleocin) may be applied directly to the skin. The drugs reduce inflammatory lesions, apparently by their antibiotic action; but the mechanism is uncertain, since too little of the drug is absorbed to have systemic effects. Another mechanism involves the reduction of fatty acids in skin lesions.

The problem with antibiotic therapy is that prolonged or repeated use of the drugs can render antibiotics less effective when they're needed for infections. It can also result in bacterial or fungal overgrowths of nonsusceptible organisms, producing secondary infection. The risk of fungal *Candida* infection may outweigh the benefits of the antibiotics, since *Candida* can actually cause skin problems.[7] Long-term low doses of antibiotics have also been linked to chronic diseases like interstitial cystitis (a sort of perpetual bladder infection without bacteria).

Controlling simple acne

So what do you do for ordinary acne? To keep symptoms under control, you can take the following measures:

1. Wash with ordinary soap and water. Dr. Bronner's pure castile soap is good. Medicated cleansers are a waste of money, because the medication washes off; and granular facial scrubs work no better than a washcloth. Facial saunas can aggravate acne.

2. Change your cosmetics and facial cleaners. Avoid lanolin, which can cause skin reactions. Use either water-based cosmetics or none at all. Avoid greasy hair dressings and wear your hair away from your face.

3. Resist the urge to pick at blemishes, a habit that increases the risk of pits and scars.

4. Try garlic and parsley tablets in high doses, and supplements of zinc, beta-carotene, and vitamin E.

5. For severe outbreaks, see a dermatologist. He may prescribe drying agents like benzoyl peroxide or other remedies.[8]

6. Look for the cause and try to eliminate it.

Treating the cause

While Accutane, antibiotics, and other drug treatments treat symptoms, the ideal cure would reach the cause. Unfortunately, the cause of skin eruptions can be very hard to find.

Hormones are known to have a strong influence on the skin. Acne rages during the raging hormone years of the teens. Flare-ups tend to be worse for women the week before their menstrual periods. Many dermatologists are investigating treatments that alter these underlying hormonal changes.

An older hormonal treatment that is less used today is the birth control pill. Estrogen is thought to improve acne by suppressing the sebaceous glands' production of oil. But when the Pill was introduced in the 1960s, it contained much higher levels of estrogen than those now prescribed. Today, improvements in the complexions of Pill-takers are much less common; and many women notice a worsening of acne when they stop taking the Pill. Oral contraceptives also have other side effects and risks, which far outweigh any benefits to the skin (see chapter 31).

Another hormonal therapy being tried by some dermatologists is small doses of corticosteroids. These drugs can be dangerous, however, since they blunt the response of the adrenal gland to stress (see chapter 7). They should be used only where conventional acne treatments have failed.[9]

In some cases, the problem is traced to drugs the sufferer is already taking. In fact, drug eruptions are among the most common skin disorders encountered by the dermatologist. Even common over-the-counter drugs can be responsible. A 1988 article in the medical journal *Dermatologica* reports the case of a woman whose skin eruptions were traced to a daily aspirin habit.[10]

In the introduction to this book, we discussed a woman's complexion problems that were traced to the fluoride in her city's water. Fluoridation of the public water supply has long been controversial. As far back as 1977, the National Toxicology Program (NTP) was ordered to determine whether fluoride causes cancer. In February of 1990, the NTP finally released data showing that rats given fluoridated water have a significantly increased incidence of a rare bone cancer called osteosarcoma. This data rekindled an issue long thought settled.[11]

The link between fluoride and acne could be even harder to trace. If this woman's sharp dermatologist hadn't spotted it in her case, her serious complexion problems would probably have been treated as an infection, with tetracycline or other antibiotics. The fluoride connection was proved when she switched to bottled water and unfluoridated tooth products. Her skin cleared up dramatically.

There is no scientific proof that chocolate, nuts, or colas trigger acne outbreaks, but anecdotal evidence suggests they do. Since these foods have no redeeming dietary virtues, cutting them out can't hurt.

A macrobiotic diet has been reported to work miracles for some people. Skin problems may also be caused by hidden food allergies. To find them, try an elimination diet, systematically eliminating foods that are potential offenders.[12] (See chapter 26.)

DRUGS FOR AGING SKIN AND HAIR: RETIN-A, MINOXIDIL, AND SUNSCREENS

[Dr. Albert Kligman, discoverer of Retin-A] says some of his patients are so enthusiastic about Retin-A that they come back to him just a few weeks after starting treatment and tell him they look much younger and prettier. But as the saying goes, beauty is often in the eye of the beholder. "I'll be damned if I can see it," he says. [1]

—*Washington Post Health* (1988)

Hopes of the fountain of youth were revived and a run on available supplies was precipitated by a much-publicized study published in the *Journal of the American Medical Association* in 1988. It reported the effectiveness of Retin-A, or retinoic acid, in removing wrinkles. Retin-A is approved by the FDA only for the treatment of acne, but once a drug is on the market, a physician can write a prescription for it for any reason. The study found that in 14 of 15 subjects, the daily application of Retin-A over a four-month period decreased wrinkles, improved the texture of the skin, and gave it a rosy "pinkness." [2]

By the second week after the study came out, the drug's manufacturer had added a second shift to fill orders; and women were reportedly traveling as far as Mexico to get the drug. Retin-A is available there over-the-counter at a tenth the high American prescription price.

Alas, wonder drugs are rarely everything they're promoted to be. As one dermatologist noted, improved appearance needn't be the result of deep changes in the skin. Wrinkles can also disappear as a result of increased skin swelling. Over 90 percent of the study subjects using Retin-A experienced swelling and redness where the cream was applied. Ten patients withdrew before the end of the trial, three due to severe dermatitis caused by the drug. Eleven of the fifteen remaining subjects required strong steroid creams to relieve this symptom.

A doctor consulting for the *Medical Letter* reported that his cosmetic results with the drug were disappointing, and that a few of his patients developed red blotches and brown areas on their faces after using the drug.

More serious than irritation to the skin may be another side effect: extreme sensitivity to the sun. It results when Retin-A peels away the outer layer of skin. There is some evidence that the drug may actually help prevent skin cancer, by interfering with the growth of tumors. But its long-term effects are still unknown. In hairless albino mice, retinoic acid has *increased* the incidence of cancers induced by sun exposure.

Another question mark is birth defects. None have yet been reported; but retinoic acid is chemically similar to isotretinoin, which produces birth defects as often as 50 percent of the time.[3]

Even for satisfied customers, the skin is liable to get worse before it gets better; and improvement may take as long as six months. Further, maintaining a youthful look probably means taking the drug for life, an expensive proposition.

Other options for aging skin

Another new product for aging skin that has received none of the fanfare of Retin-A, but which may be equally effective with fewer side effects, is a lactic acid preparation called Epilyt. According to Dr. Howard Baden, professor of dermatology at the Harvard Medical School, Epilyt can alter the surface of the skin in a way that makes it look younger, with far less irritation than Retin-A. Any topical preparation containing lactic acid will have this effect; and if the cream contains less than 6 percent lactic acid, it can be obtained without a prescription.[4]

The best way to preserve the skin, however, is to avoid the causes of skin damage. Tobacco use is one. Sunshine is another. In fact sun damage, rather than aging itself, is responsible for most of the age-related changes of the skin. This damage, called "photo-aging," can be controlled by avoiding the sun, wearing hats, and using sun-screens.[5]

Sunscreens

Photo-aging isn't the worst thing that can happen from exposure to the sun. The most dire result is skin cancer. Skin cancers due to ultraviolet radiation are the most common form of cancer. They include basal cell and squamous cell carcinomas, which are usually curable; and melanoma, which is much less common but much more serious, often ending in death.

Experts estimate that half of our total lifetime exposure to ultra-violet (UV) radiation generally occurs before we're eighteen. Reducing exposure during the early years can significantly reduce the effects of the sun that show up later in life—sagging, leathery, blotchy skin; wrinkles; and skin cancer. Regular use of a sunscreen for the first eighteen years of life has been estimated to decrease the lifetime incidence of basal and squamous cell carcinomas by 78 percent.

The most prudent thing to do is to keep your children and yourself out of the sun between 10 A.M. and 3 P.M., the hours of greatest UV intensity. But that can be difficult, especially for children who attend summer camp or day-care centers. Sending them with broad-brimmed hats can help, but children don't always keep their hats on. The other option is to send them off lathered in a long-acting sunscreen, with a note to the counselor requesting reapplication after swimming, sweating, or extended periods in the sun.

Sunscreens are most effective when applied thirty to sixty minutes before sun exposure, so they can penetrate into the skin. They should be reapplied often. Even those marked "water-resistant" will come off with towel-drying or sweating.

What "Sun Protection Factor" (SPF) should you buy? The SPF value is the time required to produce minimal sunburn with the product, divided by the time required to produce the same sunburn without the product. In other words, a sunscreen with an SPF of 2 doubles the time it takes to get a modest burn. Reapplication, however, doesn't prolong the period of protection. The value relates to each time the product is applied and isn't additive. If you get sunburned in an hour without sunscreen and you use a product with an SPF of 2, you'll get sunburned in two hours, no matter how many times you apply the product. SPF values go as high as 50, but a value higher than 15 is rarely needed.[6]

How thick you apply the sunscreen is important. In a recent study, fifty people were asked to apply the products as they normally would. In general, the layer thickness they applied was only half the suggested recommendation; and the average protection provided by the products was found to be only half the SPF designated by the manufacturer.[7]

Unfortunately, like all drugs, sunscreens aren't without their own perils. Some of them can, themselves, cause photosensitivity reactions, as well as an inflammation of the skin on contact. Allergic reactions have also been reported. Sunscreens that block ultraviolet light also block the skin's synthesis of vitamin D, which is necessary for proper bone strength. Elderly people, particularly, can end up with vitamin D deficiency from regular sunscreen use.

Another shortcoming of sunscreens is that they may not prevent the photosensitivity reactions caused by other drugs. Accutane and Retin-A are two drugs that cause an increased sensitivity to sunlight, but there are many others (see table 40). Even brief exposure to sunlight in warm or cold weather can cause intense skin reactions in people who have used these agents, and some continue to be sensitive to the sun long after they stop using them.[8]

The most popular sunscreens are aminobenzoic acid esters, benzophenones, cinnamates, salicylates, and anthranilates. They generally have their peak absorption in the midrange of ultraviolet light

(UVB). UVB is the type of radiation that reaches the earth mainly between 10 A.M. and 3 P.M., and it's the major cause of sunburn.

There is, however, another type of ultraviolet radiation—long-range ultraviolet, or UVA—which remains fairly constant throughout the day. It can cause sunburn after an hour's exposure, and it also contributes to aging and skin cancer. UVA is what causes most drug-induced photosensitivity reactions. Among sunscreens that are commonly used, only those containing benzophenones and anthranilates absorb UVA; and their absorption is far from complete. Photoplex, which contains butyl methoxydibenzoylmethane, is the first of a new class of broad spectrum sunscreens that absorb both UVB and UVA.[9]

Even chemical sunscreens that block UVA, however, may not prevent the photosensitivity reactions caused by drugs. And those containing cinnamates, oxybenzone, and aminobenzoic acid and its esters can actually cause photosensitivity.[10]

Minoxidil and balding

Only one other topical medication has approached the interest generated by Retin-A. It's minoxidil (Rogaine), an antihypertensive used topically to restore hair growth. Its hair-growing potential was discovered by accident, when patients taking it in tablet form for high blood pressure observed the effect.

Unfortunately, like Retin-A, Rogaine is not a miracle cure for reversing time's ravages. In controlled trials, it produced "dense" hair growth in only 8 percent of users after a year's application; and that growth was only about a fifth as thick as normal growth. It was also only on the crown of the head. The drug had little effect on receding hairlines or balding temples. A further 31 percent experienced a thin fluff of new growth. Only 16 percent of the men in these two groups found regrowth sufficient to continue the treatment; and the other 61 percent got little or no new hair at all.

Up to eight months may be required before effects are noticeable enough to know if the drug is going to work; and like Retin-A, minoxidil has to be applied daily for life to keep up its effects. At $45 to $55 per month, this can, again, be an expensive proposition.

Although no serious side effects were noted in the trials, some men experienced severe itching; and the long-term effects of the drug are unknown. Changes in blood fat levels, for example, could take two to three years to appear. Moreover, the test group consisted of men under fifty. Older men who might be suffering from cardiovascular disease were specifically excluded. Yet older men are those most likely to be interested in the drug.[11]

Table 40. *Drugs that Can Cause Photosensitivity*[12]

Anticancer drugs
    dacarbazine (DTIC-Dome)
    fluorouracil (Fluoroplex and others)
    methotrexate (Mexate and others)
    procarbazine (Matulane)
    vinblastine (Velban)

Antidepressants
    amitriptyline (Elavil and others)
    amoxapine (Asendin)
    desipramine (Norpramin, Pertofrane)
    doxepin (Adapin, Sinequan)
    imipramine (Tofranil and others)
    isocarboxazid (Marplan)
    maprotiline (Ludiomil)
    nortriptyline (Aventyl, Pamelor)
    protriptyline (Vivactil)
    trimipramine (Surmontil)

Antihistamines
    cyproheptadine (Periactin)
    diphenhydramine (Benadryl and others)

Antimicrobials
    demeclocycline (Declomycin and others)
    doxycycline (Vibramycin and others)
    griseofulvin (Fulvicin-U/F and others)
    methacycline (Rondomycin)
    minocycline (Minocin)

nalidixic acid (NegGram)
oxytetracycline (Terramycin and others)
sulfacytine (Renoquid)
sulfadoxine-pyrimethamine (Fansidar)
sulfamethazine (Neotrizine and others)
sulfamethizole (Thiosulfil and others)
sulfamethoxazole (Gantanol and others)
sulfamethoxazole-trimethoprim (Bactrim and others)
sulfasalazine (Azulfidine and others)
sulfisoxazole (Gantrisin and others)
tetracycline (Achromycin and others)

Antiparasitic Drugs
bithionol (Bitin)
pyrvinium pamoate (Povan)
quinine (many manufacturers)

Antipsychotic Drugs
chlorpromazine (Thorazine and others)
chlorprothixine (Taractan)
fluphenazine (Permitil, Prolixin)
haloperidol (Haldol)
perphenazine (Trilafon)
piperacetazine (Quide)
prochlorperazine (Compazine and others)
promethazine (Phenergan and others)
thioridazine (Mellaril)
thiothixene (Navane)
trifluoperazine (Stelazine and others)
triflupromazine (Vesprin)
trimeprazine (Temaril)

Diuretics
acetazolamide (Diamox)
amiloride (Midamor)
bendroflumethiazide (Naturetin and others)
benzthiazide (Exna and others)
chlorothiazide (Diuril and others)
cyclothiazide (Anhydron)
furosemide (Lasix)
hydrochlorothiazide (Hydrodiuril and others)
hydroflumethiazide (Diucardin and others)
methyclothiazide (Aquatensen, Enduron)

metolazone (Diulo, Zaroxolyn)
polythiazide (Renese)
quinethazone (Hydromox)
trichlormethiazide (Metahydrin and others)

Hypoglycemics
acetohexamide (Dymelor)
chlorpropamide (Diabinese, Insulase)
glipizide (Glucotrol)
glyburide (DiaBeta, Micronase)
tolazamide (Tolinase)
tolbutamide (Orinase and others)

Nonsteroidal Anti-Inflammatory Drugs
ketoprofen (Orudis)
naproxen (Naprosyn)
phenylbutazone (Butazolidin and others)
piroxicam (Feldene)
sulindac (Clinoril)

Sunscreens
6-acetoxy-2, 4-dimethyl-m-dioxane (preservative in sunscreens)
benzophenones (Aramis, Clinique, and others)
cinnamates (Aramis, Estee Lauder, and others)
oxybenzone (Eclipse, PreSun, and others)
PABA esters (Eclipse, Block Out, Sea & Ski, and others)
para-aminobenzoic acid (PABA-Pabagel, Pabanol, Pre-Sun, and others)

Other Agents
amiodarone (Cordarone)
bergamot oil, oils of citron, lavender, lime, sandalwood, cedar (used in many
    perfumes and cosmetics, also topical exposure to citrus rind oils)
benzocaine
captopril (Capoten)
carbamazepine (Tegretol)
contraceptives, oral
disopyramide (Norpace)
gold salts (Myochrysine, Solganol)
hexachlorophene (pHisoHex and others)
isotretinoin (Accutane)
6-methylcoumarin (used in perfumes, shaving lotions, and sunscreens)
musk ambrette (used in perfumes)
quinidine sulfate and gluconate 2

VII

Drugs, Sex, and Reproduction

31

FOR WOMEN ONLY

[The finding of a fourfold increase in breast cancer risk] hits at the heart of our philosophy that patients should be on estrogen and progestin.
—Jonathan S. Berek, M.D.[1]

Some women are afflicted with premenstrual tension, and all are eventually hit with menopause. For the most part, women also carry the burden of contraception. All attempts at a contraceptive pill for men have failed. Pharmacies supply a range of products addressed to these and other female problems.

Estrogen replacement after menopause

The loss of estrogen at menopause is blamed for a variety of midlife feminine ills. The pharmaceutical answer to the ravages of time is estrogen replacement therapy (ERT). Experts estimate that one-third to one-half of all postmenopausal American women are now taking ERT; and among upper-middle-class women, the percentage is higher yet. In wealthy Marin County, California, the figure may be as high as 75 percent.[2] ERT is promoted as relieving many midlife problems, including the hot flashes and sweating of menopause, the loss of sleep and irritability that go with them, abnormal bleeding, and, now, osteoporosis or bone loss.

Osteoporosis is a serious problem for elderly women. Four out of five hip fractures are linked to it. Between 15 percent and 34 percent of these fractures result in death within six months of the event; and for those who survive, hip fracture can mean relegation to nursing homes. A study reported in the *New England Journal of Medicine* in 1987 found that postmenopausal women who had taken estrogens at any time were only two-thirds as likely to suffer a hip fracture as those who had not; and women who had taken estrogens within the previous two years were only one-third as likely to fracture their hips.[3]

These findings are significant, but the question that hasn't yet been resolved is whether this benefit outweighs the risks of ERT. In August of 1989, Swedish researchers publishing in the *New England Journal of Medicine* reported that taking a combination of estrogen and progestin (a synthetic form of the female hormone progesterone) for six years or longer raised breast cancer rates to 4.4 times what they were in women not taking these hormones. This finding is particularly ominous given the overall incidence of breast cancer, which strikes one out of eleven women and kills thirty-seven thousand a year. The risk of endometrial cancer is also increased between fourfold and eightfold with estrogen therapy. Risks or gallbladder disease, high blood pressure, and diabetes are also higher.[4]

The Swedish study involved 23,244 women on ERT. It found that in the potent form known as estradiol used widely in Europe, estrogen alone increased breast cancer risk by 200 percent. In the conjugated form commonly used in the United States, however, estrogen alone didn't affect that risk. The finding that bodes ill for American women involved the estrogen/progestin combination, which is the form in which most American women receive ERT. This combination increased the risk of breast cancer more than fourfold. Ironically, the purpose of taking these drugs in combination is to counteract the risk of uterine cancer, which estrogen increases by as much as fourteen times when taken alone.

The Swedish women's risk of breast cancer also increased with the length of time they'd received ERT. Women who had been on it nine years or more were 70 percent more likely than other women to contract the disease. The message, according to researchers, is that women shouldn't take these powerful hormones indefinitely. Studies suggest there is no added risk in taking them for up to five years.[5]

The trouble is that to forestall bone loss, you may need to take estrogen for life. When estrogen is stopped, rapid bone loss occurs. Within four years of stopping ERT, no difference in bone mineral content has been found between women who were never treated and those who began treatment but discontinued it.[6]

Women who have had a hysterectomy need estrogen replacement, but they don't need progestin. They can do without its protection against cancer of the uterus, since they don't have uteruses. If they want to stop taking estrogen, they can do so at about age 45, when the estrogen produced by the ovaries would have declined anyway.[7]

If you definitely need estrogen replacement, the latest in delivery systems is a transdermal patch called Estraderm. The drug goes directly to the blood, avoiding gastrointestinal effects; doses are much lower; and serum concentrations more closely resemble those found naturally before menopause. Nausea is also less frequent than with oral estrogen, although other side effects are similar, and skin irritation may result from the patch. Whether transdermal estrogen is safer than oral forms remains to be determined.[8]

Nondrug options

Fortunately, ERT isn't the only way to cut the risk of fracture-causing falls. About the same reduction would result from eliminating the tranquilizers and sleeping pills many older people take routinely. A recent study found that drugs causing dizziness, sedation, and fuzzy thinking are a major cause of falls leading to hip fracture in the elderly. Older people were about twice as likely to suffer hip fractures if they were taking tranquilizers with long half-lives, like flurazepam (Dalmane); tricyclic antidepressants, including amitriptyline (Elavil), doxepin (Sinequan), and imipramine (Tofranil); or antipsychotics, including thioridazine (Mellaril), haloperidol (Haldol), and chlorpromazine (Thorazine).[9]

Another factor contributing to bone loss is faulty diet. Calcium is a critical variable; but whether increasing calcium intake can repair already-dissolving bones is a controversial question, which we'll look at in chapter 36.

Anomalously, women in Third World countries eating grain- and vegetable-based diets don't suffer increased rates of hip fracture after menopause, although their calcium intakes are far below American women's. The pivotal difference seems to be their protein intake, which is also far below ours. A too-high protein intake has been shown to leach calcium from the bones. American Seventh-Day Adventist women, who avoid meat consumption for religious reasons, are also reported not to be afflicted with osteoporosis. The minimum daily requirement of protein for women is only 44 grams, about half the average American intake. The unnecessary half imposes a significant drain on calcium stores, which can be preserved with a low-protein, plant-based diet.[10]

Contraception

Estrogen is also popular with younger women, in the form of oral contraceptives. The Pill is the most popular reversible method of contraception among American women and the second most popular contraceptive method after sterilization. The second most popular reversible method is the one most often recommended by pharmacists: the condom. After these come spermicides, withdrawal, the diaphragm, periodic abstinence, and the intrauterine device (IUD). The diaphragm, which ranks fourth, is first in popularity among women physicians.[11]

After sterilization, the Pill is not only the most popular, but also the most reliable method of preventing pregnancy. Other methods, however, get more reliable as you get older. How effective a contraceptive method is varies directly with your age, your socioeconomic status, and your level of education. Younger, poorer, less educated women are more likely to conceive by mistake. Table 41 shows the comparative effectiveness of various contraception methods during the first year of use for all married women, and for married women over thirty who made over $30,000 a year during the years 1970–75.[12]

Table 41. *First-Year Contraceptive Failures During 100 Woman/Years of Use*

Method	All Women	Women Over 30 with Higher Incomes
Sterilization	0	0
Oral contraceptive	2.5	0.8
IUD	4.8	1.5
Condom	9.6	0.9
Diaphragm	14.4	6.4
Spermicide	17.7	6.1
Rhythm	18.8	8.3

The Pill

Over fifty million women have used oral contraceptives since they first came on the market in the 1960s. During this time, dosage and dosing schedules have changed, making the Pill safer and subject to fewer side effects. The original fixed-dose combinations were replaced first by sequential dosing. The latest innovation is the "multiphasic" oral contraceptive, in which the dose of progestin is varied during the menstrual cycle so that the total steroid dose per month is reduced. Multiphasics containing norethindrone (Ortho-Novum 7/7/7, Tri-Norinyl) seem to be the most effective while having the least impact on the body.[13]

Even the updated Pill, however, can have side effects, including dizziness, headaches, tiredness, depression, hypertension, and edema (water retention). More serious is the possibility of pulmonary embolism (a blood clot lodged in the pulmonary artery).[14]

On the plus side, users of the Pill have a lower incidence of endometrial cancer, ovarian cancer, premenstrual syndrome, iron-deficiency anemia, and spinal bone loss.

On the minus side, users of the Pill have an increased risk of cervical cancer, and certain groups of users may have an increased risk of breast cancer. The evidence on this point is contradictory. A study published in the *New England Journal of Medicine* in August of 1987 found no increased breast cancer risk; but a Swedish study published in the British medical journal *The Lancet* found a highly increased risk among teenage Pill users.[15]

Older studies found an increased risk of heart attack and stroke from the Pill, but this risk hasn't been documented with the newer formulations except in women over 35 who smoke or have preexisting cardiovascular problems. Women who smoke heavily and take the Pill are over twenty times more likely to have a heart attack than other women. Oral contraceptives result in a mild elevation of blood pressure in most women and in overt hypertension in about 5 percent of them. Also, adverse changes in HDL and LDL cholesterol levels are produced by all the progestins currently used in oral contraceptives available in the United States. Multiphasic formulations using norgestrel (Triphasil, Tri-levlen)—although not those using norethindrone—can also cause a deterioration in glucose tolerance, predisposing a woman to diabetes.

The Pill has the further drawback of delaying conception when it is desired. Ultimately, however, Pill users seem to conceive as frequently and successfully as users of other contraceptive methods.[16]

Many drugs reduce the effectiveness of oral contraceptives and increase the incidence of breakthrough bleeding when taken with them, including barbiturates, phenytoin, ifoniazid, neomycin, penicillin, tetracycline, chloramphenicol, griseofulvin sulfonamide, nitrofurantin analgesics, tranquilizers, antihistamines and anti-migraine drugs.

The IUD

Another convenient but hazardous contraceptive method is the IUD. It significantly increases the risk of pelvic inflammatory disease (PID), an infection that can damage the fallopian tubes and lead to infertility. The *Journal of the American Medical Association* called PID "one of the most widespread and debilitating diseases affecting women today" and predicted that its costs, including those of tubal pregnancy and infertility, could total $3.5 billion a year by 1990. IUDs also increase menstrual blood loss and iron-deficiency anemia; and itching and allergic dermatitis have been reported.

The earliest successful IUD was the Dalkon Shield. It was developed in 1967, and sales began worldwide in 1971. They were halted in 1974—but only in the U.S.—after the device was associated with painful and sometimes lethal PID in women who became pregnant while wearing it. Of the 2.3 million women who used the device in the early 1970s, tens of thousands suffered permanent uterine damage. The manufacturer, A.H. Robins, filed for bankruptcy in 1975 after having settled 9,500 claims for a total of $530 million. To date, 330,000 claims have been filed, and more are expected. A.H. Robins, which also manufactures Chap Stick and Robitussin, has been ordered by the court to put $2.48 billion into a trust for claimants.

G.D. Searle & Co. began selling the Copper-7 and the Tatum-T in 1974. These two devices have also now been voluntarily withdrawn by the manufacturer, following increasing numbers of product-liability lawsuits. About 1,300 Copper-7 lawsuits have been filed, and over 400 are still pending. In one case, a federal jury in St. Paul awarded $8.7 million to a woman who claimed the Copper-7 had made her infertile. This is more than a tenth of the nearly $80 million the drug generated in the twelve years it was on the market.

The IUDs currently available are the Progestasert, which gradually releases progesterone, and the new Copper-T, the only available nonchemical IUD. The Copper-T is somewhat more effective than earlier versions, but it may cause more bleeding and pain. Pregnancy rates seem to be lower than the already-low rates for earlier models, but removals for bleeding or pain are high—about one in four by the end of four years' use.

Women who should particularly avoid the IUD are those with multiple sex partners, those with a history of PID, those under 25 who have never had children, and those who want children in the future.[17]

Barrier methods

"Barrier" contraceptive methods—condoms and diaphragms—aren't as convenient as the Pill or the IUD. However, they have the advantages that they don't affect how you feel or cause unwanted long-term side effects; and they reduce the transmission of sexually transmitted diseases, especially when used with spermicides.

Barrier methods also aren't as reliable for preventing pregnancy, but they get more reliable with age and practice. In one recent study, first-year failure rates for condoms used by couples under the age of 25 were between 10 percent and 33 percent. This rate dropped to a low 1–4 percent when the users passed the thirty-year mark.[18]

One thing that can cause condoms to fail is the wrong lubricant. A 1989 study released by the University of California, Los Angeles, found that the lubricants most widely used with condoms can cause the rubber to rupture within a mere sixty seconds after application. The dangerous lubricants were all oil-based, including body and hand lotions, products containing mineral oil, vegetable-based cooking oils, shortenings, and butter. The safest lubricants were the water-based variety, including KY Jelly and contraceptive gels.[19]

Condoms and diaphragms put a damper on spontaneity; but an older barrier method, the cervical cap, is seeing a resurgence of interest. The Prentif cap was approved for marketing by the FDA in 1988. It's a rubber device much smaller than a diaphragm, which covers the cervix like a thimble. The cap can be left in place longer than the diaphragm (up to forty-eight hours) and is more comfortable. It requires more training for use, but once mastered, pregnancy rates are about the same as for the diaphragm. The cervical cap may, however, adversely affect cervical tissue. Only women with normal Pap smears should use it, and follow-up Pap smears are recommended.[20]

Spermicides

Carefully controlled studies have shown that spermicides don't cause birth defects in fetuses who happen to be concealed in the womb during their use. However, science and the law aren't always in agreement. In 1987, a United States District Court upheld a $5 million settlement of a claim against Ortho Pharmaceutical Corporation brought by the parents of a severely deformed baby who, the parents alleged, got that way as a result of Ortho's spermicide.[21]

A spermicidal method gaining in popularity is the contraceptive sponge. It is effective for twenty-four hours without reinsertion. It's failure rate is only slightly (but still significantly) higher than that of the diaphragm. However, the contraceptive sponge shouldn't be used during menstruation or left in for more than twenty-four hours, due to the risk of toxic shock syndrome. This condition results when bacteria are allowed to breed and release potentially fatal toxins.

Incidentally, the leading cause of toxic shock syndrome is the tampon; and the blame has now been pinned on the tampon's absorbency, rather than the materials from which it's made. To help avoid the syndrome, use the minimum absorbency necessary for your flow; or switch to feminine napkins.[22]

Premenstrual tension

Before the question was addressed by controlled studies, premenstrual syndrome, or PMS, was thought to be all in women's heads. Then, in the 1950s, a British gynecologist found that nearly half of the women admitted to a hospital for accidents or psychological illness were in their premenstrual week. Other studies showed that about half the crimes for which women were responsible were committed during this period. These studies looked good for PMS but bad for equal employment, since employers began to question whether women were stable hires. However, other investigations showed women performed as well in the throes of PMS as otherwise.[23]

Closely related to PMS is dysmenorrhea, or painful periods. Both conditions can produce weight gain, pain, and emotional trauma. If you have really disabling pain and other symptoms, you should see your doctor, who has access to new prescription drugs that may be effective.

For milder cases, over-the-counter remedies are available. They may not, however, be effective.

Ibuprofen is the analgesic most likely to give short-term relief of pain. However, some women report that if they use it one month, the next month their cramps are worse.

Most premenstrual symptoms are due to water retention and

bloating. Diuretics, or water pills, effectively stimulate the kidneys to eliminate excess water. However, diuretics can cause the elimination of important minerals and chemicals at the same time, creating harmful imbalances in the body. This is why most diuretics are prescription drugs. In fact, PMS is the *only* condition for which their use is approved without a prescription; and that's only because the pills are taken for just a few days each month. Before you resort to these risky drugs, try drinking less the week before menstruation and avoiding salt and salt-rich foods that cause you to retain water.

Another ingredient popular in over-the-counter menstrual remedies is caffeine. Like diuretics, caffeine stimulates the kidneys to expel water. However, you can get the same effect from an aspirin and a cup of coffee as from the expensive women's remedies containing these ingredients.

Antihistamines may be another menstrual-remedy component. They seem to help, but it's not clear why. The FDA is dubious about the manufacturer's claim that PMS discomfort is caused by the release of histamine, which antihistamines block. Antihistamines cause drowsiness and have mild numbing and pain-killing properties, which may explain their effects.

Other ingredients in menstrual remedies include smooth-muscle relaxants, herbs, and vitamins. All of these are judged by the FDA to lack evidence of effectiveness.

Nondrug remedies for cramps include hot compresses, exercise, massage, and hot baths.

Dietary change may also help. The ratio between the levels of two female hormones, estrogen and progesterone, play an important role in PMS. Progesterone reduces stress and relaxes smooth muscles. Its level can be brought up by bringing the estrogen level down. This can be done by decreasing the amount of fat in the diet and by losing weight in general. Studies show women eating high-fat diets have menstrual periods that are longer, heavier, and more painful than women on low-fat diets.[24]

High-carbohydrate diets may relieve premenstrual symptoms for another reason: starches increase the brain's level of serotonin, a natural "upper" that mediates depression. Researchers at MIT recently found that women who binged on high-carbohydrate foods before menstruation experienced relief of depression, anger, tension, tiredness, moodiness, and other PMS symptoms. British researchers have also shown that a low-fat, high-carbohydrate diet can relieve premenstrual breast pain.[25]

Another effective remedy for premenstrual symptoms may be biofeedback relaxation techniques.[26]

Douching

Responding to ads about preserving feminine hygiene, American women spend millions of dollars a year on vaginal douching products. These products are not only unnecessary but may be dangerous. A study published in 1987 linked them to ectopic or tubal pregnancy, a condition that is potentially life-threatening. Women who douched at least once a week had twice the risk of ectopic pregnancy of women who didn't.

Why isn't clear, but one possibility is that douching increases the risk of spreading bacteria or other infectious agents past the cervix into the uterus and fallopian tubes. This increases the risk of pelvic inflammatory disease, which increases the risk of ectopic pregnancy.

Douching should be avoided particularly by women who are pregnant or think they might be, since some douches contain chemicals that could be absorbed and become serious risks to the fetus.[27]

Drugs to dry up breast milk

Breast-feeding is becoming increasingly popular. In 1971, 75 percent of new mothers chose not to nurse their babies. By 1987, this figure had dropped to 45 percent.

For women electing not to nurse, drugs used to be given routinely to dry up breast milk. These drugs were usually in the form of estrogen, androgen, or testosterone. Today, the most popular drug is bromocriptine (Parlodel). It acts directly on the pituitary gland from which prolactin, the hormone that produces milk, is secreted.

Bromocriptine was used by some 700,000 new mothers in 1987, or 10 percent of those who gave birth. The drug has come under federal scrutiny, however, following 53 reports of serious and, in rare cases, fatal problems associated with its use. These problems include hypertension, heart attack, stroke, seizures, and psychosis.

Less serious but more common problems are also associated with bromocriptine. In nearly half the women who take it, it does not prevent, but only delays, the production of milk and the painful engorgement of the breasts. Rebound engorgement and lactation occur as soon as the drug is stopped. Bromocriptine may also have short-term side effects that can be as annoying as the symptoms it's intended to suppress. They include nausea, vomiting, heartburn, low blood pressure, and dizziness.

Fortunately, the drug isn't really necessary. Engorgement in women who don't breast-feed lasts only a few days, and 90 percent don't complain of significant discomfort.

Alternative treatments include ice packs, binding or massaging the breasts, or pressing them to release small amounts of milk. Aspirin or other analgesics can relieve pain. The safest alternative for both mother and baby, of course, is to take no drugs and to breast-feed.[28]

Table 42. *Estrogen*[29]

Generic name	Brand name
conjugated estrogen	Premarin
diethylstilbestrol	Stilphostrol
estropipate, estradiol	Ogen, Estraderm (transdermal patch)
Uses:	To relieve menopausal symptoms, supplement estrogen production, treat certain cancers and infertility, relieve painful swelling of the breast, dry up breast milk
Side effects:	Nausea and vomiting (oral forms only), skin irritation (patch only), breast tenderness or lumps, vaginal discharge, abnormal blood clotting (predisposing to stroke, heart attack, pulmonary embolus, thrombophlebitis), fluid retention (which may worsen asthma, epilepsy, migraine, heart disease, kidney disease), increased facial and other skin pigment,

glucose intolerance, elevated triglycerides, hypertension, headache, dizziness, depression. May increase the risk of gallbladder disease and of endometrial and uterine cancer.

Should be avoided by women with:	Carcinoma of the breast or endometrium, hereditary deafness, pregnancy, active liver disease, history of thromboembolic disease
Risky for women with:	Hypertension, liver dysfunction, jaundice, gallbladder disease, fibroids, endometriosis, diabetes, family history of breast cancer or arterial disease, history of liver disease, obesity, heavy tobacco consumption

Table 43. *Progestins*

Generic name:	*Brand name:*
medroxyprogesterone	Provera
norethindrone	Micronor, Norlutate
norgestrel	Ovrette
Uses:	To correct menstrual disorders, prevent pregnancy, treat certain cancers
Side effects:	Breast tenderness, fluid retention, rash, acne, increased facial hair, increased blood clotting, abnormal vaginal bleeding, changes in menses, jaundice, depression, high blood pressure, premenstrual tension, change in sexual desire, change in appetite, headache, nervousness, dizziness, tiredness, backache, hair loss. Blood clots in the brain, veins of the leg, lung, or blood vessels of the eye can be life-threatening.
Should be avoided by women with:	Poor liver function, abnormal vaginal bleeding, or a history of cancer of the breast or genitals, stroke, embolism or thrombophlebitis, nursing babies
Risky for women with:	Diabetes, epilepsy, asthma, migraine, depression, heart or kidney problems

Table 44. *Estrogen/Progestin Combinations*

Brand name:	*Active ingredients:*	*Comments:*
Demulen	ethynodiol diacetate + ethinyl estradiol	monophasic (high progestin, low estrogen)

Ovulen	ethynodiol diacetate + mestranol	monophasic (high estrogen, high progestin)
Triphasil 21 & 28	levonorgestrel + ethinyl estradiol	triphasic (low estrogen, low progestin)
Brevicon, Loestrin, Loestrin FE, Modicon, Norinyl (1+35) Norlestrin, Norlestrin FE, Ortho-Novum (1/35, 10/11, 7/7/7), Ovcon	norethindrone + ethinyl estradiol	monophasic except Ortho-Novum 10/11 (biphasic) and 7/7/7 (triphasic); low estrogen, low progestin
Ortho-Novum (1/50, 1/80, 2), Norinyl (1+50, 1+80, 2)	norethindrone + mestranol	monophasic (low estrogen, low or intermediate progestin)
Enovid	norethynodrel + mestranol	monophasic (low estrogen, low progestin)
Lo/Ovral, Nordette, Ovral	norgestrel + ethinyl estradiol	monophasic (low estrogen, low progestin)

Uses:	To prevent pregnancy, supplement hormone production, relieve PMS
Side effects:	High blood pressure, irritability, headache, depression, masculinization, facial hair growth, rash, visual disturbances, joint and muscle pains, fluid retention, breast tenderness, irregular menses, general discomfort
Should be avoided by women with:	History of stroke, heart disease, blood clots, cancer of the breast or reproductive organs, liver problems, abnormal vaginal bleeding, heavy tobacco use
Risky for women with:	Cystic breast disease, endometriosis, high blood pressure, asthma, epilepsy, diabetes, migraine, uterine tumors, depression, gallbladder disease

32

IF YOU ARE EXPECTING

You are the bows from which your children, as living arrows, are sent forth.

—Kahlil Gibran

The thalidomide tragedy of the 1950s underscored the damage drugs can do to the developing fetus. In every pregnancy, there is a 1 percent to 5 percent risk of major malformations, and drugs taken by the mother can substantially increase this risk. Here, we'll look at some drugs of concern to expectant mothers.[1]

Analgesics

Aspirin is one of the drugs most frequently used by pregnant women. It hasn't been shown to harm the fetus in early pregnancy, but in late pregnancy—especially within a week of delivery—aspirin taken by the mother can cause blood disorders in the newborn. In one study, 12 out of 17 (71 percent) of newborns exposed to aspirin developed intraventricular bleeding, compared to 41 of 91 newborns (45 percent) who were not exposed to the drug.[2] Aspirin taken in late pregnancy can also have ill effects on the mother, including an increased risk of hemorrhage, delayed delivery, and prolonged labor. These effects are caused by aspirin's suppression of prostaglandin synthesis.

At low doses, acetaminophen is thought to be safe; but the effect of very high doses hasn't been studied.

In one reported case, a woman took 1.3 grams (four tablets) of acetaminophen daily throughout her pregnancy to treat headaches and nausea. She developed serious anemia (iron deficiency) and required blood transfusions. In the fifth month, the infant died from severe kidney failure. The death was attributed to the mother's daily acetaminophen habit.[3]

Codeine, a widely used narcotic painkiller, hasn't been associated with birth defects, but its use in large doses near delivery can cause a narcotic withdrawal syndrome in the newborn.

Drugs to combat nausea

Thalidomide was given to pregnant women to suppress morning sickness. The tragic results, and the threat of expensive litigation, prompted manufacturers of morning sickness remedies to withdraw their products. As a result, nothing is currently available that is effective for morning sickness.

Bendectin, a combination of doxylamine and pyridoxine, is an antiemetic that had promise. But soon after it came out, reports of defectively developed limbs in the newborns of mothers who took the drug resulted in some expensive legal action against the manufacturer. The risk of congenital defects wasn't borne out in controlled studies, but the company removed the product from the market to avoid the anticipated costly litigation and bad press.

Laxatives

Laxatives are popular drugs among the pregnant. Most seem to have no adverse effects on the fetus, but a few cathartics, like agar and cottonseed oil, have produced skeletal changes in the fetuses of animals. When laxatives are used in large doses throughout pregnancy, they can also cause a loss of magnesium in both mother and child. And castor oil can bring on labor. It should not be used at any time during pregnancy.

Antibiotics and other antimicrobials

Some antibiotics may cause birth defects, and some should be avoided by pregnant women for other reasons.

The evidence linking tetracyclines to birth defects is contradictory; but you shouldn't take them while pregnant in any case, because they can be deposited in your baby's newly-forming teeth and turn them a permanent yellowish brown.

The evidence that erythromycin causes birth defects in animals is also contradictory; but the form called erythromycin estolate should be avoided anyway, because it increases the risk of hepatitis.

Sulfonamides haven't been implicated as causing birth defects, but they too should be avoided, at least in late pregnancy. They can cause high bilirubin levels in the blood of the newborn, a forerunner of jaundice.

The risk of birth defects from the antimicrobial metronidazole seems to be low. However, two children born to mothers who took it during pregnancy were reported to have facial defects, and the drug has caused cancer in rats. It should be avoided at least during the first three months of pregnancy.[4]

Antifungals haven't been shown to pose a threat to the human fetus, but both griseofulvin and flucytosine have caused multiple birth defects in animals. No antifungal should be applied vaginally after the amniotic membranes have ruptured (the water has broken).

The antiviral drug acyclovir shouldn't be used by women who are pregnant or who might become pregnant.

Cold remedies

The active ingredients in nasal decongestants are sympathomimetic drugs like phenylephrine and pseudoephedrine. In an early study, sympathomimetic drugs taken by pregnant women during the first three months of pregnancy were linked to minor birth defects. These results weren't confirmed in later studies. However, sympathomimetic drugs are known to cause birth defects in animals.

The antihistamine brompheniramine (Dimetane, Dimetapp) has been implicated in causing birth defects in humans. In one study, 10 of 65 women exposed to the drug during the first three months of pregnancy had malformed children.

Diphenhydramine (Benadryl, Benylin) was at one time thought to increase the risk of cleft palate, but that association hasn't been confirmed.

Benzodiazepines

Valium was similarly associated with cleft palate in newborns in early studies, but later studies failed to confirm the association. However, a single large dose (more than 30 mg) taken by the mother can lead to the "floppy infant syndrome" in the baby. This condition is characterized by floppy limbs, difficulty breathing and suckling, and a low body temperature.

Like Valium, chlordiazepoxide (Librium) was implicated in causing birth defects in early studies, but later studies failed to confirm the link. The suspected associations were with congenital heart disease, cleft palate, and other malformations.

Asthma remedies

Corticosteroids are used in pregnancy to treat various conditions, including asthma, arthritis, kidney disease, and inflammatory bowel disease. They can produce birth defects in animals but, again, this association hasn't been shown in humans. In some cases, the complications resulting from untreated asthma attacks can outweigh the low risk of birth defects from the drugs. However, it is best to avoid these drugs unless you're desperate.

Another asthma drug, albuterol (Proventil, Ventolin), hasn't been linked to birth defects, but it can cause a fast heart rate in the baby and high blood sugar in the mother, resulting in increased serum insulin and potential low blood sugar after delivery. Moreover, no studies have covered its use during the first three months of pregnancy.

Other drugs

A single course of a general anesthetic seems to be safe in early pregnancy. However, cumulative exposure to anesthetics inhaled on the job can be hazardous to the developing fetus. Lignocaine, a local anesthetic, has been associated with skeletal defects and cataracts in animal offspring, but it hasn't been shown to have this effect in humans.

Estrogen, progestin, or combinations of them may cause birth defects and should be avoided during pregnancy. Since oral contraceptives are composed of these hormones, you should notify your doctor immediately if you suspect you may be pregnant while on them.

Accutane should not be taken by anyone who either is, or might become, pregnant while using it. In a study we looked at earlier involving women who took the drug while pregnant, the odds of having a child with major malformations were about fifty-fifty. Spontaneous abortions were also common.[5] Isotretinoin (Retin-A) hasn't yet been shown to cause birth defects, but it is structurally related to Accutane, and the possibility is there.

Many antihypertensive drugs have been linked to birth defects. These include the two most popular antihypertensive categories, thiazide diuretics and beta-blockers; as well as calcium channel blockers, and clonidine. These drugs should be avoided at least during the first three months of pregnancy. However, it's dangerous to stop taking them suddenly, so if you're on them and get pregnant, ask your doctor for help.[6]

Antimalarial drugs including quinine, primaquine, pyrimethamine with dapsone (Maloprim), and pyrimethamine with sulphadoxine (Fansidar) can cause abortion. If you're faced with the threat of malaria during pregnancy, chloroquine is your best option.[7]

Incidentally, in a 1988 study, a significantly increased risk of miscarriage was also found for women who used visual display terminals during pregnancy. Women who sat at display terminals for twenty hours a week or more were nearly twice as likely to miscarry as those not using them.[8]

A direct link between caffeine and birth defects hasn't yet been found, but the possibility hasn't been eliminated either. Pregnant women and nursing mothers are advised to limit their intake to a couple cups of coffee daily.[9]

Drastic weight-loss diets, particularly the liquid-diet variety, can be harmful to the developing fetus. Toxic waste products, including ketones released from the metabolism of fat, can find their way to the baby. Your safest dietary course is to avoid junk food and concentrate on whole, natural foods.

Alcohol can also be harmful to the developing fetus. Alcohol abuse by the mother can result in fetal alcohol syndrome in the baby, and has been associated with retarded fetal growth and structural malformations.[10]

"Recreational" drugs are also, of course, something you want to avoid. Even the smoking of marijuana, considered the least harmful of these drugs, has now been shown to result in shorter and lighter babies, and is thought to stunt fetal growth.[11]

Another thing you should avoid if you're expecting is your cat litter box. It can carry toxoplasmosis, a cat-borne parasitic disease. The condition is rarely serious in older children or adults, but it can be disastrous to the unborn and to very small children. It puts them at risk for defects that show up at birth or later in childhood, including eye problems, liver and blood disorders, brain involvement, and convulsions. About 7,500 babies are born in the United States each year with toxoplasmosis contracted in the womb.[12]

33

DRUGS, IMPOTENCE, AND INFERTILITY

Lechery, sir, it provokes and it unprovokes; It provokes the desire, but it takes away the performance.
—Shakespeare
Macbeth

One drug side effect you may be embarrassed to ask your doctor about, but which may take on major importance when you experience it, is sexual dysfunction. Antihypertensives are notorious for it, but many other drugs can cause sexual dysfunction as well. They can cause it in both men and women, although until recently most studies focused only on men. In women, sexual dysfunction includes inhibited sexual desire (once ungraciously referred to as "frigidity"), inhibited sexual preparation (vaginal lubrication and relaxation), and inhibited orgasm.

The effect of drugs on your sexual functioning may not be immediate. It may show up only after months or years. If you're having this problem, take a hard look at your medicine cabinet, ask your doctor about the side effects of any drugs he has prescribed, and see if you can wind down on possible offenders or switch to something else.

There are few well-controlled studies on the subject of drug-induced sexual problems, and the reported results vary widely. This chapter focuses on drugs for which reasonably good research is available, but many more have been blamed.[1] We'll also look at drugs used for the treatment of impotence and infertility.

Antihypertensives

The drugs best known for affecting sexual performance are those used to treat high blood pressure. In men, it's easy to picture the relationship, since erections are created by bursts of blood pressure. The reported incidence of erectile difficulty associated with diuretics varies from 5 percent to 32 percent. With methyldopa, it varies from 3 percent to 80 percent; with guanethidine, from 4 percent to 100 percent; with reserpine, from 2 percent to 46 percent; with clonidine, from 4 percent to 70 percent. With propranolol, it varies from 0 percent to 28 percent at lower doses, and from 18 percent to 100 percent at higher doses. Timolol and other beta-blockers used as eye drops in the treatment of glaucoma can also have this effect.

Not only performance but desire can be affected. Reduced libido, or sexual drive, is a reported side effect of most antihypertensives; and this one affects both sexes.

The problem may be alleviated by switching to ACE inhibitors or calcium channel blockers, which are less likely to inhibit sexual performance. However, any medication that lowers blood pressure will have some effect in men, since lowered blood pressure necessarily reduces the force of the blood going into the penis.

Psychotropic drugs

Another category of drugs known for their inhibitory effects on sexual performance are the psychotropic drugs—those that affect your mood. These include antidepressants, sedatives, stimulants, and tranquilizers. Antidepressants are particularly high on the list, and MAO inhibitors are the worst. The desire and initial performance may be there, but the goal is frustrated. Reported problems include decreased libido and failure to reach orgasm in both men and women, and inhibited and painful ejaculation and problems achieving erection in men.

One of the few studies that looked specifically at orgasm in women reported inhibitory effects from all of the following: the major tranquilizers thioridazine (Mellaril) and trifluoperazine (Stelazine), the tricyclic antidepressants amoxapine (Asendin) and amitriptyline (Elavil, Amitril, Limbitrol), the MAO inhibitors, phenelzine, isocarboxazid, and tranylcypromine.

Statistically significant differences between different antidepressants haven't been verified, except that the antidepressant desipramine (Norpramin) is associated with *increased* libido in women and with an abnormal, persistent erection in men. Another antidepressant, bupropion, seems to enhance both libido and sexual performance; but it's no longer on the market. It was withdrawn due to a high risk of seizures (see chapter 26). The drug didn't work as an aphrodisiac on everyone, and it took two or three weeks to have this effect when it did.

The major tranquilizers generally depress sexual response. However, many of these drugs are also associated with abnormal, persistent erection. In some studies, more than 50 percent of patients on major tranquilizers have reported sexual problems. The most common was decreased libido.

On the plus side, MAO inhibitors, which delay ejaculation, have been used to treat premature ejaculation; and fluphenazine, an antipsychotic, has been used to dull excess libido in sexual criminals.

Most of the commonly-used antianxiety medications haven't been available long enough to draw conclusions from the data. But medicines that have been in longer use, like the barbiturates, are known to have opposing effects on sexual function: increased libido at low doses, and decreased libido at high doses. The benzodiazepines, like Valium, also have a two-phase effect. At low doses, they release inhibitions and increase excitement. At high doses, they cause drowsiness and deaden performance.

Drugs of abuse

The same is true for drugs of abuse, although they're generally thought to enhance sexual performance. They can, in fact, have the opposite effect: the well known willing-spirit, weak-flesh syndrome.

Alcohol and marijuana, which are often indulged in for their desire-enhancing abilities, are reported to have the long-term effect in chronic abusers of reducing desire and arousal. Cocaine, too, has this effect at high doses and with long-term use. Opiates will do it even after short-term use.

Impotence or reduced sexual drive, or both, are found in 70–80 percent of chronic alcoholics. Alcoholics also tend to have much lower levels of testosterone (the main male hormone) and higher levels of estrogen (a female hormone). This can result in certain acquired female characteristics.[2]

Anabolic steroids, the male hormones taken illicitly by athletes to enhance performance on the field, have the opposite effect on performance in the bedroom. They make women more masculine and can cause the growth of facial hair. They don't, however, make men more masculine. Rather, the drugs can shrink the testicles, enlarge the breasts, diminish sex drive, reduce the sperm count, and cause impotence. Anabolic steroids also pose dangerous risks to the heart and immune system, and they can cause hair loss, mood swings, uncontrolled aggression, acne, liver problems, and prostate troubles.[3]

Other drugs

Sexual problems can also be caused by the stomach medications cimetidine (Tagamet), ranitidine (Zantac), and metoclopramide (Reglan, an antinausea drug). These drugs are linked to a failure of desire and erection. Tagamet is also associated with enlarged breasts and breast pain in both sexes. If you're having these problems and you need a drug for ulcers, sucralfate (Carafate) may be a better option.

Anticancer drugs are associated with a decline in sexuality, but this may be merely because the patient is too sick to be interested.

Oral contraceptives are reported to cause sexual problems of an undefined nature.

Anticonvulsants lower libido in some patients.

Even antibiotics can interfere with sexual function in women.

Broad-spectrum antibiotics like tetracycline can wipe out friendly intestinal bacteria along with unfriendly ones, allowing yeasts to take over. The resulting vaginitis (inflammation of the vagina) and painful intercourse can cause a loss of libido.

Antihistamines can also interfere with female sexual function, by drying out the vaginal tissues.

Aphrodisiacs and drugs to treat impotence

Spanish fly doesn't work and can have dangerous side effects. Vitamin E is safe but doesn't work. What of other drugs touted as aphrodisiacs and impotence remedies? According to the FDA, no oral aphrodisiacs are effective, and none should be sold over-the-counter; but the agency hasn't actually banned their sale.

According to impotence researcher Dr. Irwin Goldstein of Boston University, no oral medication has been shown to change the ability to achieve or sustain an erection. One drug, called papaverine, works by causing vasodilation, increasing blood flow to the penis. However, to get this effect, it has to be injected into the penis before intercourse.[4]

Drugs to treat infertility

Some drugs can cause infertility even in people whose spirit is willing and flesh is strong. There are also drugs that may help correct this problem.

More than five million American couples of child-bearing age, or about one in seven, are infertile. In up to a third of infertile women, the problem has been traced to overproduction of the hormone prolactin by the pituitary gland. The result can be the cessation of menstruation and ovulation.

One cause of the overproduction of prolactin is interference with dopamine, the natural substance that inhibits prolactin release. Dopamine can be shut down by certain drugs, including the tricyclic antidepressant imipramine (Tofranil), and the major tranquilizers chlorpromazine (Thorazine) and trifluoperazine (Stelazine).

There is also a drug that can correct the condition. It is bromocriptine (Parlodel), the same drug given to new mothers to dry up breast milk. Some 80–90 percent of women who are infertile from this cause regain normal ovulation and menstruation after taking it. The drug's side effects are generally mild, but they can include nausea, headache, dizziness, abdominal cramps, and sometimes a drop in blood pressure on standing.[5]

For women having trouble ovulating from other causes, there are also other drugs. The newest of this type, called urofollitropin (Metrodin), is useful for women with low estrogen activity. Its most serious side effect is enlargement of the ovaries. Symptoms can range from slightly enlarged and tender to extremely enlarged, with fluid retention, difficulty urinating, abdominal swelling, and fluid in the lungs. About one in five Metrodin-induced births also produces multiple babies.

For women with natural estrogen activity, the drug of choice is clomiphene (Clomid, Serophene). In appropriate cases, it induces ovulation about 80 percent of the time and pregnancy about 30–40 percent of the time. Again, its most serious side effect may be enlargement of the ovaries, but this happens less often than with Metrodin, and multiple births result only 10 percent of the time.[6]

Another cause of infertility may be low thyroid activity. To compensate for this problem, natural thyroid hormones or synthetic hormones like levothyroxine (Synthroid) are often given. The downside of this alternative is that your body will compensate for the additional hormones by reducing its own hormone production. That means once you start on these drugs, you are liable to be on them for life.

34

DRUGS FOR THE SEXUALLY ACTIVE

I've watched too many sicken in a month and die by Christmas, so that a fatal sort of realism comforts me more than magic.

—P. Monette, *On Borrowed Time: An AIDS Memoir*[1]

It's not easy being single these days. It used to be that all you risked with promiscuity was gonorrhea, and that could be cleared up with a quick round of antibiotics. Now it's not only hard to find an antibiotic that will work; you risk diseases that will be with you for life, or that can bring your life to an abrupt end.

According to the Centers for Disease Control, sexually transmitted diseases (STDs) were reported at higher rates in 1988 than in previous years. Syphilis was up from 35,147 cases in 1987 to 40,200 cases in 1988. Gonorrhea has actually dropped; but the antibiotic-resistant kind is steadily rising, from 110 cases in 1976 to 25,714 cases in 1988.[2] AIDS is up from 291 cases in 1981 to 20,100 cases in 1988.[3]

Unfortunately, you can't avoid these diseases simply by avoiding sexual contact with people known to have them. Since a high percentage of cases are without symptoms, you can contract them from people unaware of being carriers. There may be as many as a million asymptomatic carriers of gonorrhea. That is roughly equivalent to the number of cases reported each year. Up to 70 percent of all female contacts of males with nongonococcal urethritis (including chlamydia) are thought to be asymptomatic carriers, as well as 10–15 percent of women with genital herpes infections. At one time, it was thought that only 1 percent of male cases of herpes were symptom-free, but that figure is now suspected to be much higher.

When the bacteria ascend into the uterus or fallopian tubes, both gonorrhea and nongonococcal urethritis can result in pelvic inflammatory disease. Blockage of the fallopian tubes can cause infertility. In the worst case, the result can be death.

Women with these vaginal infections who are able to get pregnant can transmit the disease through the birth canal to their babies. This can happen even if the woman has no symptoms and is unaware of the disease. This is the reason for the irritating silver nitrate drops that are routinely placed in babies' eyes at birth, whether or not the mother has evidence of vaginal infection. Even asymptomatic infection can result in blindness in the newborn.[4]

AIDS

The worst-case scenario is to contract AIDS, a condition generally considered fatal. Only one prescription medicine is approved for its treatment, the antiviral drug zidovudine (AZT). Unfortunately, AZT is not a cure for active AIDS. At best, it slows the replication of the HIV virus. It can't restore an AIDS patient's immune system once destroyed. It also has many side effects, including nausea, insomnia, severe headaches, muscle pain, reduction in white blood cells, and increased anemia. Suppression of the growth of bone marrow cells results in a lack of red blood cells, producing anemia, and in a lack of white blood cells, increasing susceptibility to infection. As many as half of all AIDS patients can't take AZT because of these side effects. Liver damage has also been documented. One man developed jaundice and liver dysfunction within a week of taking the drug. When he quit taking it, his liver recovered. Another drawback of the drug is its cost, which comes to around $7,000 or $8,000 per patient, per year.

A study reported in August of 1989 was hailed as "a turning point in the battle to change AIDS from a fatal disease to a treatable one." It found that AZT delayed the development of AIDS in people who have the virus but have no symptoms, a category believed to include several hundred thousand Americans. The study involved 3,200 HIV-infected volunteers who received either AZT or a placebo for two years. Only 4 percent of those taking AZT developed AIDS, compared to 9 percent taking the placebo.

However, this good news was tempered by studies reported by the manufacturer several months later. They linked high doses of AZT to vaginal cancer in rats. For people who already have AIDS, this risk is of small consequence, since their life expectancy is typically only a year or two after their first hospitalization. But for people who are infected with the virus but are asymptomatic, the ill effects of the disease may not be felt for years. Cancer could affect them before AIDS does.[5] The significance of the finding is uncertain, and it did not prevent FDA approval of the drug for sale to this much broader consumer base.

Many drugs besides AZT are used by AIDS patients. Because AIDS seriously impairs immunity, patients end up highly vulnerable to attack from opportunistic organisms, particularly "P. carinii" pneumonia (PCP); and to such malignancies as lymphoma and Kaposi's sarcoma, a once-rare form of cancer that attacks the endothelial cells lining the blood vessels. Medications used in the treatment of these infections and malignancies are listed in Table 45.[6]

For desperate AIDS patients, alternative therapies may be as good as or better than orthodox treatment. A Chinese practitioner in Melbourne, Australia, for example, reports the elimination of active symptoms in pre-AIDS cases with the use of acupuncture.[7] Many AIDS patients are using a combination of therapies, conventional and alternative.[8]

What about a vaccine against AIDS? Scientists had been working on this possibility without success until a recent breakthrough, published in *Science* in December of 1989. Researchers reported that a vaccine for the monkey version of AIDS prevented development of the disease in nine rhesus monkeys after their exposure to the active virus, at least for the length of the nine-month experiment. There are, however, problems in applying this research to humans. One is that monkey AIDS is not the same as human AIDS. Another problem is that the vaccine was the dangerous live-virus version, which can cause, as well as prevent, the disease.[9]

Table 45. *Medications Used for AIDS-Related Conditions*

Drug:	*Used against:*
acyclovir	Epstein-Barr virus, Herpes simplex virus, Varicella-zoster virus
amphotericin	Cryptococcal meningitis
bleomycin	Kaposi's sarcoma
clofazimine	*P. carinii* pneumonia
clotrimazole	Oral candidiasis
dapsone	*P. carinii* pneumonia
doxorubicin	Kaposi's sarcoma
Fansidar	*P. carinii* pneumonia
flucytosine	Cryptococcal meningitis
ganciclovir	Cytomegalovirus
Drug:	*Used against:*
interferon	Kaposi's sarcoma
ketoconazole	Oral candidiasis
nystatin	Oral candidiasis
pentamidine	*P. carinii* pneumonia
pyrimethamine	Toxoplasmosis
trimethoprim and sulfamethoxazole	*P. carinii* pneumonia
vincristine	Kaposi's sarcoma
zidovudine (AZT)	HIV

Chlamydia

The leading sexually transmitted disease in 1988 was actually one of the lesser known varieties. Called chlamydia, this low-profile disease is 2–4 times as prevalent as gonorrhea; and its cost in suffering may actually be higher than for AIDS. While only about 150,000 cases were reported in 1988, the actual incidence is estimated at *three to four million.* The problem is that the disease can exist without symptoms.

Untreated, chlamydia can lead to sterility in men and to pelvic inflammatory disease in women, resulting in infertility, ectopic pregnancy, and sometimes death. Chlamydia bacteria can also be responsible for a chronic eye inflammation called trachoma, which is one of the world's leading causes of blindness.

Drug treatment for chlamydia is usually with tetracycline antibiotics. Penicillin won't work; and even tetracycline may fail as much as 40 percent of the time. Treatment failures are often due to re-infection by an untreated sexual partner. Cultures for chlamydia are expensive and are not always positive, even when the bacteria are present. Preventive measures include sexual abstention, the proper use of condoms and, for the sexually active, regular checkups by a physician.[10]

Genital warts

Another little-known but fast-rising STD is genital warts. These warts can occur, among other places, on the anus, penis, urethra, vulva, vagina, or cervix. If you get them, you may have trouble tracing the source, since they may not show up for 18–24 months after exposure.

Genital warts are caused by infection with the human papilloma virus (HPV), which is linked to genital cancer. In one study of women aged 15–50, HPV was found in 10 percent of those with normal "Pap" results and in 35–40 percent of those with abnormal smears.

There is no foolproof method for treating genital warts. All methods are associated with a high rate of recurrence. Most also have serious side effects that can be quite disabling. Adequately controlled trials comparing different approaches haven't been done, and the long-term safety of these treatments is unknown.[11] As with chlamydia, your best defenses are abstention, condoms, and regular checkups.

Syphilis

Cases of syphilis rose from 20,000 in 1977 to 30,000 in 1982, and fell to about 25,000 cases a year after that. More than 70 percent of these cases appear in men, and nearly 40 percent of these men are homosexual.

The syphilis bacteria is one that hasn't yet developed resistance to antibiotics, so the disease usually responds to penicillin. Drug treatment is often accompanied by fever, chills, headaches, worsening of lesions, and a general feeling of ill-health. However, this complication is not an allergic response to the drug. It is the result of the rapid release of antigens from the suddenly-killed syphilis bacteria.[12]

Gonorrhea

Reported cases of gonorrhea exceeded one million in the early 1980s and fell to about 850,000 by the mid-80s. However, the actual annual incidence is estimated at over three million. Homosexual men are again at highest risk. Of those who visit VD clinics, 30 percent are found to have the infection.

One complication of the disease is gonococcal arthritis, the most common form of arthritis caused by an infectious agent. The first symptoms are fever, chills, and body aches. If left untreated, the condition develops into full-blown arthritis, with rapid destruction of cartilage and bone.[13]

Gonorrhea was once easily treated with penicillin, but antibiotic-resistant strains have increasingly frustrated standard treatment. (See chapter 3.) In many areas, only one or two effective drugs are available, and these may soon be obsolete. Whether science or the bacteria will prevail in the race between the development of new drugs and antibiotic-resistant strains remains to be seen.

Genital herpes

The Herpes simplex virus belongs to the group of large DNA viruses that includes varicella-zoster virus, Epstein-Barr virus and cytomegalovirus. There is no effective cure for genital herpes. Lesions can be quite painful, and in many cases they keep coming back. The disease can promote cervical cancer in women and can kill infants who contract it from their mothers at birth. Half the victims of neonatal herpes die, and half the survivors develop serious brain damage or blindness.

Herpes symptoms can be reduced by an expensive drug called acyclovir (Zovirax); but the drug doesn't prevent recurrences. It works best when used on the first attack.

The most important preventive measure is to recognize a recurrence when it hits, and to studiously avoid sexual contact while the lesions are present. Herpes lesions are painful blisters that break and form crusty sores, shedding viruses that are extremely contagious. Unfortunately, the viruses may emerge before the blisters do; but there is often a feeling of tingling, itching or general ill-health that warns of an impending outbreak.

Genital herpes lesions should be kept clean and dry. Although they can be very painful, anesthetics should be avoided if possible, since they can counteract the desired drying effect.

For patients with frequent recurrences, acyclovir is sometimes given orally three to five times a day and topically up to every three hours. This regimen can reduce the frequency of recurrences by as much as 75 percent, but its long-term safety and effectiveness are unknown. Acyclovir shouldn't be used by women who are pregnant or who might become pregnant.[14]

There is some evidence that herpes recurrences can be avoided by keeping a positive attitude. Controlled studies recently confirmed anecdotal evidence linking these outbreaks to psychological stress. In one study, the stress of taking a medical school exam was found to activate latent herpes. Another study found that men who were anxious, depressed or lonely had higher levels of herpes antibodies in their blood than men who were in better spirits. Since antibody levels go up during periods of reactivation, higher levels are thought to reflect a depressed immune system that is unable to keep the virus under control.[15]

Other herpes infections

Genital herpes is usually caused by the Herpes simplex virus-2 (HSV-2), but increasingly it's also caused by the virus that causes cold sores, HSV-1. HSV-2, in turn, can be responsible for blisters on the mouth.

Cold sores (fever blisters) and canker sores (aphthous ulcers) are two of the most common infections of the mouth. An important difference is that canker sores aren't contagious, while cold sores are. Cold sores may be accompanied by fever, swollen neck glands and a general achy feeling. Canker sores are rarely accompanied by fever or other signs of illness.

With cold sores, it is important to keep hands away and to avoid kissing. Touching the sores can result in spreading the virus to new sites on the body or to other people.

Once you get oral herpes, the virus remains in a nerve near the cheekbone, and outbreaks can recur. Like with genital herpes, oral herpes outbreaks have been linked to emotional stress, as well as to fever, illness, injury, and overexposure to sun.

Furthermore, as with genital herpes, no effective drug is available to treat the condition. However, the FDA is currently considering approval of acyclovir as a remedy for symptomatic relief. Some preparations may ward off discomfort, but they do not affect healing time or delay recurrences. A soft, bland diet is recommended to avoid irritating the sores.

For canker sores, mouthwashes containing tetracycline are available, but they can permanently stain the teeth if given to young children or pregnant women. Oral steroids and immunosuppressive drugs are also available, but they are strong medicines that can have undesirable side effects. The cause of canker sores is unknown, but they may be due to allergy, nutritional deficiencies or defects in the immune system. If you contract them, avoid acidic and spicy foods or any foods to which you may be allergic.

Another common sexually-transmitted virus in the herpes family is cytomegalovirus (CMV). While it generally causes no symptoms, it can cause severe infections and even death in infants of infected mothers, who may not even know they have the disease. There is no effective treatment. Again, the best option is prevention, through abstinence or condoms and regular physician checkups.[16]

Trichomoniasis

This common protozoan infection affects about a quarter of all sexually active women, or about 2.5 million yearly. Its symptoms include vaginal itching, burning, and a yellow or creamy-white vaginal discharge with a strong odor.

The usual treatment is metronidazole. This drug should not be taken with alcohol, since the combination can result in nausea, vomiting, flushing and breathing difficulty. It also shouldn't be taken by pregnant women, due to the risk of cancer.[17]

VIII

Special Topics

35

TRENDS IN SELF-TESTING

Medicine has traditionally been a priestly function. Physicians were the high priests, and hospitals the temples. But the home thermometer and other devices moved medicine out of its traditional setting and, in doing so, demystified it. We peeked behind the curtain at the great physician Oz fiddling with knobs and such. And we realized that at least some of what he was doing . . . we can do for ourselves.[1]

—F. Samuel Jr. (1989)

People are increasingly seeking to take charge of their own health care. Aiding this trend are new self-testing products to assess and monitor their conditions. Much routine testing is moving out of the laboratory and into the home.

The trend began with the thermometer, a simple device that helped mothers determine the honesty of children who complained they were too sick for school. From this modest beginning, the self-testing market mushroomed to $618 million in 1986 and is expected to reach $2.2 billion by 1995.

The latest in home testing includes products that help diagnose conditions with or without symptoms (like pregnancy and colon cancer), and that help monitor existing conditions (like high blood pressure and diabetes). Self-testing products that are currently, or soon to be, marketed include those for blood glucose, urine glucose and ketones, blood pressure, serum cholesterol, pregnancy, ovulation prediction, drugs of abuse in the urine, hidden blood in the stool, impotence, tooth status (plaque and cavities), visual status (acuity and color blindness), lung function, strep throat, urinary tract infections, and therapeutic drug monitoring.

As with testing by professional laboratories, a crucial limitation on the usefulness of these tests is the competence of the person reading the results. To develop the skills necessary to use them properly, you need to read the product information carefully. You may also need to consult your pharmacist or your doctor. Remember that a single positive result isn't proof that you're ill, and a single negative result isn't proof that you're well. Home tests should supplement, not replace, professional medical care.[2]

Tests for occult blood

Self-testing techniques for detecting potentially cancerous lumps in the breast or moles on the skin are well known. Now there are also self-testing kits that make it possible to detect potential colon cancer in the privacy of your own bathroom.

The telltale sign of the condition is blood in the stool. But this blood isn't always visible to the eye, and what *is* visible may be caused by hemorrhoids or menstruation rather than the more ominous cancer. Chemical kits can distinguish between them.

Two new kits use anal wiping for specimen collection. One can be read at home (Early Detector). The other is returned to the physician for developing (HemaWipe). Two other new tests use pads that are dropped into the toilet bowl (ColoScreen Self-Test, EZ-Detect). Other brands of home tests include Hemoccult Home Test, Fleet Detecatest, and ColoScreen III/VPI.

Accurate home use requires following the directions carefully. Dietary restrictions may be required, since many foods and vitamin supplements can cause false results. No published studies have tested the effectiveness of the kits when used at home by patients, so the results should be considered suggestive rather than conclusive.[3]

Blood pressure monitoring

Fifteen years ago, blood-pressure monitors were considered the exclusive domain of health professionals. They can now be purchased at most community pharmacies. Their sales reached $100 million by 1986, and several million families now have them.

Home blood-pressure monitoring devices are particularly useful for making the decision to start treatment in patients with only mild hypertension. Some patients suffer from "white coat" hypertension that shows up only in the doctor's office. Relaxing at home, their blood pressures are normal.

Different types of home blood-pressure monitoring kits are available, with different strengths and weaknesses. The mercury sphygmomanometer is the most accurate and durable, but it's also the most difficult to use. Electronic models are easy to use but are fragile and less accurate, and their cost tends to be high. Finger oscillometric monitors offer the latest in technology and are very easy to use, but they're the least accurate of the available models, and their cost is also high. The aneroid sphygmomanometer is the cheapest model. It's durable, manageable, and fairly accurate.[4]

Tests for planning and detecting a pregnancy

A rapidly expanding segment of the self-testing market is the home pregnancy test. Sales reached $72 million in 1987, doubling in only three years. The test allows a woman to determine her condition early and to alter her lifestyle accordingly. She can ingest the healthful, avoid the harmful, and seek prenatal care from the beginning of her pregnancy.

While the home pregnancy test has been available for a decade, the ovulation prediction kit is new in the prenatal testing field. It helps couples plan a pregnancy. The kit is particularly useful for those having trouble conceiving, since the ovum remains alive and subject to fertilization only 12–24 hours after it drops. Knowing the hour of ovulation allows for precise encounter by sperm.

Again, for accurate results, the test needs to be performed exactly according to the manufacturer's instructions. Timing of the test is crucial. A clock with a second hand may be required.

Unfortunately, the kits aren't reliable for preventing conception. Since sperm can live for three days, they can already be lurking in wait when the ovum drops.[5]

Diabetes monitoring

The largest share of the self-testing market goes to products for diabetes control. Sales in this area increased from $129 million in 1983 to $205 million in 1986.

Urine glucose monitoring has been around for at least forty years, but it's not very accurate. Home blood glucose monitoring is a new tool allowing accurate, immediate feedback. Automatic spring-driven disposable lances have made home blood-letting easier. Results can be read either visually, by comparison with color strips, or by a meter that reads the color automatically.

Products for the self-monitoring of blood glucose include the Glucometer, Accu-Chek, One-Touch, and ExacTech. The latest of these devices include meters with memories that keep track of blood glucose levels at various times of day. One such product is the Glucometer-M. The meter can be hooked up to a computer to get printouts of information. This makes it much easier to coordinate food intake with insulin doses, so blood glucose levels can be kept normal.

Another new testing kit for diabetics allows the accurate screening of family members for the disease. This product, called Biotel/ Diabetes, is also recommended to any overweight middle-aged person who wants to know if he may have diabetes.

Other products for diabetics include Tes-Tape or Diastix, which can be used to determine whether "diet" soft drinks are really sugar-free; products to test for ketones in the urine; and products to treat insulin reactions.[6]

Therapeutic drug monitoring

Millions of people routinely take drugs for chronic conditions such as asthma, angina, and seizures. Like diabetics, these people need to monitor their drug levels; and kits to help them do it should be arriving soon. Medications most likely to be watched are theophylline, digoxin, and phenytoin.[7]

36

VITAMIN AND MINERAL SUPPLEMENTS: HEALTH IN A BOTTLE?

Allow not nature more than nature needs.
                              —Shakespeare,
                              King Lear

In 1987, the American Medical Association's Council on Scientific Affairs, the American Dietetic Association, and the National Council Against Health Fraud, Inc., published reports finding that healthy adults eating normal varied diets don't need vitamin supplements. The exceptions were certain high-risk groups: pregnant women, nursing mothers, and people on restricted diets. Despite these findings, recently compiled statistics show that in 1983, consumers spent about $3 billion for these pills.[1]

The vitamin and mineral craze was stirred first by evidence discovered by Linus Pauling that vitamin C cures the common cold, and more recently by evidence that calcium supplements may ward off osteoporosis (bone loss). In the single year 1985–86, sales of calcium supplements increased by a third, to $166 million; and by 1988, they had jumped to $318 million. This increase followed a 1984 National Institutes of Health recommendation that calcium intake be increased to 1,000 mg per day for all Americans, and to 1,500 mg per day for postmenopausal women, to prevent osteoporosis.[2]

Unfortunately, later studies have failed to confirm either that calcium prevents osteoporosis or that vitamin C cures colds.[3]

The evidence for calcium supplements is tenuous at best. In one of many studies that have raised professional eyebrows, bone density was measured over an average period of nearly five years in 107 women aged 23–88. The women's calcium intakes ranged from 269 to 2,000 mg/day, but they stayed the same over the test period for each woman. No correlation was found between calcium intake and bone loss—"not even a trend." This was true even when other variables (age, menopause status, estrogen level) were controlled. When comparison was limited to women with very high intakes (over 1,400 mg/day) and very low intakes (under 500 mg/day), bone loss in the two groups was still essentially the same.[4]

Whether calcium intake is related to hip fracture is also unclear. A 1988 study found an inverse association between dietary calcium and the risk of hip fracture.[5] But in two studies reported in 1989, one in Britain and one in the United States, hip fracture showed no significant relation to calcium intake. What did prove to be significant was exercise. In the American study, the risk of hip fracture was only half as great for people who exercised regularly as for those who didn't.[6]

Epidemiological studies also fail to support a relation between dietary calcium and the incidence of fractures. Anomalously, fractures are actually *less* common in populations with low intakes of calcium.[7]

The World Health Organization and the Food and Agriculture Organization suggest a practical calcium allowance of 400–500 mg/day, only half the American recommendation; and some studies have found a requirement of less than 300 mg/day.

After reviewing the evidence, researchers writing in the *British Medical Journal* in January of 1989 concluded that all normal diets contain sufficient calcium, and that supplements for healthy people have no demonstrated value.[8]

Not only is it unclear whether these supplements do any good; they can do harm. Excess calcium can cut off vitamin D, which is necessary for cellular activation of bone cells; can cause extraskeletal calcification and kidney stones; and can increase iron and zinc requirements. Calcium supplements also interfere with the absorption of manganese; and manganese, like calcium, is important for building bones. In laboratory animals, osteoporosis increases when there is too little manganese in the diet. Magnesium balance, too, can be upset by too much calcium. A too-high calcium/magnesium ratio can contribute to cardiovascular damage and functional abnormalities.[9]

Similar problems are seen with megadoses of vitamin C. Once thought to be harmless, this vitamin is now known to be toxic at high levels. It also increases the tendency to form kidney stones in susceptible people, and it is antagonistic to vitamin E, copper, and vitamin B_{12}. This means increasing your vitamin C intake can make you deficient in those other nutrients. In one study, when men took 500 mg of vitamin C three times a day with their meals, they developed secondary iron-deficiency anemia.[10]

Pregnant women need to be especially careful with vitamin C, because large doses can create a dependency in their infants. Infants having normal vitamin C intakes whose mothers took as little as 400 mg of the vitamin daily during pregnancy have wound up with "rebound scurvy." The same problem has been reported with vitamin B_6. Infants whose mothers took large doses of it while pregnant have become B_6-dependent, resulting in seizures.[11]

Other vitamins can be poisonous in large doses. This includes the fat-soluble vitamins, A, D, E and K. These vitamins aren't excreted but are stored in body fat, where they accumulate and can produce toxic symptoms. Overdoses can actually be lethal; and in lesser amounts, they can cause nausea, vomiting, headache, extraskeletal calcification, tiredness, anorexia, and irritability. Vitamin A can be toxic at doses of only five times the adult RDA. It can cause liver damage and, possibly, birth defects. Vitamin B_6 can cause numbness in the fingers and toes in doses as low as 200 mg and can eventually lead to nerve damage and paralysis. Selenium is toxic at doses as low as 1 mg, and it can be fatal in larger doses. All of these minimum toxic doses can be found in single pills that are available over-the-counter.[12]

Excess iron can also kill, and in lesser amounts it can interfere with the absorption of copper, zinc, and manganese. Less serious, but no less annoying, it can be very constipating.[13]

Many vitamins and minerals are antagonistic, so that increasing one inhibits the absorption of the other. Vitamin E is antagonistic to iron and to vitamin K. Vitamins A and E are antagonistic to each other. Zinc is antagonistic to copper, which is often deficient to start with and can't be spared. Excess zinc can also have adverse effects on the immune system, and can increase LDL and decrease HDL cholesterol levels.[14] Calcium is antagonistic to iron, zinc, and manganese. Vitamin C is antagonistic to copper and vitamins E and B_{12}. Interference with vitamin B_{12} absorption has been demonstrated with regular vitamin C doses as low as 500 mg a day.[15] Vitamin B_{12} requirements can also be increased by thiamine and nicotinamide, copper, vitamin E, and iron, not to mention smoking, alcohol, and certain drugs.[16]

Pernicious anemia results from vitamin B_{12} deficiency, but it can also be produced by the very vitamin supplementation designed to avoid it. Virtually all synthetic B_{12} supplements contain breakdown products of the vitamin which can interfere with its action. These "B_{12} analogues" are like keys that fit a lock but don't turn it, and that keep the correct key out. That means they can block the normal binding of B_{12} to "intrinsic factor," a substance present in gastric secretions that is required for B_{12} absorption.[17] There is also evidence that B_{12} supplements increase the symptoms of atherosclerosis.[18]

Theoretically, you could remedy the antagonistic-nutrient problem by taking a "balanced" nutritional formula. Unfortunately, no one really knows what a balanced formula is. Vitamin, mineral, and trace substance requirements and interactions haven't been established with certainty. Recommendations vary not only from one year to another but from one organization to another. The current Canadian recommended dietary allowance for zinc, for example, is 9 mg, but it's 15 mg in the United States. The Dutch recommendation for iron is less than half that recommended by the U.S. National Academy of Sciences. Further, the Academy has revised the U.S. recommended dietary allowances every four or five years since 1941.[19]

Despite these cautions, if your diet is laden with junk food, you may be better off with vitamin pills than without them. The safer alternative, however, is a diet liberally balanced with whole plant foods—grains, greens, fruits, and beans. These foods can satisfy nutrient requirements without help from the drug industry.[20]

What about nutritional supplements for children?

Children are especially likely to favor junk food over greens. Yet a 1985 Canadian survey showed that the risk of nutritional deficiency in children without supplements was less than the risk of overdose with them. The only supplement recommended in Canada is vitamin D for breast-fed infants; and this recommendation is to protect only a very small percentage of the breast-feeding population.

A much larger percentage of the toddling population is exposed to the unnecessary risk of vitamin overdose. In a study in Ontario, poisonings among children from accidental overdose proved to be a regular occurrence. Thirty-five percent of these cases involved a particular cartoon-character preparation (the Flintstones). The children managed to eat these vitamins like candy, even though they came packaged in child-resistant containers.

The appealing cartoon-character format alone, however, wasn't responsible for the overdoses. In fact, two cases involved cod liver oil. The researchers observed that "children are capable of ingesting anything they can get their hands on." They concluded:

The extent of multiple-vitamin use . . . demonstrates the public's preoccupation with micronutrients. Unfortunately, the use of vitamin supplements will not address the major problems confronting children: excess energy intake in inactive children, and excess intake of salt and sugar. Adequate fibre intake, fibre being the most commonly deficient dietary component, will only be provided by a varied, well-balanced diet. Food rather than pills should continue to be emphasized in all forms of nutrition education.[21]

Overdoses of vitamins A and D are of particular concern, because they can lead to toxicity. The *Journal of the American Medical Association* reported the case of a four-year-old boy diagnosed as having minimal brain dysfunction. He had reportedly been given large doses of vitamin A by his grandmother, who owned a health food store. The boy was irritable, feverish, and had bone pain—classic signs of vitamin A overdose. The researchers stated that about one out of ten children they saw with "minimal brain dysfunction" had been treated by their parents with large amounts of vitamins.[22]

If you want to make sure your children are getting enough vitamin A, the best sources are foods like carrots, sweet potatoes, apricots, orange squash, cheese, and milk.

Vitamin D supplementation may be necessary for children in smoggy northern industrial areas who don't get sufficient sunlight. But for most children, the sun is the safer and more reliable option. This is also true for the elderly, who may not drink the milk that is the food chosen nationally for vitamin D fortification. A Tufts University study in Boston found that a mere ten to fifteen minutes of exposure of the hands, arms, and face to the sun three times a week in the summertime was sufficient to meet the vitamin D requirements of elderly people.[23]

Overdoses of minerals can also be dangerous to children. A study reported in the *British Medical Journal* in May of 1989 associated a high iron intake in infants with sudden infant death syndrome. High dietary iron can damage fat membranes, increase susceptibility to infection, and inhibit intestinal absorption of other trace elements such as zinc and magnesium. In countries that don't share our enthusiasm for fortifying infant formulas and cereals with iron to prevent anemia, "crib deaths" are much less frequent than in the United States and Great Britain. Vegetarian Asian families in Britain also have a low incidence of this mysterious condition. British researchers suggest it's because their blood iron levels tend to be low.[24]

What about calcium supplements for children whose diets are low in it? Studies show these supplements generally have no effect on the speed of children's growth. In fact, a complete array of vitamin, mineral, and protein supplements given to pregnant Taiwanese women who were nutritionally at risk didn't appreciably affect the growth and development of their offspring.[25]

A study published in 1981 found that megavitamin therapy could raise the low IQs of mentally retarded children. However, a 1989 repeat of the study was unable to duplicate the results.[26]

Supplements for other special groups

Some elderly people can't eat a balanced diet, for reasons ranging from illness to dentures that don't fit. They may need supplements. A Tufts University study, for example, showed that vitamin E supplements enhanced the normally depressed ability of elderly people to fight off infection. However, elderly people should limit their multivitamin/mineral intake to no more than 100 percent of the recommended daily allowances, since more can result in toxic overdose.[27]

Athletes consume large amounts of vitamin and mineral supplements, but studies have failed to show this practice improves their physical performance. In a 1988 study, trained male runners received either supplements or a placebo for three months, then the reverse for three months (after a three-month washout period). No discernible difference was found in various physiologic measures, including maximum uptake peak running speed, blood lactate turnpoint, and peak postexercise blood lactate level. With or without supplementation, blood vitamin and mineral levels were normal throughout the study. This study and others have dispelled the myth that heavy exercise increases the need for vitamins and minerals.[28]

Many reports suggest that beta-carotene, a vitamin A precursor, is protective against cancer. Supplementation with the vitamin, however, isn't necessary. The evidence supporting the protective effect of beta-carotene is based on the consumption of normal amounts of the fruits and vegetables that contain it.[29]

Choosing a supplement

If you've decided to take nutritional supplements, which should you buy?

According to conventional wisdom, "natural" vitamins are no better than synthetic ones. But while they may be chemically identical, the natural versions often contain other nutrients that render the vitamins more bioavailable (available for use by the body). A study reported in the *American Journal of Clinical Nutrition* in 1988, for example, found that 500 mg of a natural citrus extract containing bioflavonoids, proteins, and carbohydrates was 35 percent more absorbed by fasting human subjects than synthetic ascorbic acid (vitamin C) alone.[30] Minerals that have been chelated, or changed into their digestible form, are also more available for use by the body than unchelated forms. Further, synthetic substances can provoke reactions in chemically sensitive people, where the natural versions don't.[31]

One problem with vitamins from natural sources, however, is their size. In some cases, the amount of natural material required for therapeutic doses would be too great to swallow. For this reason, nutritionists who use vitamin and mineral supplements often compromise and use the synthetic variety.[32]

Calcium tablets vary substantially in their bioavailability. The calcium in many of them never makes it to your bones. Ironically, the least available tend to be those with the highest concentrations of calcium: supplements made of calcium carbonate. As larger and larger amounts of calcium are squeezed into smaller and smaller pills, it gets harder and harder for the acid in the stomach to break them down.

Calcium carbonate tablets made by the major suppliers (OS-Cal, Caltrate-D, Tums) are probably okay. But private brands made by small companies (Medicine Shoppe Cal.-D, General Nutrition Center Calcium-D 600, Ames Calcium-D 600) are suspect. The problem for smaller companies is that they can't afford to formulate and test their products as well. If you're not sure which is which, ask your pharmacist. Another way to find out, suggested by Dr. Ralph Shangraw of the University of Maryland School of Pharmacy, is to drop a tablet in a glass of vinegar, stirring occasionally. In half an hour, a proper formulation should be three-fourths dissolved.

"Starch-free" calcium tablets, while less likely to provoke a reaction in the starch-sensitive, aren't the best options for most people, because starch can actually aid in the pills' disintegration.[33]

A brand that seems to have high bioavailability is the calcium hydroxyapatite crystalline form sold by Mutagenics. It's more easily absorbed because the calcium is bound to protein.

For iron, Fero-Grad 500 is less constipating than other formulations. You pay more for this benefit, but it's likely to be worth the money.

If you're pregnant, nursing, or suspect actual vitamin or mineral deficiencies (which, in fact, are very rare), you should consult your doctor for advice on what supplements, if any, are appropriate.

37

DRUGS, VITAMINS, AND FOOD: BAD COMBINATIONS

[I]ncreasingly we are finding that considerable damage is being done to the way the human body functions by the regular prescription of drugs.
—Dr. Andrew Waxman, research biochemist[1]

Vitamin and mineral deficiencies are rare in normal people eating normal diets. They can, however, be induced by drugs. Not only can drugs affect what you get from what you eat, but what you eat can affect what drugs do to you. Many drugs also make poor bedfellows with each other. We'll look at some of these bad chemical mixes in this chapter.

Drugs and vitamins

Drugs alter the metabolism of the body, changing the way vitamins and minerals are absorbed. Some are vitamin thieves. Others affect vitamin and mineral balance.

The Food and Nutrition Research division of the Agricultural and Medical Research Council recently published a 203-page report on this problem. It found that drug use can interfere with the metabolism of vitamins and minerals by acting as a barrier that prevents them from being absorbed. This was true not only of long-term but of short-term drug use. Some leading offenders are set forth in table 46.

Interference with nutrient absorption may be one factor leading to the depression that is a side effect common to many drugs. The feeling of malaise produced by diuretics, for example, is linked to the loss of potassium, a mineral necessary to various normal activities of cells.[2]

Antibiotics can decrease the absorption of vitamins A, K, B vitamins, and folic acid. Vitamin K isn't one you hear much about, but it's actually essential for the synthesis of at least four of the proteins required to make blood clot. The reason you don't hear much about it is that you don't normally need to get it in your diet. The bacteria in your intestines can make it themselves. But antibiotics destroy the intestinal bacteria that make vitamin K. The result can be serious bleeding disorders. In a study reported in the *Journal of the American Medical Association* in 1988, 42 patients at a hospital in Texas were found to have bleeding disorders tied to vitamin K deficiency. Ten of them died. All had received antibiotics intravenously.[3]

Other drugs that deplete the body of vitamin K are the cholesterol-lowering drug Questran and the anticoagulants, including aspirin. If you are regularly taking any of these drugs, you should be sure to get 70–140 mg of vitamin K in your diet every day. Dark, leafy green vegetables are the best source.

Aspirin can also deplete body stores of vitamins C, B_1, and folic acid.

Another vitamin thief is the birth control pill. It can rob the body of vitamin B_6, other B vitamins, vitamin C, and zinc. The result can be anemia, irritability, anxiety, tiredness, weight gain, leg cramps, and blood vessel problems. If you're taking aspirin or anticonvulsants along with the Pill, these effects can be magnified.

Of the minerals, the one most likely to be depleted by drugs is potassium. Diuretics are notorious for this effect. Other drugs that can cause it are cortisone, steroids, strong laxatives, and antacids. Kidney and blood pressure problems can result.

Laxatives and antacids can also interfere with the absorption of nutrients and fluids in general. One essential mineral impaired by antacids is calcium. Calcium can be absorbed only in its soluble ionized form, which requires a low pH in the stomach. Antacids neutralize stomach acid, raising the pH.

Steroids increase the body's requirements for vitamins C and D, calcium, and potassium. One side effect of the drugs can be retarded growth in children. This effect may be reduced by supplementation with vitamin C, vitamin D, and calcium.[4]

Vitamin supplementation may also help patients with drug-induced diseases. In a study at Columbia University, patients with tardive dyskinesia, a movement disorder caused by drugs, showed significant improvement when they were given 1,200 mg of vitamin E daily. The vitamin was useful as well in treating Parkinson's disease.[5]

Table 46.   *Selected Drugs that Are Vitamin and Mineral Thieves*[6]

Nutrient:	*Status impaired by:*
vitamin A	cholestyramine, mineral oil, neomycin
vitamin B₁ (thiamine)	antibiotics, oral contraceptives, aspirin
vitamin B₂ (riboflavin)	antibiotics
vitamin B₆ (pyridoxine)	steroids, cortisone, oral contraceptives, antihypertensives, anti-tuberculosis drugs
vitamin B₁₂	antibiotics, oral diabetes drugs, antituberculosis drugs, oral contraceptives, cholestyramine, colchicine
biotin (a B vitamin)	antibiotics, sulfa drugs
folic acid (a B vitamin)	oral contraceptives, diuretics, aspirin, anticonvulsants, cholestyramine, triamterene, trimethoprim
inositol (a B vitamin)	antibiotics
vitamin C	aspirin, steroids, oral contraceptives, tetracycline
vitamin D	anticonvulsants, steroids, cholestyramine, mineral oil, irritant laxatives
vitamin E	oral contraceptives
vitamin K	antibiotics, anticoagulants, aspirin, Questran, cholestyramine, mineral oil
calcium	steroids
copper	oral contraceptives
potassium	diuretics, steroids
zinc	oral contraceptives

Drugs and food

Food and drugs can also interfere with each other. For example, if you take aluminum-containing antacids with orange juice—or with any other citrus fruit or juice—you can increase the absorption of aluminum into your blood stream by a factor of fifty.[7] The result can be both brain damage and bone loss (see chapter 21).

If you combine acidic foods with aspirin, the result can be excess stomach acid, leading to ulcers.

Antidepressants taken with caffeine can cause water and sodium retention, raising the blood pressure. Taking the antibiotic tetracycline with milk can cancel out the effect of the drug. Other products containing calcium can also have this effect, and so can antacids. Tetracycline should be taken at least an hour before, or two hours after, these foods or products.[8]

The anti-infective metronidazole taken with alcohol can result in nausea, vomiting, flushing, and difficult breathing.[9]

Food in general affects theophylline absorption, and the effect varies with the formulation of the drug. With one product, food may cause toxic amounts of theophylline to be dumped into the blood. With another, drug levels may drop too low if food is taken first. Due to this variability and uncertainty, theophylline is one of those drugs for which substitution between products isn't recommended. You should start with one and stay with it.[10]

The extreme case is cheese and MAO inhibitors. This combination can result in a sudden increase in blood pressure, producing severe headache, stroke, heart failure, and death. The culprit in cheese is tyramine, an amine that has an effect on the body similar to epinephrine (adrenalin). Other foods containing tyramine can also have this effect in combination with MAO inhibitors; and so can other drugs.[11]

The tyramine in food can also increase the hypertensive effects of the sympathomimetic drug phenylpropanolamine (PPA), found in popular nasal decongestants, cough remedies, and diet aids.[12]

Drugs can affect your nutritional status in another way: by suppressing your appetite. Digitalis drugs are major offenders here.[13]

Drugs and drugs

Drugs can also adversely affect the absorption and effects of other drugs. Possible adverse drug interactions are legion and constitute the subject matter of numerous medical texts. Adverse interactions can occur not only between prescription drugs but with the over-the-counter variety that unwary consumers pop routinely.

While your doctor should warn you of the interference with drug absorption caused by the prescription anti-ulcer drug Tagamet (see chapter 22); you're on your own with over-the-counter antacids, which can have the same effect. Drugs with which antacids are likely to interact are listed in table 47.[14] To alleviate this problem, take antacids at least thirty minutes before or after meals and other medications. Better yet, avoid taking antacids.

Over-the-counter remedies for allergies, nasal congestion, or insomnia containing antihistamines or anticholinergic drugs (those that block the parasympathetic nervous system) can enhance the effects of tricyclic antidepressants and antipsychotic drugs (the major tranquilizers). The result can be oversedation or delirium. Over-the-counter products containing alcohol can cause oversedation when combined with antihistamines, tranquilizers, or more alcohol. Tranquilizers also interact with many other drugs. Tagamet is particularly likely to increase the toxic effects of tranquilizers.[15]

People taking tricyclic antidepressants or MAO inhibitors can wind up with high blood pressure if they mix these drugs with sympathomimetic amines found in over-the-counter cough and cold remedies and diet aids. Examples are the pseudoephedrine in Sudafed and the phenylpropanolamine in Sine-off and Dexatrim. These over-the-counter remedies can also cause hypertension in people predisposed to the condition, without help from other drugs.

Over-the-counter products that contain caffeine can reduce the effects of antihypertensives, antiarrhythmics, and antianxiety drugs.

Table 47. *Drug/Antacid Interactions*

Drug	Aluminum salts	Calcium salts	Antacid Magnesium salts	Sodium bicarbonate	Magnesium aluminum combinations
allopurinol	−				
appetite suppressants				+	
benzodiazepines	+		−	−	−
captopril					−
cimetidine					−
corticosteroids	−		−		−
diflunisal	−				
digoxin	−		−		
flecainide				+	
iron	−	−	−	−	−
isoniazid	−				
ketoconazole				−	−
levodopa					+
lithium				−	
penicillamine	−		−		−
phenytoin		−			−
quinidine		+	+		+
quinolones					−
ranitidine	−				−
salicylates		−		−	−
sulfonylureas				−	
sympathomimetics				+	
tetracyclines	−	−	−	−	−
tranquilizers (major)	−		−		−

+ Effect increased by antacids.
− Effect decreased by antacids.

Aspirin increases the effects of oral diabetes drugs. Both aspirin and acetaminophen increase the effects of anticoagulants. Acetaminophen can also increase the risk of liver damage from overindulgence in alcohol.[16]

If your doctor has prescribed drugs and you're taking several at once, make sure he's aware of all of them—over-the-counter as well as prescription. Ask him about the possible adverse drug interactions of the medications he has prescribed. And read drug labels and inserts.

This is particularly important for elderly people. They not only take more drugs, in more combinations, than younger people; they metabolize and eliminate drugs less efficiently. Nursing home patients are typically on four to nine medications a day. Older people also take the lion's share of psychotropic drugs, including antidepressants, sedatives, and tranquilizers. These drugs are responsible for nearly half the adverse drug interactions suffered by elderly patients.[17]

Studies have shown that prescription drugs are taken by 95 percent of elderly patients living in nursing homes and by 84 percent of those living at home. Seventy percent of elderly patients use over-the-counter drugs in combination with these prescription products without first consulting their doctors or their pharmacists.

Senior citizens are the number-one target of the medical/industrial complex. They are also the patron class most likely to have trouble participating with their doctors in informed treatment decisions. We'll look at their unique drug problems in the next chapter.

38

DRUGS AND THE ELDERLY

The long habit of living indisposeth us for dying.
—Sir Thomas Browne (1605–82)

Fully 30 percent of our multimillion dollar Medicare budget goes for care of the terminally ill—patients who will die anyway within a year of treatment.[1] Nobody wins in these cases but the industries the treatments support. Yet the medical/industrial complex isn't necessarily at fault. Supply merely meets demand. The frightened older patient and the people who love him demand the best and most expensive the system can provide, and insurance unflinchingly foots the bill. It's up to the elderly consumer and his relatives to be informed of the benefits and risks of treatment before either demanding it or acquiescing to it. It is important for them to realize that heart disease and cancer, the major killers, are also Big Business.

Take the coronary bypass operation, which is now very popular with surgeons; it grosses about $25,000 an operation, and an efficient surgeon can perform three of them in a day. The exorbitant but "customary" fee, paid by insurers at a flat rate, was set at a time when the surgery was a lot trickier than it is now. What the patient needs to ask is whether the surgery is likely to make him live any longer. In fact, it only rarely extends life or improves the quality of the short one remaining.[2]

Another thriving business revolves around the cardiac pacemaker. The recent popularity of this device was described in a 1988 *New England Journal of Medicine* editorial as "pacemaker mania."

Researchers reporting in the same issue found that less than half the pacemaker implants investigated were clearly appropriate. In 36 percent, the indications were questionable, and in another 20 percent, the devices definitely weren't indicated.[3] A 1982 report from the U.S. Senate Special Subcommittee on Aging concluded that up to half of Medicare's outlay for pacemaker implants was unjustified.[4] Worse than the dollar cost may be the cost in health. Pacemakers can aggravate symptoms, become infected, produce cardiac arrhythmias and, like any mechanical equipment, fail to function properly.

So why the push to install them? The commentators offered three possible explanations. One was inadequate knowledge on the part of physicians. Symptoms are overestimated, leading doctors to conclude implants are indicated when they're not. A second consideration was legal. Mounting medical malpractice awards have rung in the era of "defensive medicine," in which doctors feel compelled to overtest, overprescribe, and overtreat. The most obvious factor, however, was economic. Pacemakers mean high sales commissions to the industry, as well as about $10,000 each to the hospital and $2,000 to the doctor.[5]

Drug problems of the elderly

The profits made by the pacemaker industry from the elderly pale in comparison to those accruing to the drug industry. Retirees make up only 12 percent of the population, yet they're the largest consumers of all medications, prescription and nonprescription. Their average prescription rate is thirteen per patient per year. One study found that over 90 percent of older people took an average of five prescription drugs and three over-the-counter drugs daily. The total annual drug bill footed by the elderly, their insurers, or Medicare is $3 billion.[6]

Unfortunately, this largest class of consumers is also the group least able to handle drugs. Older people are particularly susceptible to adverse drug reactions and interactions, not only because they take so many drugs but because their systems are less well equipped to deal with the ones they take. Their drug clearance (the time it takes for medication to pass through their systems) is often greatly reduced. Kidney function is lower and so is blood flow to the liver. The older patient has less body water and more body fat. This means water-soluble drugs become more concentrated, while fat-soluble drugs stay around longer and accumulate in the tissues. Moreover, older people have been accumulating these drugs for years. Sedatives and hypnotics linger and cause confusion. Drug doses that have been tested on younger people can easily sedate the elderly brain or drop the elderly blood pressure, causing dizziness and fainting. Dosage errors are more likely because the older patient can't see well to read the label or hear the doctor's directions or remember what was said.

Not only prescription but nonprescription drugs can result in dangerous reactions and interactions. Seduced by inflated advertising claims, older people use great quantities of both. Toxic effects occur in the elderly at lower doses than in younger people, but the symptoms of toxicity are often attributed to old age and overlooked.

Studies show that fully 12 percent of the elderly wind up in the hospital with a drug-induced illness. Aspirin and other NSAIDs are the drugs most often implicated in these admissions.[7] Because drugs tend to linger longer and be more concentrated in their bodies, the elderly can wind up with salicylate poisoning at lower doses than younger people. Older people with chronic pains (arthritis, backaches, and headaches) are also the most likely victims of analgesic nephropathy from overuse of aspirin or acetaminophen. Aspirin can cause allergic reactions, irritation and bleeding in the stomach, and anemia through imperceptible iron loss. It can also alter blood coagulation and lower body temperature. "Feeling cold" is a common senior-citizen complaint.

Antacids are another over-the-counter favorite of the elderly. Antacids affect the absorption of other drugs and nutrients; and repeated use of those containing calcium carbonate can result in chronic constipation. Antacids can also affect bone mineral metabolism, weakening the bones.

Other drugs that can inhibit bowel function include tricyclic antidepressants, antihistamines, antiparkinson drugs, iron, and tranquilizers.

Chronic constipation, in turn, can lead to chronic laxative use. As many as 30 percent of the elderly have acquired the laxative habit. The result of this can be abnormally low blood potassium levels and other electrolyte imbalances.

Over-the-counter cough and cold preparations can alter blood pressure, cause psychiatric problems, and exacerbate glaucoma. Over-the-counter sleep remedies can also exacerbate glaucoma, and overuse of over-the-counter insomnia and stomach remedies containing bromides can lead to dependence, confusion, and depression.[8]

Drugs and nursing-home admissions

Even the enormous drug bill of the elderly pales in comparison to the cost of their institutionalization. The Mayo Clinic estimates that the price of long-term care for elderly Americans will be as much as $60 billion in 1990. Reducing these costs means finding ways of reducing admissions to nursing homes. One way is to reduce medications, which are related in a major way to nursing-home admissions.

Leading reasons for nursing-home admission include hip fracture, urinary incontinence, senility, and the inability to self-administer medications correctly.[9] All are linked to over-medication.

An Oregon study found that the most important trait distinguishing older people in nursing homes from those able to maintain themselves at home was the inability to manage their medications properly.[10] As many as half the prescription medications self-administered by the elderly aren't taken correctly. The problem can be alleviated by reducing the number of medications they take. Studies show the more drugs patients must take, the less likely they are to comply with their doctor's instructions about taking them.[11]

Senility, or senile dementia, is another cause of nursing home admission. It can also be drug-induced. Symptoms like disorientation, memory loss, confusion, psychosis, and depression, which are attributed to the patient's disease, may be the result of the drugs he is taking to treat it. A 1988 report in the medical journal *Psychiatric Clinics of North America* compiled the results of many studies investigating the psychiatric side effects of drugs in the elderly. Drugs found to induce psychosis or depression in selected studies are listed in table 48. One of the first steps in evaluating the development of dementia is to review all drugs used by the patient, prescription and nonprescription, and to systematically discontinue them. Since this can result in serious withdrawal problems, however, it should be done only under the supervision of a physician.[12]

Urinary incontinence is another cause of nursing home admission. It afflicts about one-half of all nursing home residents; and it, too, can be caused by drugs. Medications that can be responsible include antihistamines, diuretics, tranquilizers, antipsychotics, antidepressants, antiparkinson drugs, opiate analgesics, antidiarrheal drugs, antiarrhythmics, and sympathetic blockers (e.g., belladonna).[13]

The other leading reason for nursing home admission is hip fracture. By far the most common cause of dizziness and falls in the elderly is a drop in blood pressure on standing. This drop is most commonly induced by antihypertensives and other drugs.[14] A recent study that we looked at earlier found that a major cause of falls leading to hip fracture in the elderly is medication that causes dizziness, sedation, and confusion. Older people were about twice as likely to suffer hip fractures if they were taking tranquilizers with long half-lives, like flurazepam (Dalmane); tricyclic antidepressants, including amitriptyline (Elavil), doxepin (Adapin, Sinequan), and imipramine (Tofranil); or antipsychotics, including thioridazine (Mellaril), haloperidol (Haldol), and chlorpromazine (Thorazine).[15] These drugs are routinely prescribed for older people, either to help them get to sleep or to manage agitation and unruly behavior.

Table 48. *Drugs Found to Induce Psychosis and Depression in the Elderly in Selected Studies[16]*

Category	Drug
Analgesics/anti-inflammatories	indomethacin
	sulindac
	aspirin
	pentazocine
Anticonvulsants	phenytoin
	primidone
	carbamazepine
Antidepressants	trazadone
	nortriptyline
	imipramine
	amitriptyline
	amoxapine
Antihypertensives/heart drugs	digoxin
	digitoxin
	quinidine
	procainamide
	mexilitine
	tocainide
	disopyramide
	nifedipine
	propranolol
	nadolol
	timolol
	methyldopa
	methyldopa hydralazine
	reserpine
	thiazide diuretics
Antiparkinson drugs	levodopa
	amantadine
	bromocriptine
Antituberculosis drugs	isoniazid
Central nervous system stimulants	methylphenidate
	diethylpropion
	fenfluramine
	phenteramine
	phenylpropranolamine
	ephedrine

Chemotherapeutic agents	cisplatin
	doxorubicin
	cyclophosphamide
	asparaginase
H2-blockers	ranitidine
	cimetidine
Sedatives/hypnotics/antianxiety agents	triazolam
	alprazolam
	diazepam
	flurazepam
	bupropion
Steroids/androgens	prednisolone
	prednisone
Miscellaneous	thyroid levothyroxine
	baclofen
	metrizamide

Drugging the elderly to sleep

Insomnia is a common problem among the over-65 set. Nearly half report chronic difficulty getting to sleep. Half the residents of nursing homes, and 10 percent of the elderly not in nursing homes, take sleep medication nightly. The most popular drugs for this purpose are the benzodiazepines—flurazepam (Dalmane), temazepam (Restoril), and triazolam (Halcion). These drugs have replaced the earlier favorites, barbiturates and chloral hydrate. The benzodiazepines are claimed to have fewer side effects and adverse drug interactions than the older options, as well as less potential for abuse and a higher therapeutic index (the difference between the amount you need to get an effect and the amount that will kill you).

However, benzodiazepines can cause significant side effects in the elderly, including daytime sedation, loss of memory, and rebound insomnia. These problems are compounded in older people because they don't eliminate drugs as well as their younger counterparts and because more of the drug accumulates in their fat cells. Tranquilizer intoxication is also much more dangerous to geriatric than to younger patients. The condition is four times as likely to be fatal to the old as to the young.

The elderly are also large consumers of the major tranquilizers

(Thorazine, Taractan, Prolixin, Haldol, Loxitane, Serentil, Moban, Trilafon, Mellaril, Navane, Stelazine). In younger people, these drugs are used to treat psychotic symptoms like hallucinations and delusions. In the elderly, their most common use is to manage agitation, unruly behavior, and wandering.[17]

Again, these drugs can have serious adverse reactions and interactions with other drugs; and the effects are magnified in the elderly because of their decreased ability to metabolize drugs, and their increased intake of drugs in general. The MAO-inhibitor antidepressants are particularly likely to interact adversely with other drugs. The major tranquilizers, MAO inhibitors, and tricyclic antidepressants all cause a fall in blood pressure, which can intensify the effects of antihypertensive drugs. They all cause sedation, intensifying the sedative effects of benzodiazepines and antihistamines. They can also cause constipation, urinary retention, confusion, and memory loss.[18]

When antidepressants or tranquilizers are used by older people, the dose should be reduced. Intakes of other drugs should be slashed to a minimum. And the doctor should be kept informed of all drug use, over-the-counter as well as prescription. If older people need benzodiazepines, the drugs should be reserved for short periods of particular stress, not exceeding four to six weeks. This is the ideal; but one problem with benzodiazepines is that it's hard to get off them once you're on them, due to a severe rebound-insomnia effect (see chapter 24).

Barbiturates aren't recommended for the elderly, because they produce an unsteady gait that's liable to result in falls and fractures. Older people are also more likely to experience adverse side effects and drug interactions from barbiturates, and the drugs have a high addiction potential. If used by older people at all, barbiturates should be limited to two weeks' use.[19]

For some patients, old-fashioned chloral hydrate may still prove to be the best option.

Common-sense measures for ensuring sound sleep include a warm, comfortable bed in a well-ventilated room; the avoidance of caffeine, alcohol, and cigarettes at bedtime and during the night;

and minimal drinking of liquids near bedtime, so the urge to urinate doesn't disturb sleep.

The quality of life after eighty

It seems the best way for older people to avoid adverse drug reactions and keep out of nursing homes is to slash their drug intakes to a minimum. This means cutting both the number of medications and the dose. It takes nerve; but Jane Brody describes one woman who had the temerity to try it, with excellent results.

Dr. Mary Calderone, a woman in her eighties, had been debilitated by extreme sleepiness, loss of balance, loss of memory, weakness, trouble concentrating, depression, and tiredness. Dizziness and instability caused her to take several serious falls. Her doctors could find no explanation. These symptoms were, after all, normal for her age. But Dr. Calderone wasn't willing to accept that. She decided to try abandoning her drugs. The major offender in her case turned out to be Elavil, a brand-name form of the antidepressant amitriptyline. She'd been taking it in small doses for years to help her get to sleep. When she quit, she got back her energy, her memory, her balance, and her ability to think clearly.[20]

Life after eighty needn't be the sickly, weak, and confused state of patients in modern nursing homes; but there is more to preserving clarity of mind and suppleness of limb in old age than merely avoiding sedatives and tranquilizers. One secret was divulged by Luigi Cornaro, a fifteenth-century centenarian who described himself at the age of 95:

[T]hough at this great age, I am hearty and content, eating with a good appetite, and sleeping soundly. Moreover, all my senses are as good as ever. . . . How different from the life of most old men, full of aches and pains, and forebodings, whilst mine is a life of real pleasure. . . .

His secret was a "regular life," which he described as follows:

By a regular life I mean, that a man shall ascertain for himself, how small a quantity of food and drink is sufficient to supply the daily wants of his nature and having done this, and found out the kinds of food and drink best suited to his constitution, he shall . . . strictly adhere to his resolutions and principles . . . taking care always to avoid excess. . . . [B]y regular living, he destroys every seed of sickness, and thus, by removing the cause, prevents the effect.

Appendix

Interchangeable Drugs Evaluated by the FDA as Therapeutically Equivalent (1988)[1]

Brand Name	*Generic Equivalent*
Achromycin V	tetracycline HCL
Aldactazide	spironolactone; hydrochlorothiazide
Aldactone	spironolactone
Aldoclor	methyldopa; chlorothiazide
Aldomet	methyldopa
Aldoril	methyldopa; hydrochlorothiazide
Alupent	metaproterenol sulfate
Aminophyllin	aminophylline
Amoxil	amoxicillin
Amphicol	chloramphenicol
Antepar	piperazine citrate
Antivert	meclizine HCL
Anturane	sulfinpyrazone
Apresazide	hydralazine HCL; hydrochlorothiazide
Apresoline	hydralazine HCL
Aralen	chloroquine phosphate
Aristocort	triamcinolone acetonide
Artane	trihexyphenidyl HCL
Atarax	hydroxyzine HCL
Ativan	lorazepam
Atromid-S	clofibrate
Azulfidine	sulfasalazine
Bactocill	oxacillin sodium
Bactrim	sulfamethoxazole; trimethoprim
Bancap	acetaminophen; butalbital

[1] From GPIA Generic Pharmaceutical Industry Association, *GPIA Guide to Interchangeable Drugs* (Port Washington, N.Y.: Schein Pharmaceuticals, 1988). List does not reflect the FDA's 1989 re-evaluations, the results of which have not yet been published (see chapter 2).

Benadryl	diphenhydramine HCL
Benemid	probenecid
Bentyl	dicyclomine HCL
Butazolidin	phenylbutazone
Butisol Sodium	butabarbital sodium
Cafergot	ergotamine tartrate w/caffeine
Calan	verapamil HCL
Catapres	clonidine HCL
Centrax	prazepam
Chlor-Trimeton	chlorpheniramine maleate
Chloromycetin	chloramphenicol
Choledyl	oxtriphylline
Cleocin	clindamycin HCL
Cloxapen	cloxacillin sodium
Cogentin	benztropine mesylate
Combipres	chlorthalidone; clonidine HCL
Compazine	prochlorperazine maleate
Coumadin	warfarin sodium
Cyclapen	cyclacillin
Dalmane	flurazepam HCL
Danocrine	danazol
Darvocet-N	propoxyphene napsylate; acetaminophen
Darvon	propoxyphene HCL
Decapryn	doxylamine succinate
Deltasone	prednisone
Demerol	meperidine HCL
Depakene	valproic acid
Desoxyn	methamphetamine HCL
Desyrel	trazodone HCL
Dexedrine	dextroamphetamine sulfate
Diabinese	chlorpropamide
Diamox	acetazolamide
Dilantin*	phenytoin sodium, extended
Dimetane	brompheniramine maleate
Diprosone	betamethasone dipropionate
Ditropan	oxybutynin chloride
Diucardin	hydroflumethiazide
Diuril	chlorothiazide

* Prompt release dosage form not therapeutically equivalent.

Doriden	glutethimide
Dyazide	hydrochlorothiazide; triamterene
Dymelor	acetohexamide
Dynapen	dicloxacillin sodium
E.E.S.	erythromycin ethylsuccinate
Elavil	amitriptyline HCL
Endep	amitriptyline HCL
Enduron	methyclothiazide
Equagesic	aspirin; meprobamate
Equanil	meprobamate
Erythrocin	erythromycin stearate
Esidrix	hydrochlorothiazide
Eskalith	lithium carbonate
Fastin	phentermine HCL
Fiorinal	butalbital w/aspirin and caffeine
Flagyl	metronidazole
Folvite	folic acid
Furadantin	nitrofurantoin
Gantanol	sulfamethoxazole
Gantrisin	sulfisoxazole
Garamycin	gentamicin sulfate
Haldol	haloperidol
Hycodan	homatropine methylbromide; hydrocodone bitartrate
Hydergine	ergoloid mesylates
HydroDIURIL	hydrochlorothiazide
Hygroton	chlorthalidone
Ilosone	erythromycin estolate
Inderal	propranolol HCL
Inderide	propranolol HCL; hydrochlorothiazide
Indocin	indomethacin
Indocin SR	indomethacin CR
INH	isoniazid
Ionamin-30	phentermine resin complex CR
Ismelin	guanethidine monosulfate
Isoptin	verapamil HCL
Isordil	isosorbide dinitrate
Keflex	cephalexin
Kenalog	triamcinolone acetonide
Kwell	lindane

Larotid	amoxicillin
Lasix	furosemide
Librium	chlordiazepoxide HCL
Limbitrol	amitriptyline HCL; chlordiazepoxide
Lioresal	baclofen
Lioresal DS	baclofen
Lomotil	diphenoxylate HCL w/atropine sulfate
Loniten	minoxidil
Loxitane	loxapine succinate
Ludiomil	maprotiline HCL
Macrodantin	nitrofurantoin macrocrystalline
Maxzide	hydrochlorothiazide; triamterene
Meclomen	meclofenamate sodium
Medrol	methylprednisolone
Megace	megestrol acetate
Mellaril	thioridazine HCL
Midamor	amiloride HCL
Miltown	meprobamate
Motrin	ibuprofen
Mycifradin	neomycin sulfate
Mycostatin	nystatin
Mysoline	primidone
Nalfon	fenoprofen calcium
Navane	thiothixene
NegGram	nalidixic acid
Nembutal Sodium	sodium pentobarbital
Neotrizine	trisulfapyrimidines
Nicolar	niacin
Norflex	orphenadrine citrate
Norgesic	aspirin; caffeine; orphenadrine citrate
Norinyl 1+35	norethindrone; ethinyl estradiol
Norinyl 1+50	mestranol: norethindrone
Norpace	disopyramide phosphate
Norpace CR	disopyramide phosphate CR
Norpramin	desipramine HCL
Oretic	hydrochlorothiazide
Orinase	tolbutamide
Ortho Novum 1/ 35	norethindrone; ethinyl estradiol

Ortho Novum 1/ 50	mestranol; norethindrone
Paraflex	chlorzoxazone
PBZ	tripelennamine HCL
Pentids	penicillin G potassium
Pen·Vee K	penicillin V potassium
Percocet	acetaminophen; oxycodone HCL
Percodan	aspirin; oxycodone HCL; oxycodone ter-ephthalate
Periactin	cyproheptadine HCL
Placidyl	ethchlorvynol
Plegine	phendimetrazine tartrate
Polycillin	ampicillin/ampicillin trihydrate
Polycillin-PRB	ampicillin trihydrate; probenecid
Ponstel	mefenamic acid
Principen	ampicillin/ampicillin trihydrate
Pro-Banthine	propantheline bromide
Procan	procainamide HCL
Procan SR	procainamide HCL CR
Prolixin	fluphenazine HCL
Proloprim	trimethoprim
Pronestyl	procainamide HCL
Prostaphlin	oxacillin sodium
Quinaglute	quinidine gluconate
Quinora	quinidine sulfate
Redisol	cyanocobalamin
Reglan	metoclopramide HCL
Restoril	temazepam
Ritalin	methylphenidate HCL
Ritalin-SR	methylphenidate HCL CR
Robaxin	methocarbamol
Robaxisal	methocarbamol w/aspirin
Robinul	glycopyrrolate
Saluron	hydroflumethiazide
Seconal Sodium	secobarbital sodium
Septra	sulfamethoxazole; trimethoprim
Serax	oxazepam
Sinequan	doxepin HCL
Slow-K	potassium chloride
Soma	carisoprodol

Stelazine	trifluoperazine HCL
Surmontil	trimipramine maleate
Symmetrel	amantadine HCL
Synalar	fluocinolone acetonide
Tegopen	cloxacillin sodium
Tegretol	carbamazepine
Temaril	trimeprazine tartrate
Tenuate	diethylpropion HCL
Terramycin	oxytetracycline HCL
Tetracyn	tetracycline HCL
Tofranil	imipramine HCL
Tolinase	tolazamide
Tranxene	clorazepate dipotassium
Triavil	perphenazine; amitriptyline HCL
Trilafon	perphenazine
Trimpex	trimethoprim
Tylenol w/Codeine	acetaminophen; codeine phosphate
Urecholine	bethanechol chloride
V-Cillin K	penicillin V potassium
Valisone	betamethasone valerate
Valium	diazepam
Vancocin HCL	vancomycin HCL
Velosef	cephradine
Vibramycin	doxycycline hyclate
Vicodin	acetaminophen; hydrocodone bitartrate
Vicoprin	aspirin; hydrocodone bitartrate
Vistaril	hydroxyzine pamoate
Wellcovorin	leucovorin calcium
Wygesic	acetaminophen; propoxyphene HCL
Zyloprim	allopurinol

Brand Name Drugs not Available as Generics

Aventyl HCL	Cinobac	Glucotrol
Blocadren	Clinoril	Halcion
Calderol	Corgard	Imodium
Capoten	Dolobid	Lo/Ovral
Cardizem	Feldene	Lopressor
Ceclor	Flexeril	Micronase

Minipress	Parlodel	Tenormin
Minizide	Proventil	Timoptic
Moduretic	Seldane	Xanax
Naprosyn	Sinemet	Zantac

Notes

Chapter One   Your Medicine Cabinet: Friend or Foe?

1. See A. Melville, C. Johnson, *Cured to Death* (New York: Stein and Day, 1982), p. 5; C. Inlander, E. Weiner, "You can say 'no' to a hospital stay," *Whole Life Times* (September 1985), p. 16.
2. T. Preston, *The Clay Pedestal* (Seattle: Madrona Publishers, 1981), quoted in C. Inlander, et al., *op. cit.*
3. See M. Kapp, "Placebo therapy and the law: Prescribe with care," *American Journal of Law and Medicine* 8(4):371 (1982); P. Sanberg, Richard Krenna, *Over-the-Counter Drugs: Harmless or Hazardous?* (New York: Chelsea House, 1986), pp. 96–98; F. James, "Doctors don't tell all on drugs' effects," *Wall Street Journal* (May 20, 1988), p. 27.
4. See N. Davis, M. Cohen, *Medication Errors: Causes and Prevention* (Philadelphia: George F. Stickley Co., 1981), pp. 1–2 (citing studies in eight different hospitals using conventional drug distribution methods); D. Harney, *Medical Malpractice* (Indianapolis: Allen Smith Co., 1973), p. 321.
5. *Ibid,* pp. 134, 193.
6. *Howell v. Outer Drive Hospital,* 66 Mich. App. 142, 238 N.W.2d 553 (1975).
7. *Malone v. Sunnyvale Medical Clinic,* Docket No. 201229, Superior Ct., Santa Clara County, Cal., April 11, 1972.
8. *McKinley v. Vize,* 563 S.W.2d 505 (Mo. App. 1978).
9. *Hair v. County of Monterey,* Docket No. 67538, Superior Ct., Monterey County, Cal., 1971.
10. A. Melville, et al., *op. cit.,* pp. 136–40.
11. E. Hess, "Drug-related lupus," *New England Journal of Medicine* 318(22):1460–62 (1988).
12. "Hazards of non-practolol beta blockers," *British Medical Journal* 1(6060): 529 (1977); A. Melville, et al., *op. cit.,* pp. 136–40.
13. See chapter 11.
14. *National Disease and Therapeutic Index,* I.M.S. (Ambler, Pennsyl-

vania, 1983), cited in S. Wolfe, et al., *Worst Pills, Best Pills* (Washington, D.C.: Public Citizen Health Research Group, 1988), p. 343.

15. See K. Butler, L. Rayner, *The Best Medicine* (San Francisco: Harper & Row, 1985), p. 446.

16. See L. Ponte, "The bugs that bug us: What you should know about colds," *Reader's Digest* (October 1987), pp. 85–89.

Chapter Two   The Generics Scandal and the Drug Approval Process

1. Quoted in S. Martin, "Generic drug scandals raise questions about safety," *American Pharmacy* (October 1989), pp. 23–24.

2. J. Scott, "Generics: Are they as good?", *Los Angeles Times* (August 30, 1989), p. 1.

3. See GPIA Generic Pharmaceutical Industry Association, *GPIA Guide to Interchangeable Drugs* (Port Washington, N.Y.: Schein Pharmaceuticals, 1988); M. deCourcy Hinds, "The battle over generic drugs heats up," *New York Times* (March 4, 1989), p. 35.

4. From *GPIA Guide to Interchangeable Drugs, op. cit.,* p. 20.

5. B. Strom, "Generic drug substitution revisited," *New England Journal of Medicine* 316:1456–62 (1987); J. Scott, *op. cit.*

6. "The capsules that flunked," *Time* (September 11, 1989), p. 59.

7. S. Martin, *op. cit.;* S. Nightingale, "From the Food and Drug Administration: Action on generic drug products," *JAMA* 262(14):1916 (1989); R. Koenig, "SmithKline still suffering from Dyazide side effects," *Wall Street Journal* (August 9, 1989), p. B2.

8. R. Rose, "Eli Lilly workers submitted false data on drugs, FDA investigators report," *Wall Street Journal* (September 21, 1989), p. A4.

9. E. Feldmann, "The 'weak link' in new drug research," *Journal of the Pharmaceutical Association* 72:463 (1983).

10. S. Martin, *op. cit.;* A. Kibbe, "The generic drug issue: A scientist's perspective," *American Pharmacy* (November 1989), pp. 22–23.

11. J. Scott, *op. cit.*

12. L. Hendeles, "Slow-release theophylline: Do not substitute," *American Pharmacy* (March 1989), p. 22; P. Kramer, "Slow-release theophylline: Substitute only AB-rated products," *Ibid.,* pp. 23–24.

13. "Generic topical corticosteroids," *Medical Letter* 30(765): 49–50 (1988).

Chapter Three   *Antibiotics: The Exploitation of a Wonder Drug*

1. K. Butler, L. Rayner, *The Best Medicine* (San Francisco: Harper & Row, 1985), p. 446.
2. *Ibid.;* A. Burger, *Drugs and People* (Charlottesville, Va.: University Press of Virginia, 1986), pp. 118–19.
3. J. Bennett, "Human infections: Economic implications and prevention," *Annals of Internal Medicine* 89 (Part 2):761–63 (1978); K. Butler, et al., *op. cit.* Concerning vaccines, see chapter 9.
4. J. Boslego, et al., "Effect of spectinomycin use on the prevalence of spectinomycin-resistant and of penicillinase-producing *Neisseria gonorrhoeae,*" *New England Journal of Medicine* 317(5):272–78 (1987).
5. J. Zenilman, et al., "Penicillinase-producing *Neisseria gonorrhoeae* in Dade County, Florida: Evidence of core-group transmitters and the impact of illicit antibiotics," *Sexually Transmitted Diseases* 15(1):45–50 (1988).
6. R. Pallares, et al., "Risk factors and response to antibiotic therapy in adults with bacteremic pneumonia caused by penicillin-resistant pneumococci," *New England Journal of Medicine* 317(1):18–22 (1987); M. Lappé, *Germs That Won't Die: Medical Consequences of the Misuse of Antibiotics* (Garden City, NY: Anchor/Press Doubleday, 1982), p. 15.
7. J. Spika, et al., "Chloramphenicol-resistant *Salmonella newport* traced through hamburger to dairy farms," *New England Journal of Medicine* 316:565–70 (1987).
8. M. Diamant, B. Diamant, "Abuse and timing of use of antibiotics in acute otitis media," *Archives of Otolaryngology* 100:226–32 (1974).
9. K. Sunakawa, et al., "Clinical superinfection and its attendant symptomatic changes in pediatrics," *Infection* 13(Supp. 1):S103–11 (1985); W. Crook, "Pediatrics, antibiotics, and office practice," *Pediatrics* 76(1):139–40 (1985).

Chapter Four   Antibiotic and Antimicrobial Options

1. L. Simonsen, "Top 200 drugs of 1988," *Pharmacy Times* (April 1989), p. 40; M. Lappé, *Germs That Won't Die* (Garden City, N.Y.: Anchor/Press Doubleday, 1982), p. 21.
2. M. Parry, "The penicillins," *Medical Clinics of North America* 71(6):1093–1112 (1987); K. Butler, L. Rayner, M.D., *The Best Medicine* (San Francisco: Harper & Row, 1985), pp. 448–55.
3. S. Norrby, "Adverse reactions and interactions with new cephalosporin and cephamycin antibiotics," *Medical Toxicology* 1:32–46 (1986); D. Goldberg, "The cephalosporins," *Medical Clinics of North America* 71(6):1113–33 (1987).
4. K. Sunakawa, et al., "Clinical superinfection and its attendant symptomatic changes in pediatrics," *Infection* 13(Supp. 1):S103–11 (1985).
5. S. Bryant, et al., "Increased frequency of doxyclycline side effects," *Pharmacotherapy* 7(4):125–29 (1987); E. Francke, H. Neu, "Chloramphenicol and tetracyclines," *Medical Clinics of North America* 71(6):1155–75 (1987); J. Riond, J. Riviere, "Pharmacology and toxicology of doxycycline," *Veterinary and Human Toxicology* 30(5):431–38 (1988).
6. D. Brittain, "Erythromycin," *Medical Clinics of North America* 71(6):1147–54 (1987); K. Butler, et al., *op. cit.; Drug Facts and Comparisons* (St. Louis, Mo.: J.B. Lippincott Co., 1989), p. 1514.
7. H. Beaty, R. Petersdorf, "Iatrogenic factors in infectious disease," *Annals of Internal Medicine* 65(4):641–56 (1966).
8. E. Francke, et al., *op. cit.*
9. M. Foltzer, R. Reese, "Trimethoprim-sulfamethoxazole and other sulfonamides," *Medical Clinics of North America* 71(6):1177–95 (1987); P. Berg, P. Daniel, "Co-trimoxazole-induced hepatic injury —an analysis of cases with hypersensitivity-like reactions," *Infection* 15(5):S259-S263 (1987).
10. J. Allan, "Antibiotic combinations," *Medical Clinics of North America* 71(6):1079–91 (1987).
11. *Yetton v. Desert Hosp. District of Palm Springs,* Docket No. 92756, Superior Ct., Riverside County, Cal. 1972; *Bochum v. Sherman Hosp.,* Docket No. 70L, Circuit Ct., Kane County, Ill. 1973.
12. *Kong v. Clay-Grant Pharmacy,* Docket No. 619350, Superior Ct., San Francisco County, Cal. 1972.

13. "Current concepts in tuberculosis (II)," *American Pharmacy* NS28 (5):37–42 (1988).
14. K. Butler, et al., *op. cit.*
15. J. Rosenblatt, R. Edson, "Metronidazole," *Mayo Clinic Proceedings* 62:1013–17 (1987).
16. "Topical metronidazole for rosacea," *Medical Letter* 31 (798):75–76 (1989).
17. See W. Crook, *The Yeast Connection* (Jackson, Tenn.: Professional Books, 1985), pp. 291–92.
18. See G. Cawood, et al., *Prescription Drug Encyclopedia 1989–90* (Peachtree City, Ga.: FC&A Publishing, 1989).

Chapter Five Antibiotics for Common Ailments: Ear Infections and Strep

1. F. Disney, "Pediatricians, antibiotics, and office practice," *Pediatrics* 74(6):1135 (1984).
2. G. Gates, et al., "Effectiveness of adenoidectomy and tympanostomy tubes in the treatment of chronic otitis media with effusion," *New England Journal of Medicine* 317(23):1444–51 (1987); W. Crook, "Pediatricians, antibiotics, and office practice," *Pediatrics* 76(1):139–40 (1985).
3. G. Gates, et al., *op. cit.;* J. Paradise, "Otitis media in infants and children," *Pediatrics* 65(5):917 (1980).
4. G. Gates, et al., *op. cit.;* J. Paradise, C. Bluestone, "Adenoidectomy and chronic otitis media," *New England Journal of Medicine* 318(22):1470 (1988); P. Lorentzen, P. Haugsten, "Treatment of acute suppurative otitis media," *Journal of Laryngology and Otology* 91:331–40 (1977).
5. G. Gates, et al., *op. cit.;* T. McGill, M. Goodman, "A seven-year-old Japanese-American boy with persistent right-ear drainage despite antibiotic therapy," *New England Journal of Medicine* 316:1589–97 (1987).
6. See, e.g., W. Crook, *op. cit.;* M. Diamant, B. Diamant, "Abuse and timing of use of antibiotics in acute otitis media," *Archives of Otolaryngology* 100:226–32 (1974).
7. M. Casselbrandt, et al., "Otitis media with effusion in preschool children," *Laryngoscope* 95:428–36 (1985); J. Lous, M. Fiellau-Nikolajsen, "Epidemiology of middle ear effusion and tubal dys-

function," *International Journal of Pediatric Otorhinolaryngology* 3:303–17 (1981).

8. About half the cases had been treated with antibiotics and half had not. Of those receiving antibiotics, about half got them from the first day of the disease, a third got them from the second to the seventh day, and the rest got them after the seventh day. The patients seen from the outset at the county hospital were treated according to the "timing principle": antibiotics were not administered unless, or until, the symptoms showed a direct threat of complications. This meant the hospital almost never administered antibiotics during the first week of illness. The rate of serious complications in cases treated according to the timing principle was substantially lower than expected. Most of the patients receiving antibiotics had been transferred to the hospital by other physicians. Nearly all of these transferred patients were already being treated with antibiotics, frequently from the first day of the disease; and in these cases, the hospital continued the antibiotic therapy.

9. These results can't be explained by assuming the cases receiving antibiotics from the first day of the disease were also the severest cases. To the contrary, those given antibiotics from the first day got them regardless of severity. The severest cases were generally those receiving antibiotics after the eighth day. In these patients, recurrences were 30 percent higher than in untreated patients—compared to *300 percent* higher in patients treated with antibiotics from the first day of the disease.

10. M. Diamant, et al., *op. cit.*

11. W. Crook, *op. cit.*

12. E. Mandel, et al., "Efficacy of amoxicillin with and without decongestant-antihistamine for otitis media with effusion in children," *New England Journal of Medicine* 316(8):432–37 (1987).

13. E. Cantekin, et al., "Lack of efficacy of a decongestant-antihistamine combination for otitis media with effusion ('secretory' otitis media) in children: Results of a double-blind, randomized trial," *New England Journal of Medicine* 308:297–301 (1983).

14. P. Lowry, et al., *"Mycobacterium chelonae* causing otitis media in an ear-nose-and-throat practice," *New England Journal of Medicine* 319:978–82 (1988).

15. A. Bisno, "Acute rheumatic fever: Forgotten but not gone," *New England Journal of Medicine* 316(8):476–78 (1987); see chapter 10.

16. L. Veasy, et al., "Resurgence of acute rheumatic fever in the inter-

mountain area of the United States," *New England Journal of Medicine* 316(8):421–27 (1987); "Resurgence of acute rheumatic fever," *ibid.* 317(8):507–08 (1987).

17. S. Holmberg, G. Faich, "Streptococcal pharyngitis and acute rheumatic fever in Rhode Island," *JAMA* 250(17):2307–12 (1983).

18. *Ibid.*

19. *National Disease and Therapeutic Index,* I.M.S. (Ambler, Pennsylvania, 1983), cited in S. Wolfe, et al., *Worst Pills, Best Pills* (Washington, D.C.: Public Citizen Health Research Group, 1988), p. 343.

Chapter Six   Cold and Cough Remedies: One Week With Them, Seven Days Without

1. Stanley Wohl, M.D., *The Medical Industrial Complex* (New York: Harmony Books, 1984), p. 193.

2. Consumers Union, *The Medicine Show* (New York: Pantheon Books, 1980), pp. 34–36.

3. R. Foust, et al., "Nyquil-associated liver injury," *American Journal of Gastroenterology* 84(4):422–25 (1989).

4. "Late news on the cold front," *University of California, Berkeley Wellness Letter* 5(2):4–5 (1988).

5. A. Feller, et al., "The failure of antihistaminic drugs to prevent or cure the common cold and undifferentiated respiratory diseases," *New England Journal of Medicine* 242(19):737–44 (1950).

6. E. Bravo, "Phenylpropanolamine and other over-the-counter vasoactive compounds," *Hypertension* 11(Supp. II): II-7—II-10 (1988).

7. J. Orson, L. Bassow, "Over-the-counter cough formulas," *Clinical Pediatrics* (June 1987), p. 287.

8. From E. Bravo, *op. cit.*

9. See D. Zimmerman, *The Essential Guide to Nonprescription Drugs* (New York: Harper & Row, 1983), pp. 113–25.

10. *Ibid.*

11. "Late news on the cold front," *op. cit.;* "Zinc-induced copper deficiency," *Nutrition & the M.D.* 15(4):4 (1989).

12. *Ibid.*

Chapter Seven   Drugs for Asthma and Allergies

1. Quoted in A. Buist, "Asthma mortality: What have we learned?", *Journal of Allergy and Clinical Immunology* 84 (3):275–83 (1989).
2. "The baffling rise in asthma deaths," *Newsweek* (May 22, 1989), p. 79.
3. A. Buist, *op. cit.;* B. Lanier, "Who is dying of asthma and why?", *Journal of Pediatrics* 115:838–40 (1989).
4. W. Hines, "For asthma sufferers, an encouraging view of overcoming a lifelong disorder," *Washington Post Health* (April 18, 1989), p. 6; L. Thompson, "The asthma dilemma: With better treatment available, why are more patients dying?", *ibid.* (August 25, 1987), pp. 12–14.
5. L. Thompson, *op. cit.*
6. T. Creer, et al, "Psychological problems associated with drug therapy in childhood asthma," *Journal of Pediatrics* 115:850–55 (1989); K. Butler, L. Rayner, *The Best Medicine* (San Francisco: Harper & Row, 1985), pp. 457–58.
7. T. Creer, et al., *op. cit.*
8. A. Rooklin, "Theophylline: Is it obsolete for asthma?", *Journal of Pediatrics* 115:841–45 (1989); D. DeSilver, "Powerful drugs, disturbing effects," *Vegetarian Times* (August 1989), p. 24.
9. A. Rooklin, *op. cit.;* L. Thompson, *op. cit.;* R. Henig, "The big sneeze," *Washington Post Health* (May 31, 1988), pp. 12–15; D. DeSilver, *op. cit.*
10. W. Lewis, *Medical Botany* (New York: John Wiley & Sons, 1977), p. vii.
11. S. Wynn, "Alternative approaches to asthma," *Journal of Pediatrics* 115:846–49 (1989).
12. R. Henig, *op. cit.*
13. *Ibid.*
14. See G. Maleskey, "Stuffed up? Try these natural remedies," *Prevention* (September 1984), pp. 63–66.
15. S. Squires, "Allergy season returns," *Washington Post Health* (April 18, 1989), pp. 6–7.
16. H. Sampson, S. Scanlon, "Natural history of food hypersensitivity in children with atopic dermatitis," *Journal of Pediatrics* 115:23–27 (1989).

17. R. Henig, "Who gets allergies?", *Washington Post Health* (May 31, 1988), p. 15.
18. S. Lingling, Y. Hongying, "Effect of needling sensation reaching the site of disease on the results of acupuncture treatment of bronchial asthma," *Journal of Traditional Chinese Medicine* 9(2):140–43 (1989); B. Brown, *Stress and the Art of Biofeedback* (New York: Harper & Row, 1977).
19. Adapted from *Nursing89 Drug Handbook* (Springhouse, Pa.: Springhouse Corp., 1989); G. Cawood, et al., *1989–90 Prescription Drug Encyclopedia* (Peachtree City, Ga.: FC&A Publishing, 1989).

Chapter Eight   Reducing Fever with Drugs

1. D. Jaffe, et al., "Antibiotic administration to treat possible occult bacteremia in febrile children," *New England Journal of Medicine* 317 (19):1175–80 (1987).
2. C. Jender, D. Schechter, "Reye's Syndrome: Child killer in disguise," *PTA Today* (December 1988/January 1989). Carolyn Jender is Cindy's mother and is president of the Chicago Chapter of the National Reye's Syndrome Foundation.
3. J. Meythaler, R. Varma, "Reye's syndrome in adults: Diagnostic considerations," *Archives of Internal Medicine* 147(1):61–64 (1987).
4. "Acetaminophen doesn't help chicken pox sufferers," *American Pharmacy* NS29(11):13 (November 1989).
5. See J. Dobowy, et al., "Inhibition of postpyrogenic increase of phagocytic and killing activity of neutrophils by nonsteroid antiinflammatory drugs," *Archivum Immunologiae et Therapiae Experimentalis* 36(3):295–301 (1988); E. Kiester, Jr., "A little fever is good for you," *Science* (November 1984), pp. 168–73; T. Rosenthal, D. Silverstein, "Fever: What to do and what not to do," *Postgraduate Medicine* 83(8):75–84 (1988).
6. H. Igarashi, et al., "Effects of drugs on the pyrogenicity of toxic shock syndrome toxin 1 and its capacity to enhance susceptibility to the lethal effects of endotoxic shock in rabbits," *Review of Infectious Diseases* 11 (Supp. 1):S210–13 (1989).
7. T. Rosenthal, et al., *op. cit.;* H. Kai, et al., "Heat, drugs, and radiation given in combination is palliative for unresectable esophageal cancer," *International Journal of Radiation Oncology, Biology, and Physics* 14(6):1147–52 (1988); H. Bicher, et al., "Micro-

wave hyperthermia as an adjunct to radiation therapy: Summary experience of 256 multifraction treatment cases," *ibid.* 12:1667–71 (1986); F. Storm, "Clinical hyperthermia and chemotherapy," *Radiologic Clinics of North America* 27(3):621–27 (1989).

8. Professor Werner Zabel, cited in K. Ally, "Cancer defeated by body's own defenses," *Tidskrift for Halsa* (Sept. 9, 1975).

9. J. Kruse, "Should fever be treated?", *Washington Post Health* (March 7, 1989), p. 11; T. Rosenthal, et al., *op. cit.*

10. T. Rosenthal, et al., *op. cit.;* J. Kruse, *op. cit.*

Chapter Nine   Vaccines: Benefits and Risks

1. R. Hiltner, "Vaccinations revisited," *Resonance* (September-October 1989), pp. 13–14.

2. B. Nkowane, et al., "Vaccine-associated paralytic poliomyelitis," *JAMA* 257(10):1335–40 (1987); R. Mendelsohn, *How to Raise a Healthy Child in Spite of Your Doctor* (Chicago: Contemporary Books, 1984).

3. See H. Beaty, R. Petersdorf, "Iatrogenic factors in infectious disease," *Annals of Internal Medicine* 65:641–56 (1966).

4. *Berkovitz v. U.S.;* see A. Kamen, "Court rules government liable for negligence," *Washington Post* (June 14, 1988), page A1.

5. H. Coulter, B. Fisher, *DPT: A Shot in the Dark* (San Diego: Harcourt Brace Jovanovich, 1985); D. Holzman, "Signs of cure for vaccine's troubles," *Insight* (June 6, 1988), pp. 50–52; R. Hiltner, *op. cit.*

6. "Whooping cough: The last gasp?", *Harvard Medical School Health Letter* (December 1989), pp. 3–4; R. Hiltner, *op. cit.*

7. H. Brauer, "Are we sweeping DTP contraindications under the rug?", *American Journal of Diseases of Children* 142:698 (1988).

8. See T. Gustafson, et al., "Measles outbreak in a fully immunized secondary-school population," *New England Journal of Medicine* 316(13):771–74 (1987); "Measles revaccination," *Medical Letter* 31(797):69–70 (1989); J. Siwek, "Measles in college," *Washington Post Health* (April 18, 1989), p. 19.

9. S. Crowley, et al., "Mumps, measles, and rubella vaccination and encephalitis," *BMJ* 299:660 (1989).

10. R. Hiltner, *op. cit;* R. Mendelsohn, *op. cit.*, p. 30.

11. See H. Beaty, et al., *op. cit.;* R. Mendelsohn, *op. cit.*, pp. 209–30.

12. N. Halsey, D. Henderson, "HIV infection and immunization

against other agents," *New England Journal of Medicine* 316(11):683–85 (1987).

13. R. Redfield, et al., "Disseminated vaccinia in a military recruit with human immunodeficiency virus (HIV) disease," *New England Journal of Medicine* 316(11):673–76 (1987).

14. *London Times* (May 11, 1987), discussed in J. Rappoport, "Smallpox vaccine as AIDS trigger," *L.A. Weekly* (June 5–11, 1987), p. 8.

15. H. Beaty, et al., *op. cit.;* R. Hiltner, *op. cit.,* citing R. Leviton, "Who calls the shots?", *East/West Journal* (November 1988).

16. P. Andrews, "The creation of AIDS," *Whole Life Times* (May 1989), p. 15.

17. L. Seeff, et al., "A serologic follow-up of the 1942 epidemic of post-vaccination hepatitis in the United States Army," *New England Journal of Medicine* 316(16):965–70 (1987).

18. N. Halsey, et al., *op. cit.;* R. Redfield, et al., *op. cit.*

19. R. Mendelsohn, *op. cit.,* p. 211.

20. From J. Grabenstein, "Pharmacists and immunizations: Advocating preventive medicine," *American Pharmacy* (August 1988), pp. 25–33.

Chapter Ten   Elective Vaccines

1. See R. Ornstein, D. Sobel, *The Healing Brain* (New York: Simon and Schuster, 1987), pp. 19–24; R. Mendelsohn, *How to Raise a Healthy Child in Spite of Your Doctor* (Chicago: Contemporary Books, 1984), pp. 210–11; R. Hiltner, "Vaccinations revisited," *Resonance* (September–October 1989), pp. 13–14.

2. A. Benenson, ed., *Control of Communicable Diseases in Man* (Washington D.C.; American Public Health Association, 1985), pp. 436–40.

3. K. Miller, et al., "Failures of combined chloroquine and Fansidar prophylaxis in American travelers to East Africa," *Journal of Infectious Diseases* 154(4):689–91 (1986).

4. See "Shots for grownups," *Harvard Medical School Health Letter* 13(10):1–2 (1988).

5. State Department communication.

6. A. Benenson, *op. cit.,* p. 338.

7. A 1989 New Zealand study found that the group A meningococcal vaccine used in that country produced neurological symptoms in about 300 of 130,000 vaccinated children. The reports ranged from

fever and rash to stiff neck, weakness, numbness, and muscle pain. See D. Hood, et al., "Meningococcal vaccine—do some children experience side effects?", *New Zealand Medical Journal* 102(862):65–67 (1989).

8. A. Benenson, *op. cit.*
9. L. Thompson, "Pediatricians recommend vaccine for young children," *Washington Post Health* (February 23, 1988), p. 5.
10. D. Granoff, et al., *"Hemophilus influenzae* type b disease in children vaccinated with type b polysaccharide vaccine," *New England Journal of Medicine* 315:1584–90 (1986). See also R. Pritikin, "Failure of vaccination with *Haemophilus influenzae* vaccine," *New England Journal of Medicine* 317(2):115 (1987).
11. T. Murphy, et al., "Prospective surveillance of *Haemophilus influenzae* type b disease in Dallas County, Texas, and in Minnesota," *Pediatrics* 79:173–80 (1987).
12. T. Murphy, et al., "Risk of subsequent disease among day-care contacts of patients with systemic *Hemophilus influenzae* type b disease," *New England Journal of Medicine* 316(1):5–10 (1987); M. Osterholm, et al., "The risk of subsequent transmission of *Hemophilus influenzae* type b disease among children in day care," *ibid.* 316(1):1–5 (1987).
13. M. Osterholm, T. Murphy, "More on rifampin prophylaxis against *Haemophilus influenzae* b in day-care facilities," *New England Journal of Medicine* 318(1):49 (1988).
14. J. Schiffman, "Flu outbreak is declared an epidemic; '91 vaccine is expected to be elusive," *Wall Street Journal* (January 26, 1990), p. B3; M. Beck, L. Wilson, "Feeling bad, getting worse," *Newsweek* (February 5, 1990), p. 57.
15. "Shots for grownups," *op. cit.*

Chapter Eleven   Drugs that Lower Cardiovascular Risk Factors: Reassessing the Evidence

1. A. Brett, "Treating hypercholesterolemia," *New England Journal of Medicine* 321(10):676–80 (1989).
2. See, e.g., S. Guttmacher, et al., "Ethics and preventive medicine: The case of borderline hypertension," *Hastings Center Report* 11:12–20 (1981); R. Levy, "Current status of the cholesterol controversy," *American Journal of Medicine* (May 23, 1983), pages 1–

4; J. Wikstrand, "Initial therapy for mild hypertension," *Pharma-cotherapy* 6(2):64–72 (1986).

3. See N. Freundlich, J. Weber, "Hypertension drugs: How much is hype?", *Business Week* (November 20, 1989), pp. 98–102; H. Lithell, et al., "Are effects of antihypertensive treatment on lipoproteins merely 'side-effects'?", *Acta Medica Scandinavica* 223:531–36 (1988).

4. S. Guttmacher, et al., *op. cit.;* N. Kaplan, "Non-drug treatment of hypertension," *Annals of Internal Medicine* 102:359–73 (1985).

5. N. Freundlich, et al., *op. cit.;* H. Lithell, et al., *op. cit.*

6. See R. Frentzel-Beyme, et al., "Mortality among German vegetarians: First results after five years of follow-up," *Nutrition and Cancer* 11:117–26 (1988); H. Kahn, et al., "Association between reported diet and all-cause mortality," *American Journal of Epidemiology* 119:775–87 (1984); D. Snowdon, "Animal product consumption and mortality because of all causes combined, coronary heart disease, stroke, diabetes and cancer in Seventh-day Adventists," *American Journal of Clinical Nutrition* 48:739–48 (1988); and other studies cited in E. Brown, *With the Grain* (New York: Carroll & Graf, 1990).

7. Veterans Administration Cooperative Study Group on Hypertension, "Effects of treatment on morbidity in hypertension. I. Results in patients with diastolic blood pressure averaging 115 mmHg through 129 mmHg," *JAMA* 202:1028–34 (1967); "Effects of treatment on morbidity in hypertension. II. Results in patients with diastolic blood pressure averaging 90 through 114 mmHg," *JAMA* 213:1143–52 (1970). Mild hypertension was defined as a diastolic pressure of 90–105 mm Hg.

8. W. Smith, U.S. Public Health Service Hospitals Cooperative Study Group, "Treatment of mild hypertension. Results of a ten-year intervention trial," *Circulation Research* 40 (Supp. 1)98–105 (1977).

9. New York Heart Association, "Survey on high blood pressure screening facilities" (1980); M. Alderman, et al., "High blood pressure treatment facilities," *New York State Journal of Medicine* 79(5):754–57 (1979).

10. Hypertension Detection and Follow-up Program Cooperative Group, "Five-year findings of the Hypertension Detection and Follow-up Program," *JAMA* 242(23):2562–71 (1979).

11. A. Relman, "Mild hypertension: No more benign neglect," *New England Journal of Medicine* 302(5):293–94 (1980).
12. See Medical Research Council Working Party, "MRC trial of treatment of mild hypertension: Principal results," *British Medical Journal* 291:97–104 (1985); S. Guttmacher, et al., *op. cit.*
13. Medical Research Council Working Party, *op. cit.*
14. Multiple Risk Factor Intervention Trial Research Group, "Multiple Risk Factor Intervention Trial," *JAMA* 248(12):1465–77 (1982).
15. A. Helgeland, "Treatment of mild hypertension: A five year controlled drug trial. The Oslo Study," *American Journal of Medicine* 69:725–32 (1980). See I. Holmes, et al., "Treatment of mild hypertension with diuretics: The importance of ECG abnormalities in the Oslo Study and in MRFIT," *JAMA* 251(10):1298–99 (1984).
16. Management Committee, "The Australian Therapeutic Trial in Mild Hypertension," *Lancet* (June 14, 1980), pp. 1261–67.
17. A. Amery, et al., "Mortality and morbidity results from the European Working Party on High Blood Pressure in the Elderly Trial," *Lancet* (June 15, 1985), pp. 1349–54.
18. Medical Research Council Working Party, *op. cit.;* see A. Breckenridge, "Treating mild hypertension," *ibid.* at 89–90.
19. *Ibid.*
20. Medical Research Council Working Party on Mild to Moderate Hypertension, "Adverse reactions of bendrofluazide and propranolol for the treatment of mild hypertension," *Lancet* 8246:539–43 (1981).
21. The Steering Committee of the Physicians' Health Study Research Group, "Preliminary report: Findings from the aspirin component of the ongoing Physicians' Health Study," *New England Journal of Medicine* 318:262–64 (1988).
22. S. Shapiro, "The Physicians' Health Study: Aspirin for the primary prevention of myocardial infarction," *New England Journal of Medicine* 318(14):924 (1988).
23. R. Peto, et al., "Randomized trial of prophylactic daily aspirin in British male doctors," *British Medical Journal* 296:313–16 (1988).
24. The amount of magnesium in Bufferin is small; but so is the amount in hard water, which some researchers think is responsible for the reduced incidence of heart disease and sudden death in hard water areas. See J. Landauer, "The Physicians' Health Study:

Aspirin for the primary prevention of myocardial infarction," *New England Journal of Medicine* 318(14):925 (1988).

25. Steering Committee of the Physicians' Health Study Research Group, "Final report on the aspirin component of the ongoing Physicians' Health Study," *New England Journal of Medicine* 321(3):129–35 (1989).

26. "W.H.O. cooperative trial on primary prevention of ischaemic heart disease using clofibrate to lower serum cholesterol: Mortality follow-up: Report of the Committee of Principal Investigators," *Lancet* 2:379–85 (1980).

27. Lipid Research Clinics Program, "The Lipid Research Clinics Coronary Primary Prevention Trial results. I. Reduction in incidence of coronary heart disease," *JAMA* 251:351–64 (1984).

28. M. Frick, et al., "Helsinki Heart Study: Primary-prevention trial with gemfibrozil in middle-aged men with dyslipidemia: Safety of treatment, changes in risk factors, and incidence of coronary heart disease," *New England Journal of Medicine* 317:1237–45 (1987). The difference in total deaths wasn't statistically significant.

29. See "Gemfibrozil and coronary heart disease," *New England Journal of Medicine* 318(19):1274 (1988).

30. See, e.g., M. Rosenthal, et al., "Effects of a high-complex-carbohydrate, low-fat, low-cholesterol diet on levels of serum lipids and estradiol," *American Journal of Medicine* 78:23–27 (1985); and many other studies cited in E. Brown, *With the Grain* (New York: Carroll & Graf, 1990), chapters 16–17.

31. C. Blum, R. Levy, "Current therapy for hypercholesterolemia," *JAMA* 261(24):3582–87 (1989).

32. See B. Ingersoll, "Doctors warned about prescribing heart drugs," *Wall Street Journal* (April 26, 1989); M. Cimons, "2 heart drugs are withdrawn after death rate rises," *Los Angeles Times* (April 26, 1989).

33. J. Cairns, "The treatment of diseases and the war against cancer," *Scientific American* 253(5):51 (1985).

Chapter Twelve   Conventional Blood Pressure Drugs: Diuretics and Beta-Blockers

1. Quoted in N. Freundlich, J. Weber, "Hypertension drugs: How much is hype?" *Business Week* (November 20, 1989), pp. 98, 102.

2. A. Melville, C. Johnson, *Cured to Death: The Effects of Prescription Drugs* (New York: Stein and Day, 1983), p. 159.
3. See S. Guttmacher, et al., "Ethics and preventive medicine: The case of borderline hypertension," *Hastings Center Report* 11:12–20 (1981).
4. I. Holme, et al., "Treatment of mild hypertension with diuretics," *JAMA* 251(10):1298–99 (1984).
5. J. Wikstrand, "Initial therapy for mild hypertension," *Pharmacotherapy* 6(2):64–72 (1986), citing G. Olsson, N. Rehnqvist, "Reduction of non-fatal reinfarctions in patients with a history of hypertension by chronic postinfarction treatment with metoprolol," *Acta Medica Scandinavica* (1986), and J. Wikstrand, et al., "Antihypertensive treatment with metoprolol or hydrochlorothiazide in patients aged 60–75 years: Report from a double-blind international multicenter study," *JAMA* (1986).
6. See L. Simonsen, "Top 200 drugs of 1988," *Pharmacy Times* (April 1989), pp. 40–48.
7. J. Wikstrand, *op. cit.*
8. See R. Burack, M.D., *The New Handbook of Prescription Drugs* (New York: Ballantine, 1976), pp. 228–29.
9. G. McMahon, et al., "Upper gastrointestinal lesions after potassium chloride supplements: A controlled clinical trial," *Lancet* 2:1059–63 (1982).
10. K. Khaw, E. Barrett-Connor, "Dietary potassium and stroke-associated mortality," *New England Journal of Medicine* 316(5):235–40 (1987). Advocates of drug therapy point to a significant drop in stroke deaths in the years since drug treatment has been aggressively pursued. The trouble with this theory is that the drop actually began *before* the drugs became popular. See N. Kaplan, "Nondrug treatment of hypertension," *Annals of Internal Medicine* 102:359–73 (1985). Khaw, et al., propose another explanation: the drop may be linked to the increased consumption of potassium-rich fruits and vegetables occurring at the same time.
11. G. Krishna, et al., "Increased blood pressure during potassium depletion in normotensive men," *New England Journal of Medicine* 320(18):1177–82 (1989).
12. Hypertension Detection and Follow-up Program Cooperative Group, "Five year findings of the hypertension detection and follow-up program. I. Reduction in mortality of persons with high

blood pressure, including mild hypertension," *JAMA* 242:2562–71 (1979).

13. "Magnesium in human nutrition," *Nutrition & the M.D.* 14(11):1–3 (1988).

14. M. Weinberger, "Diuretics and their side effects," *Hypertension* 11 (Supp. II):II-16—II-20 (1988), citing W. Kannel, et al., "Hypertension, antihypertensive treatment and sudden death," *CVD Epidemiol. Newsletter* 37:34 (1985), and T. Morgan, et al., "Failure of therapy to improve prognosis in elderly males with hypertension," *Medical Journal of Australia* 2:27–32 (1980).

15. H. Trowell, "Hypertension and Salt," *Lancet* (July 22, 1978), p. 204.

16. M. Weinberger, *op. cit.*

17. T. Pollare, H. Lithell, et al., "A comparison of the effects of hydrochlorothiazide and captopril on glucose and lipid metabolism in patients with hypertension," *New England Journal of Medicine* 321:868–73 (1989).

18. See D. Drayer, "Lipophilicity, hydrophilicity, and the central nervous system side effects of beta blockers," *Pharmacotherapy* 7(4):87–91 (1987).

19. J. Cunnane, G. Blackwood, "Psychosis with propranolol: Still not recognized?", *Postgraduate Medical Journal* 63:57–58 (1987).

20. R. Rosen, et al., "Beta-blocker effects on sexual function in normal males," *Archives of Sexual Behavior* 17(3):241–55 (1988); J. Fodor, et al., "A comparison of the side effects of atenolol and propranolol in the treatment of patients with hypertension," *Journal of Clinical Pharmacology* 27(11):892–901 (1987).

21. J. Wikstrand, *op. cit.*

22. M. Weinberger, *op. cit.*

23. H. Lithell, et al., "Are effects of antihypertensive treatment on lipoproteins merely 'side-effects'?", *Acta Medica Scandinavica* 223:531–36 (1988).

24. M. Weinberger, *op. cit.*

25. *Ibid.*

26. Adapted from G. Cawood, et al., *1989–90 Prescription Drug Encyclopedia* (Peachtree City, Ga: FC&A Publishing, 1989); *Nursing89 Drug Handbook* (Springhouse, Pa.: Springhouse Corp., 1989).

Chapter Thirteen   Newer Blood Pressure Alternatives

1. J. Edelson, et al., "Long-term cost-effectiveness of various initial monotherapies for mild to moderate hypertension," *JAMA* 263(3):407–13 (1990).
2. See "High blood pressure: Newer treatments," *Harvard Medical School Health Letter* 14(3):1–3 (1989).
3. R. DiBianco, "Adverse reactions with angiotensin converting enzyme (ACE) inhibitors," *Medical Toxicology* 1:122–41 (1986).
4. See M. Waldholz, "Heart-drug study favors beta-blockers over newer remedy," *Wall Street Journal* (January 19, 1990), p. B1.
5. S. Croog, et al., "The effects of antihypertensive therapy on the quality of life," *New England Journal of Medicine* 314:1657–64 (1986).
6. C. Sahler Jr., "Antihypertensive therapy and quality of life," *New England Journal of Medicine* 316(1):52 (1987); S. Benway, "Don't look back, Squibb—a giant is gaining on you," *Business Week* (October 10, 1988), pp. 68–76.
7. J. Edelson, et al., *op. cit.*
8. M. Weinberger, "Metabolic and blood pressure effects of angiotensin converting enzyme inhibitors in mild to moderate American hypertensives," *Clinical and Experimental Hypertension* 9(2–3): 643–52 (1987); J. Kayanakis, L. Baulac, "Comparative study of once daily administration of captopril 50 mg, hydrochlorothiazide 25 mg and their combination in mild to moderate hypertension," *British Journal of Clinical Pharmacology* 23 (Supp. 1):89S–92S (1987); F. Pupita, et al., "Life quality in patients under hypotensive treatment," *International Journal of Clinical Pharmacology Research* 7(1):13–7 (1987).
9. C. Muiesan, et al., "Antihypertensive efficacy and tolerability of captopril in the elderly: Comparison with hydrochlorothiazide and placebo in a multicentre, double blind study," *Journal of Hypertension* 5(5):S590–602 (1987); T. Omae, et al., "Side effects and metabolic effects of converting enzyme inhibitors," *Clinical and Experimental Hypertension* 9(2–3):635–42 (1987).
10. T. Pollare, H. Lithell, et al., "A comparison of the effects of hydrochlorothiazide and captopril on glucose and lipid metabolism in patients with hypertension," *New England Journal of Medicine* 321:868–73 (1979).

11. J. Thachil, et al., "Hypersomnolence with beta-adrenergic blockers," *Chest* 92(5):943–44 (1987).
12. R. DiBianco, *op. cit.;* P. Lamy, "Potential adverse effects of antihypertensive drugs in the elderly," *Journal of Hypertension* 6 (Supp. 1):S81–85 (1988).
13. From N. Freundlich, J. Weber, "Hypertension drugs: How much is hype?", *Business Week* (November 20, 1989), pp. 98, 102.
14. See P. Lamy, *op. cit.*
15. J. Schoenberger, "Calcium antagonists: Use in hypertension evaluation of calcium antagonists in combination with diuretics," *Angiology* 39 (1 Pt 2):87–93 (1988); J. Bochsler, et al., "Verapamil SR and propranolol LA: A comparison of efficacy and side effects in the treatment of mild to moderate hypertension," *Journal of Human Hypertension* 1(4):305–10 (1988).
16. H. Gelmers, et al., "A controlled trial of nimodipine in acute ischemic stroke," *New England Journal of Medicine* 318(4):208–14 (1988). During the next six months of follow-up, deaths were the same in both groups.
17. H. Lithell, et al., "Are effects of antihypertensive treatment on lipoproteins merely 'side-effects'?", *Acta Medica Scandinavica* 223:531–36 (1988).
18. T. Pollare, H. Lithell, et al., "Application of prazosin is associated with an increase of insulin sensitivity in obese patients with hypertension," *Diabetologia* 31:415–20 (1988).
19. N. Lasser, et al., "Effects of antihypertensive therapy on blood pressure control, cognition, and reactivity. A placebo controlled comparison of prazosin, propranolol, and hydrochlorothiazide," *American Journal of Medicine* 86(1B):98–103 (1989).
20. H. Itskovitz, et al., "The long term antihypertensive effects of prazosin and atenolol," *American Journal of Medicine* 86(1B):82–86 (1989).
21. D. Cheung, et al., "Mild hypertension in the elderly. A comparison of prazosin and enalapril," *American Journal of Medicine* 86 (18):87–90 (1989).
22. W. Louis, et al., "Comparison of pharmacokinetics and pharmacodynamics of adrenoceptor agonists and antagonists as antihypertensive agents," *Journal of Cardiovascular Pharmacology* 10 (Supp. 12):S100–03 (1987).
23. W. Frishman, et al., "Terazosin: A new long-acting alpha 1-adren-

ergic antagonist for hypertension," *Medical Clinics of North America* 72(2):441–48 (1988).
24. D. Torvik, H. Madsbu, "An open one-year comparison of doxazosin and prazosin for mild to moderate hypertension," *American Journal of Cardiology* 59(14):68G–72G (1987); P. Hjortdahl, et al., "A 24-week multicenter double-blind study of doxazosin and hydrochlorothiazide in patients with mild to moderate essential hypertension," *Acta Medica Scandinavica* 221(5):427–34 (1987).
25. R. Englert, H. Mauersberger, "A single-blind study of doxazosin in the treatment of essential hypertension when added to nonresponders to angiotensin-converting enzyme inhibitor therapy," *American Heart Journal* 116 (6 Pt 2):1826–32 (1988); U. Lindner, et al., "The addition of doxazosin to the treatment regimen of hypertensive patients not responsive to nifedipine," *American Heart Journal* 116 (6 Pt 2):1814–20 (1988).
26. A. Bartels, et al., "Doxazosin in the treatment of patients with mild or moderate hypertension and mild or moderate renal insufficiency," *American Heart Journal* 116 (6 Pt 2):1772–77 (1988); J. Rosenthal, "Control of coronary heart disease risk factors with doxazosin as monotherapy and in combination therapy," *American Heart Journal* 116 (6 Pt 2):1763–66 (1988).
27. K. Hayduk, "Efficacy and safety of doxazosin in hypertension therapy," *American Journal of Cardiology* 59(14):35G–39G (1987); P. Hjortdahl, et al., *op. cit.*
28. J. Rosenthal, *op. cit.*
29. L. Ramsay, et al., "Comparison of nifedipine, prazosin and hydralazine added to treatment of hypertensive patients uncontrolled by thiazide diuretic plus beta-blocker," *Postgraduate Medical Journal* 63(736):99–103 (1987).
30. W. Louis, et al., *op. cit.*
31. S. Franklin, et al., "Randomized, double-blind comparison of transdermal clonidine with oral propranolol," *Journal of Cardiovascular Pharmacology* 10 (Supp. 12):S244–47 (1987).
32. L. Ferder, et al., "Safety aspects of long term antihypertensive therapy (10 years) with clonidine," *Journal of Cardiovascular Pharmacology* 10 (Supp. 12):S104–08 (1987); P. Lamy, *op. cit.*
33. M. Holdiness, "A review of contact dermatitis associated with transdermal therapeutic systems," *Contact Dermatitis* 20:3–9 (1989).
34. See S. Guttmacher, et al., "Ethics and preventive medicine: The

case of borderline hypertension," *Hastings Center Report* 11:12–20 (1981).

35. G. Mancia, et al., "Effects of blood pressure measurement by the doctor on patient's blood pressure and heart rate," *Lancet* 2:695–98 (1983).

36. N. Kaplan, "Non-drug treatment of hypertension," *Annals of Internal Medicine* 102:359–73 (1985); "High blood pressure: A new look," *Harvard Medical School Letter* 12(2):1–4 (1988); "What do we really know?", *University of California, Berkeley Wellness Letter* 4(5):1 (1988). See E. Brown, *With the Grain* (New York: Carroll & Graf, 1990).

37. O. Lindahl, et al., "A vegan regimen with reduced medication in the treatment of hypertension," *British Journal of Nutrition* 52:11–20 (1984).

38. See C. Patel, K. Datey, "Relaxation and biofeedback techniques in the management of hypertension," *Angiology* 27(2):106–13 (1976).

39. *Ibid.;* K. Datey, et al., " 'Shavasan'—a yogic exercise in the management of hypertension," *Angiology* 20:325–33 (1969); N. Kaplan, *op. cit.* Simple relaxation also works, but not as well. See, e.g., R. Jacob, et al., "Relaxation therapy for hypertension: Comparison of effects with concomitant placebo, diuretic, and beta-blocker," *Archives of Internal Medicine* 146:2335–40 (1986).

40. H. Benson, M.D., *The Relaxation Response* (New York: William Morrow and Co., 1975), pp. 99–102.

41. S. Fahrion, et al., "Biobehavioral treatment of essential hypertension: A group outcome study," *Biofeedback Self Regulation* 11(4):257–77 (1986).

42. C. Patel, et al., *op. cit.;* compare R. Jacob, et al., *op. cit.* See also C. Patel, M. Carruthers, "Coronary risk factor reduction through biofeedback-aided relaxation and meditation," *Journal of the Royal College of General Practitioners* 27:401–05 (1977), a British study investigating the effects of meditation and relaxation reinforced by biofeedback. Average blood pressures dropped after six weeks from 165/101 to 156/90 in hypertensive volunteers, and from 127/83 to 117/76 in normotensive volunteers. Blood pressures increased slightly in an untreated control group during the same period. Serum cholesterol and triglyceride levels also dropped in the treated group while increasing slightly in the controls.

43. See N. Kaplan, *op. cit.*

44. *Ibid.*
45. Adapted from *Nursing89 Drug Handbook* (Springhouse, Pa.: Springhouse Corp., 1989); G. Cawood, et al., *1989–90 Prescription Drug Encyclopedia* (Peachtree City, Ga.: FC&A Publishing, 1989).

Chapter Fourteen   Drugs that Lower Serum Cholesterol

1. See chapter 11.
2. See J. Byrne, "The miracle company: Excellence in the lab and executive suite makes Merck a powerhouse," *Business Week* (October 19, 1987), pp. 84–90. See chapter 11.
3. A. Miller, et al., "Pitching to patients," *Newsweek* 113(19):40–1, 1989.
4. "Diet: The first line of defense," *University of California, Berkeley Wellness Letter* 4(3):1–2 (1987).
5. See J. Kenney, "Heart Failure? Failed thesis," *Center Post* (January 1990), pp. 1 ff., citing *Journal of Cardiac Rehabilitation* 1:99 (1981); *American Journal of Clinical Nutrition* 44:212 (1986); *Circulation Supplement* 14:11 (1988); *Archives of Internal Medicine* 148:36 (1988).
6. See, e.g., A. Keys, et al., "The diet and all causes death rate in the Seven Countries Study," *Lancet* 2:58–61 (1981) (all-cause mortality in 12,000 men under age 60 in seven countries positively associated with saturated fat intake); and other studies cited in E. Brown, *With the Grain* (New York: Carroll & Graf, 1990).
7. See C. Blum, R. Levy, "Current therapy for hypercholesterolemia," *JAMA* 261(24):3582–87 (1989); R. Ballentine, *Diet and Nutrition* (Honesdale, Penn.: Himalayan International Institute, 1982), pp. 91–95; *Dorland's Illustrated Medical Dictionary.*
8. C. Blum, *op. cit.;* " 'Fingerstick' cholesterol tests are fast but faulty," *Vegetarian Times* (May 1989), p. 12.
9. C. Blum, *op. cit.*
10. F. Oliver, et al., "A co-operative trial in the primary prevention of ischaemic heart disease using clofibrate," *British Heart Journal* 40:1069–1118 (1978).
11. M. Frick, et al., "Helsinki Heart Study: Primary-prevention trial with gemfibrozil in middle-aged men with dyslipidemia," *New England Journal of Medicine* 317(20):1237–45 (1987).
12. C. Blum, et al., *op. cit.*
13. *Ibid.*

14. *Ibid.;* M. Frick, et al., *op. cit.;* S. Siwolop, "Curbing killer choles-
    terol," *Business Week* (October 26, 1987), pp. 122–23.
15. P. Canner, et al., "Fifteen year mortality in Coronary Drug Project
    patients: Long-term benefit with niacin," *American Journal of Car-
    diology* 8:1245–55 (1986).
16. "Choice of cholesterol-lowering drugs," *Medical Letter* 30(774):81–
    84 (1988); C. Blum, et al., *op. cit.*
17. S. Siwolop, *op. cit.;* C. Blum, et al., *op. cit.*
18. A. Garg, S. Grundy, "Lovastatin for lowering cholesterol levels in
    non-insulin-dependent diabetes mellitus," *New England Journal of
    Medicine* 318(2):81–86 (1988).
19. Mevacor package insert.
20. "Choice of cholesterol-lowering drugs," *Medical Letter*
    30(774):81–84 (1988).
21. C. Blum, et al., *op. cit.*
22. "More on fish oil," *New England Journal of Medicine*
    316(10):624–28 (1987); S. Siwolop, *op. cit.* See E. Brown, *With the
    Grain* (New York: Carroll & Graf, 1990).
23. L. Nicholson, "Focus on fiber," *Center Post* 10(9):1 (1989).
24. "Psyllium and cholesterol," *Harvard Medical School Health Letter*
    13(8):1 (1988), citing *Archives of Internal Medicine* (February
    1988), pp. 292–96.
25. "Mystery of high-fiber diet unraveled," *Washington Post* (October
    26, 1987), p. A7; S. Siwolop, *op. cit.*
26. L. Nicholson, *op. cit.*
27. "Thyroid use in the elderly is often improper," *American Phar-
    macy* (October 1989), p. 13, citing *JAMA* 261:2653 (1989).
28. C. Blum, et al., *op. cit.*
29. Adapted from C. Blum, et al., *op. cit.; Nursing89 Drug Handbook*
    (Springhouse, Pa.: Springhouse Corp., 1989).

Chapter Fifteen   Before and After your Heart Attack

1. J. Scott, "Heart drugs do equally well in study," *Los Angeles Times*
   (April 4, 1989), V:1,6.
2. "Heart attacks: The first few hours," *Harvard Medical School
   Health Letter* 13(11):5–8 (1988).
3. J. Carey, "Genentech: A David that comes on like Goliath," *Business Week* (October 30, 1989), p. 165.

4. J. Scott, *op. cit.;* "Study questions value of biotech drug," *Los Angeles Times* (March 9, 1990), p. D2.
5. R. Levy, "Current status of the cholesterol controversy," *American Journal of Medicine* 74(5A):1–4 (1983).
6. T. Gordon, W. Kannel, "Premature mortality from coronary heart disease: The Framingham Study," *Coronary Heart Disease* 215(10):1617–25 (1971).
7. M. Packer, "Combined beta-adrenergic and calcium-entry blockade in angina pectoris," *New England Journal of Medicine* 320(11):709–18 (1989).
8. "Nitroglycerin tolerance," *New England Journal of Medicine* 318(2):120–21 (1988).
9. W. Heepe, "An acute double-blind placebo-controlled study of transdermal glyceryl trinitrate with 12 months' follow-up in patients with stable angina pectoris," *Journal of International Medical Research* 15(4):198–204 (1987); R. Mahapatra, et al., "Clinical experience with a transdermal nitroglycerin system," *Angiology* 38(4):277–86 (1987).
10. D. Waters, et al., "Limited usefulness of intermittent nitroglycerin patches in stable angina," *Journal of the American College of Cardiology* 13(2):421–25 (1989).
11. M. Holdiness, "A review of contact dermatitis associated with transdermal therapeutic systems," *Contact Dermatitis* 20:3–9 (1989); B. Schrader, et al., "Acceptance of transcutaneous nitroglycerin patches by patients with angina pectoris," *Pharmacotherapy* 6(2):83–86 (1986).
12. The Cardiac Arrhythmia Suppression Trial Investigators, "Preliminary report: Encainide and flecainide on mortality in a randomized trial of arrhythmia suppression after myocardial infarction," *New England Journal of Medicine* 321(6):406–12 (1989).
13. S. Kopecky, et al., "The natural history of lone atrial fibrillation," *New England Journal of Medicine* 317(11):669–74 (1987).
14. See K. Butler, L. Rayner, *The Best Medicine* (San Francisco: Harper & Row, 1985), pp. 464–71.
15. J. Justice, S. Kline, "Analgesics and warfarin: A case that brings up questions and cautions," *Postgraduate Medicine* 83(5):217–20 (1988).
16. "Aspirin after myocardial infarction," *Lancet* i:1172–73 (1980); W. Fields, et al., "Controlled trial of aspirin in cerebral ischaemia," *Stroke* 8:310–16 (1977); Canadian Cooperative Study

Group, "A randomised trial of aspirin and sulfinpyrazone in threatened stroke," *New England Journal of Medicine* 299:53–59 (1978). See chapter 11.

17. M. Packer, "Do vasodilators prolong life in heart failure?", *New England Journal of Medicine* 316(23):1471–73 (1987).

18. CONSENSUS Trial Study Group, "Effects of enalapril on mortality in severe congestive heart failure: Results of the Cooperative North Scandinavian Enalapril Survival Study," *New England Journal of Medicine* 316(23):1429–35 (1987).

19. J. Cohn, et al., "Effect of vasodilator therapy on mortality in chronic congestive heart failure: Results of a Veterans Administration Cooperative Study," *New England Journal of Medicine* 314:1547–52 (1986).

20. M. Packer, *op. cit.;* "Vasodilators for chronic congestive heart failure," *Medical Letter* 30(758):13–14 (1988).

21. See T. Smith, "Digitalis: Mechanisms of action and clinical use," *New England Journal of Medicine* 318(6):358–65 (1988); K. Butler, et al., *op. cit.*

22. S. Squires, "Heart researchers find diet alone can help," *Washington Post Health* (November 15, 1988); "It's true, you can reverse heart disease through vegetarianism," *Vegetarian Times* (February 1990), p. 18.

23. S. Squires, *op. cit.*

24. F. Ellis, T. Sanders, "Angina and vegan diet," *American Heart Journal* 93(6):803–05 (1977).

25. P. Kuo, et al., "The effect of lipemia upon coronary and peripheral arterial circulation in patients with essential hyperlipemia," *American Journal of Medicine* 26:68–75 (1959).

26. See M. Wolbers, "Angina: Handling its facts and myths," *Your Good Health* 2(5):21–23 (1984).

27. *Ibid.*

28. Adapted from G. Cawood, et al., *1989–90 Prescription Drug Encyclopedia* (Peachtree City, Ga.: FC&A Publishing, 1989); *Nursing89 Drug Handbook* (Springhouse, Pa.: Springhouse Corp., 1989).

Chapter Sixteen   Drugs for Diabetics: Assessing the Risks

1. R. Kaplan, T. Ganiats, "Trade-offs in treatment alternatives for non-insulin-dependent diabetes mellitus," *Journal of General Internal Medicine* 4(2):167–71 (1989).

2. R. Henig, "Beyond insulin," *New York Times Magazine* (March 20, 1988), pp. 50–51.

3. J. Weiner, "The pharmacist and diabetes mellitus: Today's considerations," *Wellcome Programs in Pharmacy* (Park Row Publishers, 1986).

4. G. Johnson, S. Goldfinger, *Harvard Medical School Health Letter Book* (Cambridge, Mass.: Harvard University Press, 1981), pp. 287–94; T. Pollare, H. Lithell, et al., "A comparison of the effects of hydrochlorothiazide and captopril on glucose and lipid metabolism in patients with hypertension," *New England Journal of Medicine* 321:868–73 (1989).

5. G. Johnson, et al., *op. cit.;* E. Bierman, "Diet and diabetes," *American Journal of Clinical Nutrition* 41:1113–16 (1985).

6. M. Billingham, et al., "Lipoprotein subfraction composition in non-insulin-dependent diabetes treated by diet, sulphonylurea, and insulin," *Metabolism* 38(9):850–57 (1989); R. Kaplan, et al., *op. cit.*

7. H. Lebovitz, M. Feinglos, "Sulfonylurea drugs: Mechanism of antidiabetic action and therapeutic usefulness," *Diabetes Care* 1(3):189–95 (1978).

8. D. Hadden, et al., "Myocardial infarction in maturity-onset diabetics: A retrospective study," *Lancet* 1:335–38 (1972); D. Boyle, et al., "Ischemic heart disease in diabetics: A prospective study," *Lancet* 1:338–40 (1972); N. Soler, et al., "Coronary care for myocardial infarction in diabetics," *Lancet* 1:475–77 (1974).

9. R. Kaplan, et al., *op. cit.*

10. *Ibid.*

11. K. Dahl-Jorgensen, et al., "Effect of near normoglycaemia for two years on progression of early diabetic retinopathy, nephropathy, and neuropathy: The Oslo study," *British Medical Journal* 293:1195–99 (1986).

12. DCCT Research Group, "Are continuing studies of metabolic control and microvascular complications in insulin-dependent diabetes mellitus justified?", *New England Journal of Medicine* 318(4):246–50 (1988).

13. S. Amiel, et al., "Defective glucose counterregulation after strict glycemic control of insulin-dependent diabetes mellitus," *New England Journal of Medicine* 316(22):1376–83 (1987).

14. G. Johnson, et al., *op. cit.*

15. J. Anderson, K. Ward, "High-carbohydrate, high-fiber diets for

insulin-treated men with diabetes mellitus," *American Journal of Clinical Nutrition* 32:2312–21 (1979). See also E. Bierman, *op. cit.*

16. See D. Jenkins, et al., "The diabetic diet, carbohydrate and differences in digestibility," *Diabetologia* 23:477–84 (1982).

17. L. Nicholson, "Focus on fiber," *Center Post* 10(9):1,7 (1989). See E. Brown, *With the Grain* (New York: Carroll & Graf, 1990), chapter 3.

18. A. Thorburn, et al., "Slowly digested and absorbed carbohydrate in traditional bushfoods: A protective factor against diabetes?", *American Journal of Clinical Nutrition* 45:98–106 (1987); B. Karlstrom, et al., "Effect of leguminous seeds in a mixed diet in non-insulin-dependent diabetic patients," *Diabetes Research* 5:199–205 (1987).

19. From L. Nicholson, *op. cit.*

20. G. Collier, K. O'Dea, "The effect of coingestion of fat on the glucose, insulin, and gastric inhibitory polypeptide responses to carbohydrate and protein," *American Journal of Clinical Nutrition* 37:941–44 (1983). See D. Snowdon, R. Phillips, "Does a vegetarian diet reduce the occurrence of diabetes?", *American Journal of Public Health* 75:507–12 (1985).

21. See R. Rizek, E. Jackson, "Current food consumption practices and nutrient sources in the American diet," in *Animal Products in Human Nutrition* (New York: Academic Press, 1982), pp. 150–51; C. Adams, *Nutritive Value of American Foods in Common Units* (Washington, D.C.: Agricultural Research Service, USDA 1975).

22. J. Gear, et al., "Biochemical and haematological variables in vegetarians," *British Medical Journal* 1:1415 (1980); K. West, *Epidemiology of Diabetes and Its Vascular Lesions* (New York: Elsevier North-Holland, 1978).

23. D. Snowdon, "Animal product consumption and mortality because of all causes combined, coronary heart disease, stroke, diabetes, and cancer in Seventh-day Adventists," *American Journal of Clinical Nutrition* 48:739–48 (1988). See also D. Snowdon, R. Phillips, *op. cit.*

24. J. Weiner, *op. cit.;* "Exercise and diabetes," *Nutrition & the M.D.* 14(10):3–5 (1988).

Chapter Seventeen New Treatment Options for Diabetics

1. J. Weiner, "The pharmacist and diabetes mellitus: Today's considerations," *Wellcome Programs in Pharmacy* (Park Row Publishers, 1986).
2. C. Saudek, "What is the future role of insulin delivery?", *Pharmacy Times* (April 1988), pp. 131–34; G. Johnson, S. Goldfinger, *Harvard Medical School Health Letter Book* (Cambridge, Mass.: Harvard University Press, 1981), pp. 287–94.
3. C. Saudek, et al., "A preliminary trial of the programmable implantable medication system for insulin delivery," *New England Journal of Medicine* 321:574–79 (1989).
4. R. Campbell, "Clinical use of insulin: Its types and characteristics," *Pharmacy Times* (October 1988), pp. 138–47; *Nursing89 Drug Handbook* (Springhouse, Pa.: Springhouse Corp., 1989), p. 527.
5. L. Thompson, "Problems with 'miracle' drugs," *Washington Post Health* (June 28, 1988), p. 11.
6. R. Brogden, R. Heel, "Human insulin: A review of its biological activity, pharmacokinetics and therapeutic use," *Drugs* 34:350–71 (1987); R. Campbell, *op. cit.*
7. B. Richards, "Reports of deaths among U.K. diabetics using human insulin stir concern here," *Wall Street Journal* (October 30, 1989), p. B4.
8. A. Melander, et al., "Sulphonylurea antidiabetic drugs: An update of their clinical pharmacology and rational therapeutic use," *Drugs* 37:58–72 (1989); H. Lebovitz, M. Feinglos, "Sulfonylurea drugs: Mechanism of antidiabetic action and therapeutic usefulness," *Diabetes Care* 1(3):189–95 (1978); J. Weiner, *op. cit.*
9. Adapted from J. Weiner, *op. cit.*
10. *Ibid.*
11. "Diabetes: The pill problem," *Harvard Medical School Health Letter* 13(9):7–8 (1988).
12. See "The second generation oral sulfonylureas: Glyburide and glipizide," *American Pharmacy* NS28(10):55–59 (1988); R. Campbell, "Clinical use of insulin: Side effects & dosing factors," *Pharmacy Times* (November 1988), pp. 154–63.
13. "Carteolol and penbutolol for hypertension," *Medical Letter* 31(797):70–71 (1989).

14. "Preventing diabetes complications," *U.S. Pharmacist* (August 1989), p. 22.

15. *Drug Facts and Comparisons* (St. Louis: J.B. Lippincott Co., 1989), p. 446.

16. C. Steil, "Over-the-counter product use," *Diabetes Educator* 14(1):48–49 (1988); P. Trainor, "Over-the-counter drugs: Count them in," *Geriatric Nursing* (September/October 1988), pp. 298–99.

Chapter Eighteen   Aspirin: From Headaches to Heart Attacks

1. See J. Brody, "Threading through the maze of information in the billion-dollar pain reliever market," *New York Times* (April 21, 1988), p. 24; C. Mann, M. Plummer, "The big headache," *Atlantic Monthly* (October 1988), pp. 39–57.

2. "Toxicity of nonsteroidal anti-inflammatory drugs," *Medical Letter* 25:15–16 (1983).

3. See chapter 11.

4. A. Leaf, P. Weber, "Cardiovascular effects of n-3 fatty acids," *New England Journal of Medicine* 318(9):549–57 (1988); "Fish oil pills: Jumping the gun," *University of California, Berkeley Wellness Letter* 3(5):1 (1987).

5. J. Kingham, et al., "Macular hemorrhage in the aging eye: The effects of anticoagulants," *New England Journal of Medicine* 318(17):1126–27 (1988).

6. L. Monroe, "Analgesics killing more than pain, experts fear," *Los Angeles Times* (July 25, 1989), pp. V:1–2. See J. Kaufman, et al., *Over-the-Counter Pills That Don't Work* (New York: Pantheon Books, 1983), pp. 19, 24; P. Sanberg, R. Krenna, *Over-the-Counter Drugs: Harmless or Hazardous?* (New York: Chelsea Publishers, 1986), pp. 50–51.

7. P. Barles, et al., "Adverse reaction of acetaminophen as an alternative analgesic in A.A.S. triad," *Allergologia et Immunopathologica* 16(5):321–25 (1988); G. Settipane, "Aspirin sensitivity and allergy," *Biomedicine & Pharmacotherapy,* 42:493–98 (1988); P. Fowler, "Aspirin, paracetamol and non-steroid anti-inflammatory drugs: A comparative review of side effects," *Medical Toxicology* 2:338–66 (1987).

8. L. Monroe, *op. cit.*

9. C. Mann, et al., *op. cit.;* "Pain relievers: The truth behind the ads," *University of California, Berkeley Wellness Letter* 3(12):3 (1987).

10. See J. Kaufman, et al., *op. cit.,* pp. 24–25; Consumers Union, *The Medicine Show* (New York: Pantheon Books, 1980), p. 18.

11. F. Lanza, et al., "Endoscopic evaluation of the effects of aspirin, buffered aspirin and enteric coated aspirin on gastric and duodenal mucosa," *New England Journal of Medicine* 303:135–38 (1980); J. Hoftiezer, et al., "Comparison of the effects of regular and enteric coated aspirin on gastroduodenal mucosa of man," *Lancet* ii:609–12 (1980).

12. J. Scheiman, et al., "Salicylsalicylic acid causes less gastroduodenal mucosal damage than enteric-coated aspirin," *Digestive Diseases and Science* 34 (2):229–32 (1989).

13. "Elderly users," *Vegetarian Times* (May 1989), p. 13.

14. P. Barles, et al., *op. cit.* See chapter 21.

15. See "Pain relievers: The truth behind the ads," *op. cit.*

Chapter Nineteen Arthritis: Choosing an
Anti-Inflammatory

1. See "Pain relievers: The truth behind the ads," *University of California, Berkeley Wellness Letter* 3(12):3 (1987).

2. J. Hamilton, "Why generics may not give Syntex a migraine," *Business Week* (October 10, 1988), p. 76.

3. "Top 200 drugs of 1988," *Pharmacy Times* (April 1989), p. 40; World Health Organization, *The World Drug Situation* (Geneva:WHO, 1988), p. 18.

4. D. Hussar, "New drugs of 1988," *American Pharmacy* (March 1989), pp. 25–52; G. Cowley, et al., "The promise of Prozac," *Newsweek* (March 26, 1990), pp. 38–41.

5. Adapted from D. Hussar, *op. cit.*

6. P. Fowler, "Aspirin, paracetamol and non-steroid anti-inflammatory drugs: A comparative review of side effects," *Medical Toxicology* 2:338–66 (1987).

7. "Nonsteroidal anti-inflammatory drugs," *Medical Letter* 25:15–16 (1983).

8. M. Langman, "Anti-inflammatory drug intake and the risk of ulcer complications," *Medical Toxicology* 1 (Supp. 1):34–38 (1986).

9. P. Fowler, *op. cit.*

10. J. McIntosh, et al., "Smoking, nonsteroidal anti-inflammatory

drugs, and acetaminophen in gastric ulcer," *American Journal of Epidemiology* 128(4):761–70 (1988).

11. "FDA's bimonthly update," *Pharmacy Times* (March 1989), pp. 118–24.
12. "Diet therapy for peptic ulcer disease," *Nutrition & the M.D* 14(2); 1–2, 1988.
13. E. Gall, et al., "Clinical comparison of ibuprofen, fenoprofen calcium, naproxen, and tolmetin sodium in rheumatoid arthritis," *Journal of Rheumatology* 9:402–07 (1982).
14. C. Wasner, et al., "Nonsteroidal anti-inflammatory agents in rheumatoid arthritis and ankylosing spondylitis; *JAMA* 246:2168–72 (1981).
15. J. Maliekal, "A review of current nonsteroidal anti-inflammatory drugs," *Drug Topics* (April 3, 1989), pp. 74–79.
16. P. Fowler, *op. cit.*
17. See M. Liang, "Living with arthritis," *Harvard Medical School Health Letter* 14(2):5–8 (1988).
18. *Drug Facts and Comparisons* (St. Louis: J.B. Lippincott Co., 1989), p. 2190.
19. R. Kuncl, et al., "Colchicine myopathy and neuropathy," *New England Journal of Medicine* 25 (316):1562–68 (1987).
20. See W. Robertson, et al., "The effect of high animal protein intake on the risk of calcium stone-formation in the urinary tract," *Clinical Science* 57:285–88 (1979); W. Robertson, et al., "Prevalence of urinary stone disease in vegetarians," *European Urology* 8:334–39 (1982); I. Pave, "So you thought gout was a thing of the past?", *Business Week* (October 5, 1987), p. 129.
21. L. Dunne, *Nutrition Almanac* (New York: McGraw Hill, 1990), p. 137.
22. L. Power, "Exploring the link between diet, arthritis," *Los Angeles Times* (May 6, 1986), p. 3.
23. C. Lucas, L. Power, "Dietary fat aggravates active rheumatoid arthritis," *Clinical Research* 29(4):754A (1981).

Chapter Twenty Acetaminophen and other Analgesic Alternatives

1. S. Siegelman, "Medications used by the famous," *American Druggist* (December 1989), pp. 29–33.
2. See J. Brody, "Threading through the maze of information in the

billion-dollar pain reliever market," *New York Times* (April 21, 1988), p. 24.

3. E. Gottfried, et al., "Alcohol-induced gastric and duodenal lesions in man," *American Journal of Gastroenterology* 70:587–92 (1978).

4. M. Keaton, "Acute renal failure in an alcoholic during therapeutic acetaminophen ingestion," *Southern Medical Journal* 81(9):1163–66 (1988).

5. D. Sandler, et al., "Analgesic use and chronic renal disease," *New England Journal of Medicine* 320:1238–43 (1989).

6. See T. Maugh II, "Daily use of drug linked to kidney disease," *Los Angeles Times* (May 11, 1989), pp. I:1,33; D. Sandler, *op. cit.*

7. P. Fowler, "Aspirin, paracetamol, and non-steroid anti-inflammatory drugs: A comparative review of side effects," *Medical Toxicology* 2:338–66 (1987).

8. M. Segasothy, et al., "Paracetamol: A cause for analgesic nephropathy and end-stage renal disease," *Nephron* 50:50–54 (1988).

9. A. Schwarz, et al., "Characteristics and clinical course of hemodialysis patients with analgesic-associated nephropathy," *Clinical Nephrology* 29(6):299–306 (1988); A. Schwarz, et al., "Aluminum load in patients with analgesic nephropathy," *Mineral Electrolyte Metabolism* 13:141–46 (1987).

10. L. Monroe, "Analgesics killing more than pain, experts fear," *Los Angeles Times* (July 25, 1989), pp. V:1–2.

11. R. Schrier, W. Henrich, "Nonsteroidal anti-inflammatory drugs: Caution still advised," *JAMA* 251(10):1301–02 (1984). Compare D. Fox, H. Jick, "Nonsteroidal anti-inflammatory drugs and renal disease," *JAMA* 251(10):1299–1300 (1984), finding no significant incidence of acute kidney disease in hospitalized patients who had taken NSAIDs.

12. M. Wu, et al., "Multiple myeloma in naproxen-induced acute renal failure," *New England Journal of Medicine* 317(3):171 (1987).

13. P. Fowler, *op. cit.;* C. Abrahams, N. Levin, "Analgesic nephropathy," *Lancet* 1:645 (1968); L. Prescott, "Analgesic nephropathy," *Drugs* 23:75–159 (1982).

14. See "Doctor discovers aspirin-free headache cure," *Vegetarian Times* (April 1987), p. 10.

15. F. Fulvnay, et al., "Dihydroergotamine nasal spray during migraine attacks. A double blind crossover study with placebo," *Cephalalgia* 7(2):131–33 (1987).

16. "Feverfew," *Vegetarian Times* (November 1988), p. 15.

17. B. Brown, *Stress and the Art of Biofeedback* (New York: Harper & Row, 1977).
18. "Pain control, part II: Cancer," *Harvard Medical School Health Letter* 14(9):1–3 (1989).
19. See Consumers Union, *The Medicine Show* (New York: Pantheon Books, 1980), pp. 25–26.
20. M. Kapp, "Placebo therapy and the law: Prescribe with care," *American Journal of Law and Medicine* 8(4):371 (1982).
21. See P. Sanberg, Richard Krenna, *Over-the-Counter Drugs: Harmless or Hazardous?* (New York: Chelsea House, 1986), pp. 96–98.
22. M. Kapp, *op. cit.*
23. M. Max, et al., "Association of pain relief with drug side effects in postherpetic neuralgia: A single-dose study of clonidine, codeine, ibuprofen, and placebo," *Clinical Pharmacology and Therapeutic* 43:363–71 (1988).
24. See B. Brown, *op. cit.;* H. Benson, *Beyond the Relaxation Response* (Times Books, 1984); A. Kusuma, et al., "Acupuncture analgesia in tonsillectomy," *Alternative Medicine* 1(1):69–74 (1985); "Pain control, part II: Cancer," *op. cit.*

Chapter Twenty-one   Over-the-Counter Stomach Remedies: Antacids

1. D. Taylor, "Litigious challenge," *Nature* 328:662 (1987).
2. See "What causes heartburn? What can I do about it?", *University of California, Berkeley Wellness Letter* 3(9):8 (1987); L. Altman, "Scientists track clues linking bacterium to stomach disorders," *New York Times* (January 3, 1989), p. C3.
3. See D. Zimmerman, *The Essential Guide to Nonprescription Drugs* (New York: Harper & Row, 1983), pp. 24–44; J. Kaufman, et al., *Over-the-Counter Pills That Don't Work* (New York: Pantheon Books, 1983), pp. 103–16; Consumers Union, *The Medicine Show* (New York: Pantheon Books, 1980), p. 93–105.
4. *O'Malia v. Oakes,* Docket No. 360174, Superior Court, Alameda County, Cal. 1971.
5. D. Zimmerman, *op. cit.*
6. *Ibid.*
7. D. Crapper, et al., "Brain aluminum distribution in Alzheimer's disease and experimental neurofibrillary degeneration," *Science* 180:511–13 (1973); D. Crapper, et al., "Aluminum, neurofibrillary

degeneration and Alzheimer's disease," *Brain* 99:67–80 (1976); D. Perl, A. Brody, "Alzheimer's disease: X-ray spectrometric evidence of aluminum accumulation in neurofibrillary tangle-bearing neurons," *Science* 208:297–99 (1980); J. Candy, et al., "New observations on the nature of senile plaque cores," in E. Vizi, et al., eds., *Regulation of Transmitter Function: Basic and Clinical Aspects* (Amsterdam: Elsevier Press, 1984), pp. 301–04; I. Klatzo, et al., "Experimental production of neurofibrillary degeneration. 1. Light microscopic observations," *Journal of Neuropathology and Experimental Neurology* 24:187–99 (1964); R. Terry, C. Pena, "Experimental production of neurofibrillary degeneration. 2. Electron microscopy, phosphatase histochemistry and electron probe analysis," *ibid.* 24:200–10 (1965); O. Bugiani, B. Ghetti, "Progressing encephalomyelopathy with muscular atrophy, induced by aluminum powder," *Neurobiology of Aging* 3:209–22 (1982). See P. Altmann, et al., "Serum aluminum levels and erythrocyte dihydropteridine reductase activity in patients on hemodialysis," *New England Journal of Medicine* 317(2):80–84 (1987).

8. See C. Starr, "Aluminum and Alzheimer's," *Drug Topics* (April 17, 1989), p. 30, citing *Lancet* 1:59 (1989).

9. J. Williams, et al., "Biliary excretion of aluminum in aluminum osteodystrophy with liver disease," *Annals of Internal Medicine* 104:782–85 (1986), reviewed in "Toxicologic consequences of oral aluminum," *Nutrition Reviews* 45(3):72–74 (1987).

10. "Aluminum and orange juice," *U.S. Pharmacist* (April 1989), p. 30, citing *Lancet* 2:849 (1988); A. Bakir, et al., "Hyperaluminemia in renal failure: The influence of age and citrate intake," *Clinical Nephrology* 31(1):40–44 (1989).

11. See W. Caster, M. Wang, "Dietary aluminum and Alzheimer's disease—A review," *Science of the Total Environment* 17:31–36 (1981).

12. See "Nutritional consequences of antacids for hyperacidity," *Nutrition & the M.D.* (November 1986), p. 1.

13. A. Wade, ed., *Martindale: The Extra Pharmacopoeia,* 29th ed. (London: The Pharmaceutical Press, 1989), pp. 891, 1547.

14. See M. Lane, S. Lee, "Recurrence of duodenal ulcer after medical treatment," *Lancet* (May 21, 1988), pp. 1147–49; B. Salena, R. Hunt, "The limitations of current therapy in peptic ulcer disease," *Clinical and Investigative Medicine* 10(3):171–77 (1987).

Chapter Twenty-two   Prescription Stomach Remedies:
                        The H2-Blockers

1. World Health Organization, *The World Drug Situation* (Geneva: WHO, 1988), p. 18.

2. See J. Weber, "SmithKline's case of ulcers," *Business Week* (October 10, 1988), pp. 40–41; J. Weber, R. Rhein Jr., "How Glaxo's eager beavers chewed up Tagamet's lead," *ibid.* p. 40.

3. S. Wolfe, et al., *Worst Pills, Best Pills* (Washington D.C.: Public Citizen Health Research Group, 1988), p. 287.

4. See B. Salena, R. Hunt, "The limitations of current therapy in peptic ulcer disease," *Clinical and Investigative Medicine* 10(3):171–77 (1987); M. Lane, S. Lee, "Recurrence of duodenal ulcer after medical treatment," *Lancet* (May 21, 1988), pp. 1147–49.

5. *Drug Facts and Comparisons* (St. Louis: J.B. Lippincott Co., 1989), p. 1311.

6. D. Campoli-Richards, F. Clissold, "Famotidine," *Drugs* (September 1986), pp. 197–221.

7. See M. Sax, "Clinically important adverse effects and drug interactions with H2-receptor antagonists: An update," *Pharmacotherapy* 7 (6 Pt 2):110–15S (1987); J. Gaska, K. Tietze, "Current concepts in the treatment of peptic ulcer disease . . . ," *American Pharmacy* NS29 (November 1989), pp. 48–53.

8. See E. Underwood, "How H2 antagonists have changed ulcer therapy," *U.S. Pharmacist* (April 1989), p. 53; *Nursing89 Drug Handbook* (Springhouse, Pa.: Springhouse Corp., 1989).

9. See J. Weber, R. Rhein Jr., *op. cit.;* M. Sax, *op. cit.;* J. Aymard, et al., "Haematological adverse effects of histamine H2-receptor antagonists," *Medical Toxicology* 3:430–48 (1988).

10. See S. Smith, M. Kendall, "Ranitidine *versus* cimetidine: A comparison of their potential to cause clinically important drug interactions," *Clinical Pharmacokinetics* 15:44–56 (1988).

11. *Ibid.*

12. B. Salena, et al., *op. cit.*

13. M. Driks, et al., "Nosocomial pneumonia in intubated patients given sucralfate as compared with antacids or histamine type 2 blockers: The role of gastric colonization," *New England Journal of Medicine* 317(22):1376–1382 (1987).

14. L. Altman, "Scientists track clues linking bacterium to stomach disorders," *New York Times* (January 3, 1989), p. C3.
15. J. Aymard, et al., *op. cit.*
16. B. Salena, et al., *op. cit.*
17. Compare D. Martin, et al., "Difference in relapse rates of duodenal ulcer after healing with cimetidine or tripotassium dicitrato bismuthate," *Lancet* 1:7–10 (1981); and M. Classen, et al., "Effect of sucralfate on peptic ulcer recurrence: A controlled double-blind multi-centre study," *Scandinavian Journal of Gastroenterology* 18 (Supp. 2):61–68 (1983).
18. M. Lane, et al., *op. cit.*
19. B. Salena, *op. cit.*
20. *Ibid.;* "Nutritional consequences of antacids for hyperacidity," *Nutrition & the M.D.* (November 1986), p. 1; R. Fisher, "Sucralfate: A review of drug tolerance and safety," *Clinical Gastroenterology* 3 (Supp. 2): 181–84 (1981); *Drug Facts and Comparisons* (St. Louis: J.B. Lippincott Co., 1989), p. 1291.
21. R. Lasser, et al., "The role of intestinal gas in functional abdominal pain," *New England Journal of Medicine* 293:524–26 (1975); *Federal Register* 47:486 (January 5, 1982).
22. T. Gossel, "Antiflatulence agents," *U.S. Pharmacist* (August 1989), pp. 18 ff.
23. See "Diet therapy of peptic ulcer disease," *Nutrition & the M.D.* 14(2):1–2 (1988), citing *Gut* 27:2329 (1986), *Journal of Laboratory and Clinical Medicine* 100:296 (1982), *Journal of Clinical Gastroenterology* 3 (Supp 2):45 (1981), 89:366 (1985) and 90:1617 (1986); J. Gaska, et al., *op. cit.;* A. Rydning, et al., "Prophylactic effect of dietary fibre in duodenal ulcer disease," *Lancet* (October 2, 1982), pp. 736–39 (1982); "Myth: A bland, milky diet can help prevent or cure ulcers," *University of California, Berkeley Wellness Letter* 3(10):8 (1987).
24. "Diet therapy of peptic ulcer disease," *Nutrition & the M.D.* 14(2):1–2 (1988).
25. *Ibid.;* M. Lane, *op. cit.*
26. B. Salena, et al., *op. cit.;* B. Brown, *Stress and the Art of Biofeedback* (New York: Harper & Row, 1977).

Chapter Twenty-three   Drugs for Diarrhea, Nausea, Constipation, and Hemorrhoids

1. R. Mathison, *The Shocking History of Drugs* (New York: Ballantine Books, 1958), p. 169.
2. See D. Hussar, "New drugs of 1988," *American Pharmacy* (March 1989), pp. 25–52.
3. See D. Zimmerman, *The Essential Guide to Nonprescription Drugs* (New York: Harper & Row, 1983), pp. 237–49.
4. See *Drug Facts and Comparisons* (St. Louis: J.B. Lippincott Co., 1989).
5. See M. Cullen, "A consumer's guide to laxatives," *Vegetarian Times* (March 1985), p. 49.
6. See J. Kaufman, et al., *Over the Counter Pills That Don't Work* (New York: Pantheon Books, 1983), p. 144, citing *Advertising Age* (September 9, 1982), p. 22; Consumers Union, *The Medicine Show* (New York: Pantheon Books, 1980), pp. 136–39.
7. A. Fisher, *Contact Dermatitis* (Philadelphia: Lea and Febiger, 1973), pp. 42, 312, 313; North American Contact Dermatitis Group, "Epidemiology of contact dermatitis in North America," *Archives of Dermatology* 108:537–40 (1973).
8. Consumers Union, *op. cit.;* J. Kaufman, et al., *op. cit.*
9. "Myth: Carbonated beverages relieve nausea," *University of California, Berkeley Wellness Letter* 3(4):8 (1987).
10. See K. Gannon, "What OTCs do you recommend?", *Drug Topics* (August 7, 1989), pp. 42–50.

Chapter Twenty-four   Downers: Drugs for Insomnia and Anxiety

1. Quoted in R. Mathison, *The Shocking History of Drugs* (New York: Ballantine Books, 1958), p. 218.
2. A. Melville, C. Johnson, *Cured to Death* (New York: Stein and Day, 1982), pp. 76–77.
3. P. Hager, "Mental patients allowed to refuse drugs," *Los Angeles Times* (June 24, 1989), p. I:4.
4. N. Callaghan, et al., "Withdrawal of anticonvulsant drugs in patients free of seizures for two years," *New England Journal of Medicine* 318(15):942–46 (1988); G. Johnson, S. Goldfinger, *Har-*

vard Medical School Health Letter Book (Cambridge, Mass.: Harvard University Press, 1981), p. 346.

5. See J. Bryan, *Drugs for All?* (Harmondsworth, Middlesex: Penguin Books, 1986), pp. 120–46.

6. "Top 200 drugs of 1988," *Pharmacy Times* (April 1989), p. 40.

7. See R. Greene, "The mellow market," *Forbes* (October 31, 1988), p. 106.

8. W. Leary, "F.D.A. asks stronger label on sleeping pill under scrutiny," *New York Times* (September 23, 1989), p. 6.

9. R. Greene, *op. cit.*

10. D. Greenblatt, et al., "Effect of gradual withdrawal on the rebound sleep disorder after discontinuation of triazolam," *New England Journal of Medicine* 317(12):722–28 (1987).

11. Adapted from "Choice of benzodiazepines," *Medical Letter* 30(760):26–28 (1988).

12. A. Kales, et al., "Diazepam: Effects on sleep and withdrawal phenomena," *Journal of Clinical Psychopharmacology* 8(5):340–46 (1988).

13. P. Roy-Byrne, et al., "Relapse and rebound following discontinuation of benzodiazepine treatment of panic attacks: Alprazolam versus diazepam," *American Journal of Psychiatry* 146(7):860–65 (1989).

14. M. Lader, "Assessing the potential for buspirone dependence or abuse and effects of its withdrawal," *American Journal of Medicine* 82 (Supp. 5A):20–26 (1987); D. Olajide, M. Lader, "A comparison of buspirone, diazepam and placebo in patients with chronic anxiety states," *Journal of Clinical Psychopharmacology* 7(3):148–52 (1987). See also "Buspirone: A non-benzodiazepine for anxiety," *Medical Letter* 28(728):117–19 (1986).

15. D. Gastfriend, J. Rosenbaum, "Adjunctive buspirone in benzodiazepine treatment of four patients with panic disorder," *American Journal of Psychiatry* 146(7):914–16 (1989).

16. R. Greene, *op. cit.*

17. "Buspirone reduces smoking urge," *U.S. Pharmacist* (April 1989), p. 11.

18. See P. Sanberg, R. Krenna, *Over-the-Counter Drugs: Harmless or Hazardous?* (New York: Chelsea House, 1986), pp. 76–83; J. Kaufman, et al., *Over the Counter Pills That Don't Work* (New York: Pantheon Books, 1983), pp. 159–61.

19. "Tryptophan: Natural disaster," *Harvard Medical School Health*

Letter (February 1990), pp. 1–2; B. Ingersoll, "FDA moves to embargo L-tryptophan," *Wall Street Journal* (December 6, 1989), p. B4.

20. G. Lewis, "An alternative approach to premedication: Comparing diazepam with auriculotherapy and a relaxation method," *American Journal of Acupuncture* 15(3):205–13 (1987); B. Brown, *Stress and the Art of Biofeedback* (New York: Harper & Row, 1977).

21. D. McCree, "The appropriate use of sedatives and hypnotics in geriatric insomnia," *American Pharmacy* NS29(5):49–53 (1989).

Chapter Twenty-five   Uppers: Drugs for Losing Weight and Subduing Hyperactive Children

1. S. Siegelman, "Medications used by the famous," *American Druggist* (December 1989), pp. 29–33.

2. J. McGinnis, *Fatal Vision* (New York: G.P. Putnam's Sons, 1983), reprinted in *Cosmopolitan* (January 1984), pp. 220 ff.

3. J. Horowitz, et al., "Hypertensive responses induced by phenylpropanolamine in anorectic and decongestant preparations," *Lancet* 1:60–61 (1980); P. Pentel, et al., "Myocardial injury after phenylpropanolamine ingestion," *British Heart Journal* 47:51–54 (1982).

4. E. Bravo, "Phenylpropanolamine and other over-the-counter vasoactive compounds," *Hypertension* 11 (Supp. II):II-7—II-10 (1988).

5. R. Glick, et al., "Phenylpropanolamine: An over-the-counter drug causing central nervous system vasculitis and intracerebral hemorrhage," *Neurosurgery* 20(6):969–74 (1987).

6. E. Bravo, *op. cit.*

7. See "Coffee—not guilty," *University of California, Berkeley Wellness Letter* 3(6):2 (1987); *Ibid.* 4(10):4–5 (1988).

8. North American Contact Dermatitis Group, "Epidemiology of contact dermatitis in North America," *Archives of Dermatology* 108:537–40 (1973).

9. "Will fiber make you trim?", *University of California, Berkeley Wellness Letter* 3(9):1 (1987).

10. See E. Brown, *With the Grain* (New York: Carroll & Graf, 1990).

11. R. Henig, "Courts enter the hyperactivity fray," *Washington Post Health* (March 15, 1988), p. 8; L. Williams, "Parents and doctors fear growing misuse of drug used to treat hyperactive kids," *Wall Street Journal* (January 15, 1988), p. 25.

12. L. Sroufe, M. Stewart, "Treating problem children with stimulant drugs," *New England Journal of Medicine* 289(8):407–13 (1973); M. McBride, "An individual double-blind crossover trial for assessing methylphenidate response in children with attention deficit disorder," *Journal of Pediatrics* 113:137–45 (1988).
13. L. Sroufe, et al., *op. cit.*
14. R. Barkley, C. Cunningham, "Do stimulant drugs improve the academic performance of hyperactive children? A review of outcome research," *Clinical Pediatrics* 17:85–92 (1978); K. Gadow, "Effects of stimulant drugs on academic performance in hyperactive and learning disabled children," *Journal of Learning Disabilities* 16:290–99 (1983); J. Werry, "Drugs and learning," *Journal of Child Psychology and Psychiatry* 22:283–90 (1981).
15. L. Sroufe, et al., *op. cit.;* R. Henig, *op. cit.*
16. "Methylphenidate revisited," *Medical Letter* 30(765):51–52.
17. A. Morgan, "Use of stimulant medications in children," *American Family Practice* 38(4):197–202 (1988); "Methylphenidate revisited," *op. cit.*
18. L. Williams, *op. cit.*
19. R. Henig, *op. cit.*
20. L. Sroufe, et al., *op. cit.*
21. R. Henig, *op. cit.*
22. *Ibid.*
23. See L. Moll, "The link between food and mood," *Vegetarian Times* (August 1986), pp. 28–30; R. Wunderlich, D. Kalita, "Nourishing your hyperactive child to health," *Good Health* 2(5):16–19 (1984); "Hay fever's far-reaching effects," *U.S. Pharmacist* (August 1989), p. 22.
24. R. Henig, *op. cit.,* citing a study conducted by Dr. James Satterfield, director of the National Center for Hyperactive Children in Encino, California, involving 130 hyperactive boys.
25. L. Sroufe, et al., *op. cit.*
26. See R. Mendelsohn, *How to Raise a Healthy Child in Spite of Your Doctor* (Chicago: Contemporary Books, 1984), pp. 205–06; L. Moll, *op. cit.*
27. R. Wunderlich, et al., *op. cit.*
28. A. Morgan, *op. cit.*

Chapter Twenty-six   Drugs and Depression

1. S. Fuller, E. Underwood, "Update on antidepressant medications," *U.S. Pharmacist* (August 1989), pp. 35–45; G. Cowley, et al., "The promise of Prozac," *Newsweek* (March 26, 1990), pp. 38–41.
2. S. Satel, J. Nelson, "Stimulants in the treatment of depression: A critical overview," *Journal of Clinical Psychiatry* 50(7):241–49 (1989).
3. *Ibid.;* "Advances in the diagnosis and management of depression (II)," *American Pharmacy* (February 1988), pp. 33–37.
4. G. Cowley, et al., *op. cit.*
5. S. Fuller, et al., *op. cit.*
6. "Antidepressant curbs craving for cocaine," *U.S. Pharmacist* (April 1989), p. 12.
7. Adapted from S. Fuller, et al., *op. cit.*
8. "Advances in the diagnosis and management of depression," *op. cit.;* P. Parish, *Medicines* (London: Penguin Books, 1989), pp. 75–79, 645.
9. *Ibid.;* C. Starr, "Introducing Wellbutrin, a one-of-a-kind antidepressant," *Drug Topics* (August 7, 1989); "Advances in the diagnosis and management of depression," *op. cit.;* G. Cowley, et al., *op. cit.*
10. C. Starr, "Viloxazine is for patients who get far too much sleep," *Drug Topics* (August 21, 1989), pp. 25–26.
11. B. Hardy, et al., "Pharmacokinetics of lithium in the elderly," *Journal of Clinical Psychopharmacology* 7(3):153–58 (1987).
12. S. Fuller, et al., *op. cit.;* K. Wood, et al., "Drug-induced psychosis and depression in the elderly," *Psychiatric Clinics of North America* 11(1):167–93 (1988).
13. M. Russ, S. Ackerman, "Antidepressants and weight gain," *Appetite* 10:103–17 (1988). Buproprion also doesn't seem to cause weight gain, but it's not currently available.
14. Adapted from S. Fuller, et al., *op. cit.*
15. See L. Moll, "The link between food and mood," *Vegetarian Times* (August 1986), pp. 28–30.
16. *Ibid.;* R. Ballentine, *Diet and Nutrition* (Honesdale, Pa.: Himalayan International Institute, 1982), pp. 512–14.
17. "Advances in the diagnosis and management of depression," *op. cit.*

Chapter Twenty-seven   Drugs to Repel Bugs and Relieve Itching

1. See D. Zimmerman, *Essential Guide to Nonprescription Drugs* (New York: Harper & Row, 1983), pp. 449–71.
2. "Helping the medicine go down—or in," *Business Week* (January 22, 1990), p. 84; T. Lackner, "Introduction to transdermal drug delivery systems (Part I)," *Pharmacy Times* (February 1989), pp. 100–09.
3. From T. Gossel, "OTC relief of itching," *U.S. Pharmacist* (July 1989), pp. 33–40.
4. T. Gossel, *op. cit.;* D. Zimmerman, *op. cit.*
5. T. Gossel, *op. cit.;* P. Parish, *Medicines* (London: Penguin Books, 1989), pp. 270–72.
6. From G. Cawood, et al., *1989–90 Prescription Drug Encyclopedia* (Peachtree City, Ga.: FC&A Publishing, 1989).
7. "Insect repellants," *Medical Letter* (May 19, 1989), pp. 45–46; "Are insect repellants safe?", *University of California, Berkeley Wellness Letter* (June 1988), p. 7.
8. "Prevention and treatment of insect stings," *Pharmacy Times* (April 1989), pp. 33–38; C. O'Neill, "The big sting," *Washington Post Health* (June 28, 1988), p. 22.

Chapter Twenty-eight   Eye Care

1. F. Fraunfelder, S. Meyer, "Systemic side effects from ophthalmic timolol and their prevention," *Journal of Ocular Pharmacology* 3(2):177–84 (1987).
2. G. Johnson, S. Goldfinger, *Harvard Medical School Health Letter Book* (Cambridge, Mass.: Harvard University Press, 1981), pp. 364–68.
3. P. O'Dea, "Glaucoma therapy: The pharmacist's role in compliance," *American Pharmacy* (September 1988), pp. 38–42.
4. F. Fraunfelder, et al., *op. cit.;* F. Fraunfelder, S. Meyer, "Systemic reactions to ophthalmic drug preparations," *Medical Toxicology* 2:287–93 (1987).
5. "Renin inhibitors show promise as treatment agents for glaucoma," *American Pharmacy* (October 1989), p. 15.
6. S. Boruchoff, "Effects of inappropriate use of corticosteroids in-

stilled in the eye," *New England Journal of Medicine* 316(19):1216–17 (1987).

7. *Ibid.*

8. *Kong v. Clay-Grant Pharmacy,* Docket No. 619350, Superior Ct., San Francisco County, Cal. 1972.

9. F. Fraunfelder, et al., "Systemic reactions . . ." *op. cit.*

10. *Ibid.*

11. M. Rumelt, "Blindness from misuse of over-the-counter eye medications," *Annals of Ophthalmology* 20:26–30 (1988).

12. J. Siwek, "Excess eyedrops," *Washington Post Health* (October 6, 1987), p. 21.

13. F. Warren, M. Morton, "An overview of contact lenses, cleaners, and disinfectants," *Pharmacy Times* (September 1988), pp. 142–51; "Darling . . . your contacts," *Newsweek* (October 2, 1989), p. 66.

Chapter Twenty-nine   Drugs for Blemished Skin

1. J. Trowbridge, M. Walker, *The Yeast Syndrome* (New York: Bantam Books, 1986), p. 315.

2. A. Shalita, et al., "Isotretinoin revisited," *Cutis* 42:1–19 (1988).

3. E. Lammer, et al., "Retinoic acid embryopathy," *New England Journal of Medicine* 313:837–41 (1985).

4. *Drug Facts and Comparisons* (St. Louis: J.B. Lippincott Co., 1989), p. 1886.

5. A. Shalita, et al., *op. cit.;* H. Roenigk Jr., "Retinoids," *Cutis* 39:301–05 (1987). See D. Blanc, et al., "Eruptive pyogenic granulomas and acne fulminans in two siblings treated with isotretinoin," *Dermatologica* 177:16–18 (1988).

6. A. Shalita, et al., *op. cit.*

7. *Drug Facts and Comparisons, op. cit.,* pp. 1892–93; J. Trowbridge, et al., *op. cit.*

8. "Gray hair and acne," *University of California, Berkeley Wellness Letter* 4(8):7 (1988).

9. "What's the connection between hormones and skin?", *Pharmacy Times* (May 1989), pp. 49–51.

10. S. Bharija, M. Belhaj, "Acetylsalicylic acid may induce a lichenoid eruption," *Dermatologica* 177:19 (1988).

11. S. Begley, "Don't drink the water?", *Newsweek* (February 5, 1990), pp. 60–61.

12. J. Trowbridge, et al., *op. cit.,* pp. 301–20.

Chapter Thirty   Drugs for Aging Skin and Hair: Retin-A, Minoxidil, and Sunscreens

1. R. Henig, "The war on wrinkles," *Washington Post Health* (February 23, 1988), pp. 12–15.
2. J. Weiss, et al., "Topical tretinoin improves photoaged skin," *JAMA* 259:527–32 (1988).
3. "Aging skin," *Harvard Medical School Health Letter* (May 1988), pp. 3–4; R. Henig, *op. cit.;* "Tretinoin for aging skin," *Medical Letter* 30(770):69–70 (1988).
4. R. Henig, "The other creams," *Washington Post Health* (February 23, 1988), p. 15.
5. *Harvard Medical School Health Letter, op. cit.;* R. Henig, "The war on wrinkles," *op. cit.*
6. M. Cimons, " 'There are no healthy tans,' panel insists," *Los Angeles Times* (May 11, 1989), Part I, p. 29; "Sunscreens," *Medical Letter* 30(768):61–63 (1988).
7. J. Generali, "Does the thickness of sunscreen application change the sun protection factor?", *U.S. Pharmacist* (April 1989), pp. 27–28; C. Stenberg, O. Larko, "Sunscreen application and its importance for the sun protection factor," *Archives of Dermatology* 121:1400 (1985).
8. "Drugs that cause photosensitivity," *Medical Letter* 28(713):51–52 (1986).
9. D. Hussar, "New drugs of 1988," *American Pharmacy* (March 1989), pp. 25–52.
10. "Sunscreens," *op. cit.*
11. "Myth: There's a cure for male pattern baldness," *University of California, Berkeley Wellness Letter* 5(2):8 (1988); "Minoxidil: A few of the questions you're likely to hear," *American Pharmacy* NS28(11):47–50 (1988).
12. From "Drugs that cause photosensitivity," *op. cit.*

Chapter Thirty-one   For Women Only

1. Quoted in J. Scott, "Hormones may increase cancer risk, study says," *Los Angeles Times* (August 2, 1989), pp. I:1,15.

2. See L. Monroe, "Menopause: Baby boomers' next step," *Los Angeles Times* (December 5, 1989), pp. E1–E3; J. Scott, *op. cit.*

3. D. Kiel, et al., "Hip fracture and the use of estrogens in postmenopausal women," *New England Journal of Medicine* 317(19):1169–74 (1987); L. Huppert, "Hormonal replacement therapy: Benefits, risks, doses," *Medical Clinics of North America* 71(1):23–39 (1987).

4. J. Scott, *op. cit.*; J. Scott, "Weigh hormones' risk, experts urge," *Los Angeles Times* (August 4, 1989), pp. V:1,5; L. Huppert, *op. cit.*

5. J. Scott, *op. cit.* (two articles); J. McDougall, "Balancing the estrogen issue," *Vegetarian Times* (August 1986), page 44.

6. L. Huppert, *op. cit.*

7. See L. Monroe, *op. cit.*; J. McDougall, *op. cit.*

8. "Transdermal estrogen," *Medical Letter* 28(728):119–20 (1986).

9. W. Ray, et al., "Psychotropic drug use and the risk of hip fracture," *New England Journal of Medicine* 316:363–69 (1987).

10. See E. Brown, *With the Grain* (New York: Carroll & Graf, 1990), chapters 11–15.

11. D. Mishell, "Contraception," *New England Journal of Medicine* 320(12):777–87 (1989); K. Butler, L. Rayner, *The Best Medicine* (San Francisco: Harper & Row, 1985).

12. D. Mishell, *op. cit.*, citing W. Grady, et al., "Contraceptive failure and continuation among married women in the United States, 1970–75," *Studies in Family Planning* 14:9–19 (1983), and A. Schirm, et al., "Contraceptive failure in the United States: The impact of social, economic and demographic factors," *Family Planning Perspectives* 14:68–75 (1982).

13. J. Ellis, "Multiphasic oral contraceptives," *Journal of Reproductive Medicine* 32(1):28–36 (1987).

14. D. Mishell, *op. cit.*; *Nursing89 Drug Handbook* (Springhouse, Pa.: Springhouse Corporation, 1989), pp. 512–13.

15. R. Sattin, et al., "Oral-contraceptive use and the risk of breast cancer: The Cancer and Steroid Hormone Study of the Centers for Disease Control and the National Institute of Child Health and Human Development," *New England Journal of Medicine* 315:405–11 (1986); H. Olsson, et al., "Oral contraceptive use and breast cancer in young women in Sweden," *Lancet* 1:748–49 (1985). See "Oral-contraceptive use and the risk of breast cancer," *New England Journal of Medicine* 316(3):162–64 (1987).

16. D. Mishell, *op. cit.*; J. Woods, "Oral contraceptives and hyperten-

sion," *Hypertension* 11 (Supp. II):II-11 to II-15 (1988); P. Croft, P. Hannaford, "Risk factors for acute myocardial infarction," *BMJ* 298:165 (1989).

17. D. Mishell, *op. cit.;* M. Mintz, "The selling of an IUD," *Washington Post Health* (August 9, 1988), pp. 12–16; "New copper IUD," *Medical Letter* (February 26, 1988), pp. 25–26; J. Ellis, "Monsanto and the Copper-7," *Business Week* (September 26, 1988), p. 50; S. Lang, "The Dalkon Shield," *Vogue* (August 1988), p. 234.

18. A. Schirm, et al., *op. cit.*

19. See F. Gebhart, "Condom failure? Maybe you should blame the lubricant," *Drug Topics* (April 17, 1989), p. 30.

20. "The cervical cap," *Medical Letter* (October 7, 1988), pp. 93–94; D. Mishell, *op. cit.*

21. See "Can spermicides cause birth defects?", *University of California, Berkeley Wellness Letter* (November 1987), p. 8.

22. D. Mishell, *op. cit.;* "Toxic shock and tampons revisited," *Science News* 132:136 (1987).

23. See K. Keville, "A total approach to fighting PMS," *Vegetarian Times* (August 1986), pp. 40 ff.

24. See D. Zimmerman, *The Essential Guide to Nonprescription Drugs* (New York: Harper & Row, 1983), pp. 540–56; K. Keville, *op. cit.;* J. McDougall, *op. cit.,* citing B. Goldin, *Cancer Research* 41:3771 (1981); P. Hill, "Diet and endocrine-related cancer," *Cancer* 39:1820 (1977).

25. "PMS? Let 'em eat carbs," *Vegetarian Times* (March 1990), p. 17; "Less fat, more grain can ease breast pain," *ibid.* (May 1989), p. 11.

26. B. Brown, *Stress and the Art of Biofeedback* (New York: Harper & Row, 1977).

27. See "Myth: Douching is part of good feminine hygiene," *University of California, Berkeley Wellness Letter* 3(9):8 (1987).

28. R. Henig, "Drug to dry up breast milk is under federal scrutiny," *Washington Post Health* (June 28, 1988), p. 6.

29. Adapted from G. Cawood, et al., *1989–90 Prescription Drug Encyclopedia* (Peachtree City, Ga.: FC&A Publishing, 1989); "Contraindications to use of estrogen therapy," *U.S. Pharmacist* (April 1989), p. 89; M. Rumore, J. Rumore, "Clinical therapeutics of endometriosis, Part I," *American Pharmacy* (September 1989), pp. 49–52.

Chapter Thirty-two   If You Are Expecting

1. See M. Bologa-Campeanu, et al., "Prenatal adverse effects of various drugs and chemicals," *Medical Toxicology* 3:307–23 (1988).

2. C. Rumack, et al., "Neonatal intracranial hemorrhage and maternal use of aspirin," *Obstetrics and Gynecology* 58(Supp.):525–65 (1981).

3. V. Char, et al., "Polyhydramnios and neonatal renal failure: A possible association with acetaminophen ingestion," *Journal of Pediatrics* 86:638–39 (1975).

4. J. Rosenblatt, R. Edson, "Metronidazole," *Mayo Clinic Proceedings* 62:1013–17 (1987).

5. E. Lammer, et al., "Retinoic acid embryopathy," *New England Journal of Medicine* 313:837–41 (1985).

6. See G. Cawood, et al., *1989–90 Prescription Drug Encyclopedia* (Peachtree City, Ga.: FC&A Publishing, 1989).

7. M. Bologa-Campeanu, et al., *op. cit.*

8. M. Goldhaber, et al., "The risk of miscarriage and birth defects among women who use visual display terminals during pregnancy," *American Journal of Industrial Medicine* 13(6):695–706 (1988).

9. "Are you or your children hooked on caffeine?", *Tufts University Diet & Nutrition Letter* 6(6):1–2 (1988).

10. E. Halmesmaki, "Alcohol counselling of 85 pregnant problem drinkers: Effect on drinking and fetal outcome," *British Journal of Obstetrics and Gynaecology* 95(3):243–47 (1989).

11. "Pot use may stunt fetal growth," *Los Angeles Times* (March 22, 1989), p. I:1.

12. W. Hines, "Toxoplasmosis: Its link to AIDS," *Washington Post Health* (February 23, 1988), p. 6.

Chapter Thirty-three   Drugs, Impotence, and Infertility

1. The literature is reviewed in D. McWaine, W. Procci, "Drug-induced sexual dysfunction," *Medical Toxicology* 3:289–306 (1988).

2. C. Foster, et al., eds., *Illegal Drugs and Alcohol* (Wylie, Texas: Information Plus, 1989), p. 12.

3. S. Squires, "Risks of steroid use," *Washington Post Health* (February 23, 1988), p. 5.

4. J. Randal, W. Hines, "On TV, chit-chatting about impotence," *Washington Post Health* (November 8, 1988), p. 16.
5. C. Starr, "Bromocriptine and infertility: A happy family tale," *Drug Topics* (April 3, 1989), pp. 27–28.
6. "*Metrodin* and other drugs that induce ovulation," *Medical Letter* 30(775):91 (1988).

Chapter Thirty-four   Drugs for the Sexually Active

1. P. Monette, *On Borrowed Time: An AIDS Memoir* (New York: Harcourt, Brace and Janovich 1988), quoted in P. Sanders, "Acupuncture and herbal treatment of HIV infection," *Holistic Nursing Practice* 3(4):38–44 (1989).
2. See discussion in chapter 3.
3. K. Gannon, "Preventive methods can help reduce high stats for STDS," *Drug Topics* (April 3, 1989), p. 33.
4. E. Moore, M. Ryan, "Clinical update on genital herpes, syphilis, and trichomoniasis," *Wellcome Programs in Pharmacy* (Park Row Publishers, Inc., 1986); E. Moore, M. Ryan, "Clinical update on gonococcal and nongonococcal infections," *ibid.*
5. "Zidovudine (AZT) delays appearance of AIDS symptoms," *American Pharmacy* (October 1989), p. 21; J. Lublin, "Some rodents given high doses of AZT develop cancer, AIDS drug maker says," *Wall Street Journal* (December 6, 1989), p. B4; J. Wallace, "AIDS in the workplace," *Wellcome Programs in Pharmacy* (Park Row Publishers, Inc., 1987).
6. From J. Wallace, *op. cit.*
7. L. Yi, "A report of two cases of type B AIDS treated with acupuncture," *Journal of Traditional Chinese Medicine* 9(2):95–96 (1989).
8. P. Sanders, *op. cit.*
9. "One step closer to an AIDS vaccine," *Newsweek* (December 18, 1989), p. 66.
10. K. Gannon, *op. cit.;* K. Butler, L. Rayner, M.D., *The Best Medicine* (San Francisco: Harper & Row, Publishers, 1985), pp. 209–14; E. Moore, M. Ryan, "Clinical update on gonococcal and nongonococcal infections," *op. cit.*
11. "Interferon for treatment of genital warts," *Medical Letter* 30(770):70–72 (1988).
12. E. Moore, M. Ryan, *op. cit.*

13. E. Moore, et al., "Clinical update on gonococcal and nongonococcal infections," *op. cit.*

14. K. Butler, et al., *op. cit.;* E. Moore, M. Ryan, "Clinical update on genital herpes . . . ," *op. cit.*

15. "Worried sick: Hassles and herpes," *Science News* (December 5, 1987), p. 360; H. Nelson, "Sensitive armor," *Los Angeles Times* (September 19, 1988), p. II:3.

16. L. Simonsen, "Cold sores and canker sores afflict millions of Americans," *Pharmacy Times* (February 1989), pp. 125–26; K. Butler, et al., *op. cit.*

17. E. Moore, M. Ryan, "Clinical update on genital herpes . . . ," *op. cit.*

Chapter Thirty-five   Trends in Self-Testing

1. F. Samuel Jr., "The self-care revolution: Let's make it work," *Pharmacy Times* (March 1989), pp. 31–34.

2. S. Coons, J. Fink III, "The pharmacist, the law, and self-testing products," *American Pharmacy* (November 1989), pp. 35–38.

3. "Tests for occult blood," *Medical Letter* 28(705):5–6 (1986).

4. G. Schmidt, J. Wenig, "An evaluation of home blood-pressure monitoring devices," *American Pharmacy* (September 1989), pp. 25–30.

5. J. McCombs, "Ovulation prediction kits," *Pharmacy Times* (August 1989), pp. 39–41.

6. R. Campbell, "Clinical use of insulin: Side effects & dosing factors (Part II)," *Pharmacy Times* (November 1988), pp. 154–63 (1988); J. Weiner, "The pharmacist and diabetes mellitus: Today's considerations," *Wellcome Programs in Pharmacy* (Park Row Publishers, 1986).

7. S. Coons, et al., *op. cit.;* F. Samuel Jr., *op. cit.*

Chapter Thirty-six   Vitamin and Mineral Supplements: Health in a Bottle?

1. Council on Scientific Affairs, "Vitamin preparations as dietary supplements and as therapeutic agents," *JAMA* 257(14):1929–36 (1987); M. Nelson, "Promotion and selling of unnecessary food supplements: Quackery or ethical pharmacy practice?", *American Pharmacy* (October 1988), pp. 34–36.

2. J. Shriver, "As vitamin sales pep up, so do worries on overuse," *Los Angeles Times* (March 23, 1986), Part IV, p. 1; "Not all calcium pills provide calcium," *Tufts University Diet & Nutrition Letter* 6(2):1 (1988).

3. V. Stults, "Nutritional hazards," in H. Roberts, ed., *Food Safety* (New York: John Wiley & Sons, 1981), pp. 86–87; G. Kolata, "How important is dietary calcium in preventing osteoporosis?", *Science* 233:519–20 (1986).

4. G. Kolata, *op. cit.,* citing a study by B. Lawrence Riggs of the Mayo Clinic.

5. T. Holbrook, et al., "Dietary calcium and risk of hip fracture: 14-year prospective population study," *Lancet* 2(8619):1046–49 (1988).

6. C. Wickham, et al., "Dietary calcium, physical activity, and risk of hip fracture: A prospective study," *BMJ* 299(6704):889–92 (1989); M. Farmer, et al., "Anthropometric indicators and hip fracture. The NHANES I epidemiologic follow-up study," *Journal of the American Geriatrics Society* 37(1):9–16 (1989).

7. See J. Kanis, R. Passmore, "Calcium supplementation of the diet: Not justified by present evidence," *BMJ* 298:137–40, 205–08 (1989).

8. *Ibid.*

9. G. Kolata, *op. cit.;* M. Uehling, "The calcium craze," *Newsweek* (January 27, 1986), p. 48; "Calcium supplements: Don't depend on them," *University of California, Berkeley Wellness Letter* 3(4):1 (1987); J. Sheehan, M. Seelig, "Interactions of magnesium and potassium in the pathogenesis of cardiovascular disease," *Magnesium* 3:301–14 (1984).

10. V. Stults, *op. cit.;* L. Chen, "An increase in vitamin E requirement induced by high supplementation of vitamin C in rats," *American Journal of Clinical Nutrition* 34:1036–41 (1981); "To those who fight colds with vitamin C," *Science News* 124(18):281 (1983).

11. R. Hanning, S. Zlotkin, "Unconventional eating practices and their health implications," *Pediatric Clinics of North America* 32(2):429–45 (1985).

12. V. Stults, *op. cit.,* pp. 82–87; L. Shriver, *op. cit.;* S. Vaisrub, "Vitamin abuse," *JAMA* 238:1762 (1977); B. Shaywitz, et al., "Megavitamins for minimal brain dysfunction: A potentionally dangerous therapy," *JAMA* 238:1749 (1977).

13. V. Stults, *op. cit.,* pp. 111–12.

14. *Ibid.*, pp. 83–84, 89, 113; "Take it easy with zinc, researchers warn," *Vegetarian Times* (February 1985), p. 14; "Zinc-induced copper deficiency," *Nutrition & the M.D.* 15(4):4 (1989).

15. L. Chen, *op. cit.;* V. Herbert, et al., "Low serum vitamin B12 levels in patients receiving ascorbic acid in megadoses," *American Journal of Clinical Nutrition* 31:253–58 (1978); V. Herbert, et al., "Destruction of vitamin B12 by ascorbic acid," *JAMA* 230(2):241–42 (1974); H. Hogenkamp, "The interaction between vitamin B12 and vitamin C," *American Journal of Clinical Nutrition* 33:1–3 (1980); V. Herbert, et al., "Destruction of vitamin B12 by vitamin C," *American Journal of Clinical Nutrition* 30:297–98 (1977). For a contrary view, see M. Marcus, et al., "Stability of vitamin B12 in the presence of ascorbic acid in food and serum: Restoration by cyanide of apparent loss," *American Journal of Clinical Nutrition* 33:137–43 (1980).

16. V. Herbert, et al., "Multivitamin/mineral food supplements containing vitamin B12 may also contain analogues of vitamin B12," *New England Journal of Medicine* 307(4):255–56 (1982); A. Immerman, "Vitamin B12 status on a vegetarian diet," *World Review of Nutrition and Dietetics* 37:38–54 (1981).

17. V. Herbert, et al., *op. cit.;* "Harmful B12 breakdown products in multivitamins?", *Medical World News* (September 28, 1981), pp. 12–13.

18. J. Annand, "Atherosclerosis and vitamin B12," *Lancet* 1:789–90 (1957).

19. J. Shriver, *op. cit.;* W. van Staveren, et al., "Food consumption and height/weight status of Dutch preschool children on alternative diets," *Journal of the American Dietetic Association* 85(12):1579–84 (1985).

20. See E. Brown, *With the Grain* (New York: Carroll & Graf, 1990).

21. R. Issenman, et al., "Children's multiple vitamins: Overuse leads to overdose," *Canadian Medical Association Journal* 132:781–84 (1985).

22. See G. Johnson, S. Goldfinger, *Harvard Medical School Health Letter Book* (Cambridge, Mass.: Harvard University Press, 1981), p. 16.

23. M. Holick, "Photosynthesis of vitamin D and the skin: Effect of environmental and life-style variables," *Federation Proceedings* 46:1876–82 (1987).

24. A. Moore, M. Worwood, "Iron and the sudden infant death syndrome," *BMJ* 298:1248 (1989).
25. J. Kanis, *op. cit.;* L. Adair, E. Pollitt, "Outcome of maternal nutritional supplementation: A comprehensive review of the Bacon Chow study," *American Journal of Clinical Nutrition* 41:948–78 (1985).
26. F. Menolascino, et al., "Vitamin supplements and purported learning enhancement in mentally retarded children," *Journal of Nutritional Science and Vitaminolgy* 35:181–92 (1989).
27. "Should people over 60 take supplements?", *Tufts University Diet & Nutrition Letter* 6(4):1–2 (1988); J. Brody, "New research bolsters long-held beliefs that vitamin E can provide an array of benefits," *New York Times Health* (April 27, 1989), p. B19.
28. "Vitamin and mineral supplements! The making of the athlete?", *Nutrition & the M.D.* 14(10):1 (1988), citing *American Journal of Clinical Nutrition* 47:192 (1988).
29. "Beta-carotene supplements," *Nutrition & the M.D.* 15(4):4 (1989).
30. J. Vinson, P. Bose, "Comparative bioavailability to humans of ascorbic acid alone or in a citrus extract," *American Journal of Clinical Nutrition* 48:601–04 (1988).
31. *Earl Mindell's Vitamin Bible* (New York: Rawson, Wade Publishers, 1979), pp. 18–19.
32. D. Gordon, "The doctor's forum," *Your Good Health Review & Digest* 2(5):46 (1984).
33. "Not all calcium pills provide calcium," *Tufts University Diet & Nutrition Letter* 6(2):1 (1988).

Chapter Thirty-seven Drugs, Vitamins, and Food: Bad Combinations

1. A. Waxman, *Drug and Therapeutics Bulletin,* quoted in A. Lewis, "The vitamin robbers," *Healthcrafts.*
2. A. Lewis, *op. cit.;* "High blood pressure: Newer treatments," *Harvard Medical School Health Letter* 14(3):1–3 (1989).
3. "K is for clotting," *Tufts University Diet & Nutrition Letter* (April 1988), pp. 7–8. See also K. Sunakawa, et al., "Clinical superinfection and its attendant symptomatic changes in pediatrics," *Infection* 13 (Supp. 1):S103–11 (1985).
4. K. Butler, L. Rayner, *The Best Medicine* (San Francisco: Harper & Row, 1985), p. 473.

5. J. Brody, "New research bolsters long-held beliefs that vitamin E can provide an array of benefits," *New York Times Health* (April 27, 1989), p. B19.
6. A. Lewis, *op. cit.;* "The impact of drugs on nutrition," *Townsend Letter for Doctors* (April 1990), pp. 218–19.
7. "Aluminum and orange juice," *U.S. Pharmacist* (April 1989), p. 30.
8. E. Francke, H. Neu, "Chloramphenicol and tetracyclines," *Medical Clinics of North America* 71(6):1155–75 (1987).
9. E. Moore, M. Ryan, "Clinical update on genital herpes, syphilis, and trichomoniasis," *Wellcome Programs in Pharmacy* (Park Row Publishers, 1986).
10. L. Hendeles, "Slow-release theophylline: Do not substitute," *American Pharmacy* NS29:22–24 (1989).
11. P. Parish, *Medicines* (London: Penguin Books, 1989), pp. 76–77; see chapter 26.
12. E. Bravo, "Phenylpropanolamine and other over-the-counter vasoactive compounds," *Hypertension* 11 (Supp. II):II-7—II-10 (1988).
13. A. Lewis, *op. cit.*
14. From *Drug Facts and Comparisons* (St. Louis: J.B. Lippincott Co., 1989), p. 291b.
15. "Choice of benzodiazepines," *Medical Letter* 30(760):26–28 (1988).
16. R. Abrams, G. Alexopoulos, "Substance abuse in the elderly: Over-the-counter and illegal drugs," *Hospital and Community Psychiatry* 39(8):822–23 (1988).
17. C. Sargenti, et al., "Psychotropic drug interactions in the patient with late-onset psychosis and mood disorder," *Psychiatric Clinics of North America* 11(1):235–51 (1988).

Chapter Thirty-eight   Drugs and the Elderly

1. See J. Califano Jr., *America's Health Care Revolution* (New York: Random House, 1986), p. 140.
2. "Coronary artery bypass surgery—indications and limitations," *Lancet* 2:511 (1980); R. Steinbrook, "Unnecessary cuts: Heart bypass surgery often not needed or questionable, study of 3 hospitals says," *Los Angeles Times* (July 22, 1988), p. I:3.
3. J. Kastor, "Pacemaker mania," *New England Journal of Medicine*

318(3):182–83 (1988); A. Greenspan, et al., "Incidence of unwarranted implantation of permanent cardiac pacemakers in a large medical population," *ibid.,* 318(3):158–63.

4. United States Special Subcommittee on Aging, *Fraud, Waste, and Abuse in the Medicare Pacemaker Industry* (Washington, D.C.: Government Printing Office, 1982).

5. J. Kastor, *op. cit.*

6. R. Abrams, G. Alexopoulos, "Substance abuse in the elderly: Over-the-counter and illegal drugs," *Hospital and Community Pharmacy* 39(8):822–23 (1988); R. Levy, D. Smith, "Keeping the elderly at home through improved pharmaceutical technology," *American Pharmacy* NS28(1):41–44 (1988); P. Trainor, "Over-the-counter drugs: Count them in," *Geriatric Nursing* (September/October 1988), pp. 298–99.

7. H. Colt, A. Shapiro, "Drug-induced illness as a cause for admission to a community hospital," *Journal of the American Geriatric Society* 37(4):323 (1989); M. Montagne, B. Bleidt, "How to help the elderly self-medicate," *U.S. Pharmacist* (June 1989), pp. 53–60.

8. R. Abrams, et al., *op. cit.;* P. Trainor, *op. cit.*

9. R. Levy, et al., *op. cit.*

10. L. Greene, et al., "Programs to reduce drug errors in the elderly: Direct and indirect evidence of patient education," in *Improving Patient Compliance* (Reston, Va.: National Pharmaceutical Council, 1984), p. 59.

11. R. Levy, et al., *op. cit.;* S. Wolfe, et al., *Worst Pills, Best Pills* (Washington, D.C.: Public Citizen Health Research Group, 1988).

12. G. Johnson, S. Goldfinger, *Harvard Medical School Health Letter Book* (Cambridge, Mass.: Harvard University Press, 1981), pp. 385–89.

13. R. Levy, et al., *op. cit.*

14. D. McCree, "The appropriate use of sedatives and hypnotics in geriatric insomnia," *American Pharmacy* (May 1989), pp. 49–53.

15. W. Ray, et al., "Psychotropic drug use and the risk of hip fracture," *New England Journal of Medicine* 316:363–69 (1987).

16. K. Wood, et al., "Drug-induced psychosis and depression in the elderly," *Psychiatric Clinics of North America* 11(1):167–93 (1988).

17. C. Sargenti, et al., "Psychotropic drug interactions in the patient with late-onset psychosis and mood disorder," *Psychiatric Clinics of North America* 11(1):235–77 (1988).

18. *Ibid.*

19. D. McCree, *op. cit.*

20. J. Brody, "An alert for older Americans about preventable adverse reactions to many common drugs," *New York Times* (November 10, 1988), p. B20.

21. L. Cornaro, *Discourses on the Sober Life* (Mokelumne Hill, Cal.: Health Research [undated]), pp. 36, 38–39, 67–69.

INDEX